Organizational Psychology and Health Care

Vol. 4

edited by

José Maria Peiró
Wilmar B. Schaufeli

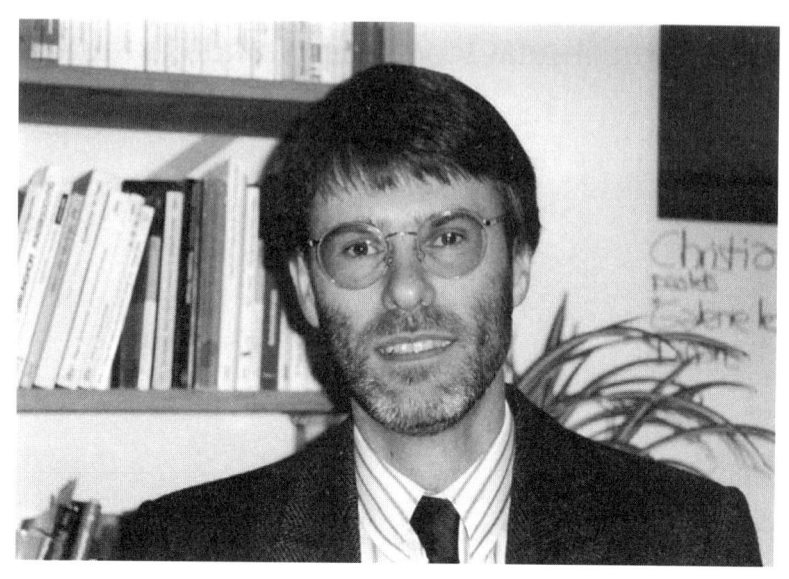

André Büssing

1950 – 2003

Christian Korunka
Peter Hoffmann
(Eds.)

Change and Quality in Human Service Work

Dedicated to the Work of André Büssing

Rainer Hampp Verlag   München und Mering   2005

Bibliografische Information Der Deutschen Bibliothek

Die Deutsche Bibliothek verzeichnet diese Publikation in der
Deutschen Nationalbibliografie; detaillierte bibliografische Daten
sind im Internet über http://dnb.ddb.de abrufbar.

ISBN: 3-87988-915-7
Organizational Psychology and Health Care: ISSN 1612-0531
1. Auflage, 2005

© 2005   Rainer Hampp Verlag München und Mering
Meringerzeller Str. 10 D – 86415 Mering

www.Hampp-Verlag.de

Liebe Leserinnen und Leser!
Wir wollen Ihnen ein gutes Buch liefern. Wenn Sie aus irgendwel-
chen Gründen nicht zufrieden sind, wenden Sie sich bitte an uns.

Table of contents

Part 2: Burnout research

Part 3: Work organization in human service work

Part 4: New Research instruments

Preface

In the last years, an acceleration of change processes is observable in the world of work. New types of work and changes in work organization appear in nearly all fields of work. Human service work is especially affected by these changes. Both, in public and private service organizations, are comprehensive changes processes carried out. Goals of these processes are typically the improvement of quality of services and cost reductions at the same time. Employees are often strongly affected by these changes.

The conference series "Organizational Psychology and Health Care", patronized by the ENOP (European Network of Organizational Psychology), focuses on human service work from a Work- and Organizational Psychology perspective. The VIII conference took place in October 2003 in Vienna, Austria. The specific topic of this conference was "Change and Quality in Human Service Work". This book presents selected papers from the Vienna conference. It is published as Volume 4 of the series "Organizational Psychology and Health Care".

The participants of the conference were invited to submit manuscripts for publication. A peer review process led finally to 21 chapters, written by scientists of 14 countries. Beside the traditional focus of the ENOP on European organizational psychology there are also chapters presented in this volume from authors of the USA and Canada.

Unfortunately, the Vienna conference was ill-fated. André Büssing, one of the founders of the ENOP conference series on Organizational Psychology and Health Care and also one of the co-organizers of the Vienna conference, died, completely unexpected, only a few days before the conference.

André was not only one of the well known organizational psychologists in Europe in the field of human service work. He was also a tireless promoter of scientific encounter and networking. He was very well prepared and happy to come to the Vienna conference to meet all his friends and colleagues. With André we lost not only an important and impressive scientist, we lost also a good colleague and friend. We will keep pleasant memories not only of the friendly and professional cooperation in preparing the conference together, but also of the good times we had together during the meetings for preparation.

We tried to act in the sense of André and we were holding therefore the conference, which was strongly shaped by his person, as previously planned together.

With this book we appreciate the scientific work of André Büssing. The book is dedicated to his work and his person. In addition to the participants of the conference we invited also some colleagues and friends of André to submit chapters for the book. We would like to emphasize the chapter of Jürgen Glaser, his coworker for many years in Munich. Jürgen gives in his chapter an overview of the work of André in the field of human service work. The influence and importance of the work of André Büssing is also noticeable by the fact of the numerous citations of his work in nearly all chapters throughout this book.

The book starts with the chapter written by Jürgen Glaser. He presents the research in Munich in the field of human service work in a chronological context, showing the compelling nature of the development of a research program and the position of Andrés' work in the field on human service work.

Denise Rousseau, currently the president of the Academy of Management, was a keynote speaker of the conference. In her chapter she points out that nurses and care personnel in health services are the essential bearers of performance. Until now, it is not succeeded fully to transfer the scientific knowledge in the field into practice. In her visionary contribution she develops a guideline for transferring scientific results into practice.

The wide range of the following chapters reflects the actual trends of organizational changes in human service work and their expression in research in organizational psychology. A strong focus on organizational change in human service work, design concepts of change management and studies of the effects of change on employees is shown by the number of chapters dealing with these subjects. Another group of papers is dealing with actual questions of burnout research. An additional focus is represented by chapters dealing with the optimization of working conditions in the field. Three chapters dealing with the development of new research instruments complete the book.

In the first chapter of the group of papers dealing with organizational change processes by Johnny Hellgren, Magnus Sverke, Helena Falkenberg and Stephan Baradi it could be shown that a privatization in human service work could also have positive effects of the working climate of physicians. The next chapter, written by Teresia Anderson-Straberg, Magnus Sverke, Johnny Hellgren and Katharina Näswall, deals with attitudes towards individualized pay systems in public health services. Padraig Mac Neela, Anne Scott and Melissa Corbally develop and test in their chapter a process oriented model to explain empowerment and commitment during organizational change processes in human service work. In the following chapter, Peggy De Prins, Erik Hendericks, Ria Janvier and Ingrid Willems show that innovative HRM strategies could lead to a reduction of the work load of employees in the health sector. In a similar vain, Ilse Cornelis and Peter Vlerick show that the perceived subjective control of organizational change processes may prevent or at least reduce negative outcomes for the employees. The chapter of Tobias

Eklund and Per Tillman deals with questions of optimal personnel selection in the field of human service work by use of assessment centers. Agnez Luhasz describes in her chapter the implementation of a program for health promotion in Hungary. Monica Nystrom analyzes in her chapter the subjective role perceptions of managers in organizational change processes. In the final chapter of this section Holger Pfaff, Jürgen Lütticke, Nicole Badura, Frank Piekarski and Peter Richter analyze organizational coping processes during organizational change. The different chapters of this section lead to a congruent picture of organizational change processes in human service work: Change processes based on the theoretical and practical scientific knowledge of work and organizational psychology have at least the potential for positive effects on the side of the employees affected by the change processes.

The chapters of the next section are dealing with actual questions of burnout research. Ronald Burke shows in a longitudinal study that personnel reduction in health services may have negative effects on the amount of burnout of current employees. Wilmar Schaufeli, Vicente Gonzales-Roma, José-Maria Peiro, Sabine Geurts and Inés Tomas analyze in their chapter the role of reciprocity processes for burnout development. Julia Hickel and Christian Korunka transfer the job-demand-support model into the field of psychotherapeutic work. Karin Proost, Karel de Witte, Hans de Witte and George Eves confirm in their study the effects of specific organizational conditions for burnout development.

The three following chapters deal with questions of work organization in human service work. Pascale Carayon, Ayse Gurses, Ann Schoofs Hundt, Phillip Ayoub and Carla Alvarado analyze in a qualitative study the promoting and hindering factors of work in health services. Nik Chmiel analyzes safety behaviour and the conditions for avoidance of accidents at the work place. Cornelia Kleindienst and Markus Schöbe analyze trust processes in the cooperation in the operating theatre.

The three final chapters of this book present new instruments for analyses in the field of human service work. Silke Pawils, Bernadette Klapper, Doris Schaffer and Uwe Koch give an overview of their comprehensive "Interkik"-tool box for analysis of communication- and change processes in the hospital. Paulino Jimenez and Wolfgang Kallus present a screening version of their recovery-stress questionnaire. Michael Trimmel and Gerlinde Rohrauer present the development of a questionnaire for the evaluation of online-counselling services.

We would like to thank all authors and co-authors for their excellent chapters. We would like to thank also the reviewers for their comprehensive and constructive comments which helped to improve the quality of the present book. We think this book shows the high quality of work- and organizational psychology research in the field of human service work. It is also an appreciate honor of the work of André Büssing in this field.

We would like to thank the ENOP (Paris) for financial support which allowed participants of Eastern European countries to participate in the conference. We would like to thank Wilmar Schaufeli and José-Maria Peiro, the editors of the book series, for the excellent cooperation and support.

For support during the conference in Vienna and the use of the conference venues we would like to thank the Vienna Chamber of Labour.

Our special thanks go to Tanja Gruber for her wonderful organizational support before, during and after the conference and to Elisabeth Höllerer for her layout work for this book.

Vienna, February 2005

Christian Korunka

Peter Hoffmann

Analysis and design of nursing work – A decade of research in different fields of health care

*Jürgen Glaser**
Chair of Psychology, Technical University Munich, Germany

The ongoing discussion about the demographic change in Germany puts health care professions more and more into the public consciousness. A declining birth-rate and a rising life-expectancy bring forth an aging society. In addition, a proceeding erosion of family structures and the growth of female employment reinforce the need for professional health care services. In former times, extended families used to care for each member, but nowadays, in the course of individualization, this task is delegated more and more to professional public or private health care providers.

According to the Federal Office of Statistics (Statistisches Bundesamt, 2003a) in 2002 health care services were offered by 2,240 hospitals, 1,388 prevention and rehabilitation centres, 9,200 nursing homes for the elderly, and 10,600 home care services. With 4,175 million employees, the health care sector has become one of the most important branches of the economy in Germany. Every tenth gainfully employed person works in this sector – more than, for example, in the German automobile industry. The development of the German labor market shows that the transition into a 'service society' is disproportionately due to employment in the health care sector. The nursing profession, with 705,000 nurses (including midwifes), represents the largest group among the 2,2 million health care professionals. Furthermore, taking into account another 229,000 assistant nurses and 277,000 nurses for the elderly, the importance of nursing for the employment in Germany is indisputable (Statistisches Bundesamt, 2003b).

The expenses for healthcare in Germany are rising inexorably and have prompted governmental reforms since the beginning of the 1990s. In 2001 these costs amounted to 226 billion Euros, which equals 10.9% of the gross domestic product or an average of 2,740 Euros per resident. Especially ex-

* *Correspondence: Jürgen Glaser, glaser@wi.tum.de*

Thanks to Severin Hornung (Chair of Psychology, TU Muenchen) for his assistance in preparing the English manuscript.

penses for nursing and therapeutical treatment have seen a strong rise in the past ten years. With a yearly growth rate of 6.1% these costs went up to 51.6 billion Euros.

The expenses for health care correspond with 17 million patients in hospitals and altogether 2,04 million persons in need of care, in the sense of the German nursing care insurance law. 81% of those in need of care are above the age of 65 years, 604,000 are living in nursing homes, 1,44 million are cared for at home, and 435,000 are in need of professional home nursing services. The number of persons in need of care has increased steadily since the nursing care insurance law was passed in 1994. Additionally, there has been a shift from persons receiving nursing allowance only, while being cared for by relatives, towards the care in nursing homes or by home nursing services. Taking into account the demographic development, it does not seem daring to forecast that the need for nursing services will continue to increase in the future.

Furthermore, there is already a nursing shortage today in several fields of the health care sector. According to a representative study by the German Institute of Applied Nursing Research there have been more than 12,000 vacant positions in hospitals and another 30,000 vacancies in nursing homes for the elderly and in home nursing services in the year 2002. On the other hand, there was only a comparably low number of job seekers with corresponding qualifications (in the year 2000 about 18,000). With an average of 2.8% the unemployment rate in nursing is extremely low (Deutsches Institut für Angewandte Pflegeforschung, 2002).

The same study also states that work stressors have increased in all fields of nursing during the past years. Rising tendencies in overtime as well as in sickness leaves can be taken as comparably 'hard' indicators for the deteriorating working conditions in nursing. This development seems particularly alarming in the light of the mentioned nursing shortage. Several federal states already suffer from a nursing shortage, especially within the areas of nursing for the elderly and home care.

Despite of societal importance, relevance for the labor market, and future needs for professional health care services, the field of nursing has been ignored for a long time by work and organizational psychologists in Germany. Several studies from the perspective of occupational medicine and safety have pointed out rather traditional work stressors (e.g., Hofmann, 1994): Shift work or hazards from harmful substances were identified as main detrimental characteristics of nursing work. However, psychological factors and their consequences, such as high demands, excessive workload, inadequate resources, dissatisfaction, stress and burnout, have rarely been taken seriously into account by research, until nursing started to gain public interest in Germany a few years ago.

Nevertheless, more than ten years ago, at the end of the 1980s, a research program was initiated by André Büssing, who recognized the need for nursing research from the perspective of work and organizational psychology. In the course of the common pioneer work of André Büssing and the author, several concepts and theory-guided methods have been developed for the analysis, evaluation, and design of nursing tasks as well as of organizational and individual conditions and consequences of person-related service work in health care systems. The purpose of this paper is to give an overview of some important milestones of this research program in memory of André Büssing.

Work analysis in nursing

Based on the 'Organization-Task-Individual (OTI)-Concept' by Büssing (1992), which formulated the need and the theoretical basis for a multi-level analysis of organizations, we began with the development of an integrated 'Work Analysis Instrument for Hospitals (TAA-KH[1])' by the end of the 1980s. The self-report version (TAA-KH-S) of the instrument was published recently (Büssing & Glaser, 2002). The final validation and publication of the expert-rating version with its two domains on organizational diagnosis and on task analysis has not been accomplished yet. The TAA-KH-S was designed specifically for nursing in hospitals and it is based on Action Regulation Theory (Hacker, 1998). The TAA-KH-S focuses on the analysis of working conditions rather than individual characteristics of workers. It differentiates between regulation demands, work stressors, and work-related resources as psychologically important characteristics of work tasks. A strong emphasis was put on testing the psychometric properties of the instrument, which complies with the criteria of objectivity in data collection, analysis, and interpretation, of reliability – as indicated by the internal consistency of the scales and inter-rater-reliability – as well as of validity – in the sense of content- and convergent validity.

Several studies have been conducted with the TAA-KH-S to analyze the working situation of nursing in hospitals. The results in the five domains of the instrument, addressing different forms of demands, stressors, and resources, have laid a solid empirical foundation, which also allows for the examination of the effects of these psychologically relevant work characteris-

---

[1] *The abbreviation 'TAA-KH' refers to the German name 'Tätigkeits- und Arbeitsanalyseverfahren für das Krankenhaus'.*

tics on the working individuals as well as for the derivation of concepts for work design in nursing. Below, a brief overview of some results is presented.

Nursing can be characterized as a job with high cognitive and motor demands. Aside from technical knowledge from the fields of medicine, psychology, social work and law, and specialized skills, which are acquired through continuous training on- and off-the-job, nursing requires physical abilities (e.g., dexterity, endurance, and strength) as well as a large amount of social abilities and social knowledge. Communicative and social competence therefore represents necessary additional core qualifications. The analysis of demands for activity and qualification has shown that – contrary to what is sometimes assumed – nursing is not a simple, undertaxing task. It rather comprises complex and demanding elements as, for example, the individual planning of the care. Furthermore, the demands for activity and qualification are determined to a large extent by the prevailing work organization. Concise differences in the demands of the tasks were found depending on the way the nursing work was organized. This link between task characteristics and the organization and design of work in nursing, which is one central issue of the OTI concept mentioned before, will be discussed in a later section of this article.

In contrast to demands, work stressors in nursing have been examined relatively often. Classical ergonomic hazards, like dangers resulting from toxic, mutagenic or allergenic substances, risks of infection, exposition to radiation, musculosceletal strain, and risks of injuries from cuts and punctures, have been examined in studies from the perspective of occupational medicine and safety. Aside from time pressure, problems of handling difficult patients, and the contact with the dying (Schlüter, 1992), psychological work stressors on the other hand have received significantly less attention. In our own studies with the TAA-KH-S we could identify several additional psychological stressors. Organizational stressors (e.g., too many admitted patients), social stressors (conflicts with patients, colleagues, and supervisors), and also most forms of regulation problems, which have been studied in industrial contexts before (e.g., Greiner, Ragland, Krause, Syme & Fisher, 1997), were found to be relevant in nursing. Regulation problems refer to circumstances that prohibit the efficient and effective regulation of work action and which can lead to additional effort and risky action. These kinds of work stressors include motor impediments (e.g., having to move beds in small, crowded rooms), informational impediments (e.g., unreadable handwritings of physicians or colleagues), interruptions by persons, by blockages or malfunctions of technical equipment, as well as time pressure and ergonomic conditions (e.g., noise), which are overtaxing the individual regulation capacity. In our studies, interruptions by persons, motor impediments, and inadequate ergonomic conditions represent the primary sources of work stressors in nursing on hospital wards.

In addition to demands for activity and qualifications and work stressors, the so-called work-related resources are systematically examined in the TAA-KH-S. The vital role of resources for coping with demands and stressors is explicated for example in the cognitive model of stress (Lazarus & Launier, 1978) as well as in the concept of salutogenesis (Antonovsky, 1987). In the context of the analysis of work tasks we have put an emphasis on activity latitudes and participation, representing important facets of autonomy at work. The instrument also assesses the transparency of the organization and of work tasks, as important prerequisites for the exertion of control, and the existing support through human, material, and social resources. The results regarding work-related resources for nursing in hospitals can be summed up as following: Transparency, activity latitudes, and social resources in the team are in a positive range; human, material, and spatial resources are dissatisfying in most cases; there seem to be deficits in leadership by the nurses in charge, resulting in inadequate feedback on performance and behavior to the nurses on many wards. Varying considerably from hospital to hospital is the quality of the cooperation with other professions and services. While an intact cooperation seems to be typical for smaller hospitals, some (larger) institutions suffer from severe interface problems between nurses, physicians, and other services, which can lead to a reduced quality of care and of the working life (e.g., Büssing, Glaser & Herbig, 2000).

The methodological standards of scientific research and the need for methods, which are applicable in practice are often incommensurate. Triggered by the observation that the full version of our TAA-KH-S as well as other established instruments for work analysis found relatively little acceptance by practitioners in hospitals, we developed an abbreviated 'screening version' of the instrument. For practitioners and decision-makers in the field – and especially in nursing – the usability and the economy, which means most of all the brevity of a survey, often seems to be more important than its psychometric properties. To meet these needs, the 'Work Load Screening TAA-KH-S' was developed out of the two domains dealing with work stressors of the full version. According to content and psychometric properties, the number of items on work stressors was substantially reduced, in order to create an economically applicable screening version.

We could show that this screening version also complies with the criteria of a reliable and valid measurement by examining the internal consistency and the intra-class-correlations, which constitute an important proof for the inter-rater reliability of condition-oriented instruments for work analysis. Construct validity was supported by conducting a convergent validation in a sample of 160 nurses from two hospitals, as well as by validating the instrument with results from expert-ratings obtained through observations (Büssing, Glaser & Höge, 2001).

The whole process for developing and testing a screening version was repeated for the remaining three domains of the full-version covering demands for activity and qualification as well as work-related resources. Complementary to the full version, we thus obtained the 'Screening TAA-KH-S' for the analysis of demands, stressors, and resources, which can be applied economically by practitioners in order to examine the working situation in nursing on hospital wards (Büssing & Glaser, 2002). As this screening version incorporates a theory-guided approach, has been shown to be objective, reliable, and valid, and also represents an economic way of obtaining information, it bridges the gap between theory and practice. It overcomes commonly reported acceptance problems of scientific instruments that often lead to the use of 'self-made' questionnaires without an examination of the common psychometric standards. The screening version can be employed completely or in a modular way in order to get a first impression of the working situation, e.g., to find out the most important work stressors. In a second step, the use of the full version can help to get more detailed and differentiated insights regarding identified problem areas.

Individual consequences of work in nursing

The disproportional high number of sickness leaves and of persons leaving the nursing profession in Germany (Becker & Meifort, 1997) can be taken as indicators that not only the psychological and physical stressors in nursing are on a high level, but that these stressors also affect the working individuals in a way, which can result in the impairment of their health and even the termination of their professional careers. As only few longitudinal studies have been able to establish an empirical connection between the working situation in nursing and effects on the psycho-physical health of nurses, however, causal explanations have to be treated cautiously and recognized as preliminary in their nature. This also holds true for models of the development of psychological stress and burnout in nursing.

In our own studies with the TAA-KH-S we drew strongly on the concept of complete work tasks (Hacker, 1998) from Action Regulation Theory. In accordance with this concept, demands and resources in nursing should – under the premise of an adequate level of qualification and expertise – have a positive effect on health, competencies, and the personality of the working persons. In early studies within our research program we could show that especially demands and possibilities for qualification contributed to an enhancement of the health and the personality of the nurses (Büssing & Glaser, 1993). Furthermore, we found out that especially activity latitudes are an important work-related resource in nursing, which leads to satisfaction at work and reduces psychological strain (Büssing & Glaser, 1991). Work-stressors on the other hand, are seen as risk factors with regard to psychological strain, burn-out, and even more far-reaching negative consequences for the health of the working individuals. Exemplary for the test of these common assumptions, results from two empirical studies will be reported in the following.

Study 1

In a research project promoted by the Federal Ministry for Education, Science, Research and Technology, we have examined the effects of work stressors on the psychological strain of nurses (Glaser & Büssing, 1996b). Work stressors were conceptualized as disturbances of the regulation of work action, which get in the way of a successful coping with work demands and therefore pose a threat to health and well-being of the working person. In our study we drew on a mediation model, in which regulation problems necessitate additional effort and can lead to risky action and a reduced quality of work, while these first order outcomes mediate the effect of regulation problems on psychological strain.

This mediator model was tested in a sample of 160 nurses working in a general hospital. By conducting stepwise multiple regressions we could show that several work stressors (obstacles to learning on the job, motor impediments, and interruptions) lead to additional effort, which, in turn, has a positive effect on irritation/strain and emotional exhaustion. Informational impediments and contradictory task goals, on the other hand, are related directly to symptoms of psychological strain. In our study the mediator model of the effects of regulation problems on psychological strain has received the first empirical support. Of particular practical relevance is the first order outcome of additional effort in the model. Additional effort can be quantified in time (e.g., in minutes or hours per work day) and thus it can be converted into an obviously economically relevant variable. Therefore, the model allows for an estimation of economic costs of work stressors and also for the calculation of economic benefits of the reduction of work stressors through work redesign. For example, on several wards of different general hospitals we found that the additional effort was in a range of up to one working hour per nurse and shift (Glaser, 1997), which could be reduced by measures of work redesign (e.g., through a diminution of interruptions at work).

Study 2

Building upon the results of study 1, a larger project on the effects of work stressors on health and well-being, in which 482 nurses in general hospitals participated, was conducted (Büssing & Glaser, 2000). In this study we used the TAA-KH-S to investigate regulation problems in nursing (informational and motor impediments, interruptions by persons, malfunctions, and block-ages) and their first order outcomes (additional effort and risky action). Additionally, we examined the degree of emotional exhaustion and depersonalisa-tion, which represent the core dimensions of the burnout-syndrome. To avoid the general problem of common method variance in questionnaire research we validated the survey results on work stressors with expert-ratings from observations.

The results of this study offer insights on two levels. First, the evaluation of work stressors obtained from survey data and from expert-rating show a strong correlation ($r = .73$), which constitutes an argument against the so-called 'methodological trap' of common method variance (Kasl, 1987). Sec-ond, the mediation of work stressors on emotional exhaustion through addi-tional effort and risky action was confirmed. Additionally, we could show that emotional exhaustion also mediated the effect of the first order outcomes of work stressors (additional effort and risky action) on depersonalisation.

This multi-stage model of the relationships between work stressors and core-symptoms of burnout was also confirmed by the results of a path analysis. Additionally, we examined the effects of activity latitudes on this model of the development of burnout. The results of this additional step in the path analysis showed that activity latitudes have a direct negative effect on work stressors, which indicates that the degrees of freedom in work are used to cope with stressors, but do not have a significant negative effect on the first or second order outcomes (additional effort, risky action, and symptoms of burnout) of work stressors.

Drawing on the results of these two exemplary studies on the causal mecha-nisms of work stressors in a health care setting, our conclusion is that forms of regulation problems do represent an important aspect of work stressors in nursing. These kinds of work stressors lead to additional effort and risky action and thus have economically quantifiable implications on working time and also on the quality of work. These first order outcomes have a negative effect on the mental health of the nurses by promoting irritation/strain and the development of burnout. Practical implications of this model exist with regard to work design, which should employ adequate forms of work organization to pursue the goal of minimizing regulation problems (e.g., interruptions at work). Furthermore, an approach of 'prospective work design' to avoid health-impairing effects of the working situation of nurses lies in the creation of activity latitudes, which – by the results of the second study – have been shown to play an important role in preventing the development of burnout in nursing.

Interaction work in nursing

Nursing can be characterized as a form of 'dialogical work', in which even simple tasks require complex processes of communication and cooperation between the nurse and the patient. Verbal and nonverbal communication does not only convey information on a factual but also on an emotional level. In nursing this applies to the working relation with colleagues in the team, with the physicians, the supervisors, and various other persons. But most of all it is important for the relationship between nurse and patient. Nursing is 'interaction work'. The social interaction with patients is a core task in nursing, it has a therapeutic value, and it makes an independent contribution to the recovery of the care receiver. Additionally, nurses act as social models for the patients, while the patients themselves are 'co-producers' of the health care service (Badura, 1995).

So far, the description and explication of work action in psychology was based mainly on a cognitive model of goal-oriented rational action. Action Regulation Theory (Hacker, 1998) systematically breaks down work action into hierarchical levels and sequential phases. This model offers a classification of the demands for the psychological regulation of tasks as well as a framework for analyzing the effects of obstacles in the regulation of work action.

However, it seems questionable whether all facets of dialogical work can be characterized comprehensively by any model of rational and goal-oriented action. As Böhle (1999) states, dialogical work can never be planned completely. Rather, it necessitates a dialogical-interactive approach, subjective understanding (empathy), and a 'feeling' for the situation. The author therefore contrasts and complements the goal-oriented, 'objectivating' model of action regulation with a 'subjectivating' model of action, which is – among others – applicable to dialogical work. As flexible responses to the condition and the reaction of patients are of utmost importance in nursing, the success of the interaction between nurse and patient largely determines the quality of the process as well as the outcome of the health care service.

One of our studies demonstrated the importance of social interaction in nursing from a slightly different perspective (Büssing & Glaser, 1999). In this project the nursing work in a general hospital was redesigned to reduce work stressors. Aside from a longitudinal questionnaire survey, we conducted qualitative interviews and group discussions with the nurses working on the restructured model wards. We included two other hospitals, in which only minor interventions of organizational development were conducted, in our study as a control group. Our main focus in this study was on work stressors, which had previously been identified as predictors of burnout (forms of regulation problems as well as social stressors). The results were surprising in some respect. First of all, we could show an improvement regarding work stressors on the model wards, which became manifest in a significantly reduced time pressure, less conflicting work goals, improved working conditions, and ways to better cope with complicated patient conditions. Judging from this positive development we expected that symptoms of work strain and burnout would decrease over time in those wards with redesigned work tasks. But contrary to our expectations, emotional exhaustion and feelings of depersonalisation even increased.

This 'paradox' result in the quantitative data, however, could be explained by taking into account the findings from the qualitative interviews and the group discussions. Although the nurses very much approved the reduction in 'traditional' work stressors as well as the increased autonomy at work, they made clear that the work redesign had also generated 'new' forms of work stressors. Social interaction between nurses and patients had intensified, responsibility for individual patients had increased considerably, and the relationship to patients had become closer, more intimate, and had more continuity. But this new situation also offered less possibilities for withdrawal from the patients. Several nurses reported that they occasionally had problems to cope with the needs and the sometimes excessive demands that patients expressed. The redesign of nursing work had thus resulted in 'new' forms of work stressors, grounded in the context of social interaction with the patients – a side-effect, which is not totally uncharacteristic for attempts to modernize work practices (Giddens, 1991). The results presented above also relate to the idea of 'detached concern', which describes the ability to maintain both emotional distance and empathy at the same time (e.g., Corcoran, 1986).

Based on the reported findings, the study of stressors resulting from social interaction and of interaction work in general became an integral part of our research program. Our interests in this area were two-fold: First, we wanted to find out how nurses deal with their own emotions, i.e., how they experience and cope with disgust, anger, sympathy, sorrow, and other emotions. Second, we wanted to know how nurses purposefully use their own emotions to better be able to fulfill their duties, i.e., to work *with* the patient instead of working *against* them. These questions led us to two research traditions in microsociology dealing with the concepts of emotional work (Hochschild, 1983), which had been well studied in the context of comparably simple service jobs like stewardesses and fast-food waiters, and with sentimental work (Strauss,

Fagerhaugh, Suczek & Wiener, 1985), which had been developed for the work in hospitals but had been relatively neglected in nursing science so far.

Our concept of 'interaction work' combines these two complementary research traditions and integrates them with elements from other fields of behavioral and psychological research (Büssing & Glaser, 2001). For analyzing interaction work we developed and validated a questionnaire dealing with interaction characteristics in terms of frequency and intensity of interaction (Morris & Feldman, 1996) as well as demands in interactions with different groups of patients (different personalities, diseases, and conditions). This instrument incorporates a condition-related approach. Additionally, we developed another questionnaire to operationalize constellations of emotional dissonance. This complementary instrument measures the states of emotional harmony, emotional dissonance (faking in good faith and faking in bad faith), and emotional deviance, as described by Rafaeli and Sutton (1987), as well as the strategies for influencing own emotions at work, which Hochschild (1983) labeled 'surface acting' and 'deep acting'.

We employed the questionnaires on interaction work in a sample of 298 nurses along with other instruments on burnout and work satisfaction in order to be able to empirically test assumptions from the integrative model of Morris and Feldman (1996) on conditions and consequences of interaction work. The obtained psychometric properties support the quality of the two developed instruments on interaction characteristics and constellations of emotional work. Stepwise multiple regressions showed that a significant amount of variance of work satisfaction and emotional exhaustion is explained by interaction characteristics and by certain constellations of emotional dissonance. With regard to the former, a difficult personality of patients turned out to be a relevant predictor of work satisfaction and emotional exhaustion.

These first findings in nursing on hospital wards raised new questions on the conditions, the adequate organizational and work design, and the most promising approaches to training for promoting quality in interaction work. Also, we had to ask ourselves what the criteria for quality and success in interaction work are and how they should be measured. To cover these issues a cooperative project on 'Interaction Work as an Innovative Approach to the Quality-Oriented Design of Service Processes' was initiated. The project is funded by the Federal Ministry for Education and Research and is currently conducted in cooperation with work sociologists and two companies. In this project a framework for analyzing interaction work was developed and operationalized. The empirical studies deal with aspects of competence and training for interaction work as well as with interaction-oriented leadership, interaction latitudes, and other conditions of interaction work. Also, the concept of sentimental work with its different facets (Strauss et al., 1985) was operationalized and investigated empirically (Büssing, Giesenbauer & Glaser, 2003).

Results of the project have shown that the analysis of interaction work adds value to the description and explanation of complex person-related service tasks. In addition to different fields of nursing, the concepts and instruments on interaction work were also validated in other service professions (e.g., teachers). By taking into account important characteristics of dialogical work tasks, the concept of interaction work complements the predominantly cognitive model of goal-oriented work action as well as the conceptualization of demands, stressors, and resources in nursing. Combined with a psychological approach to work design, the findings on interaction work can contribute to ways for improving the work-life as well as the service quality in health care systems. The next section will deal with such approaches for the field of nursing, which are based on the concepts of complete service tasks as well as on employee- and patient-orientation in nursing.

Concepts for the organization and design of nursing work

The characteristics of work tasks are largely determined by organizational structures and processes. Therefore, work design in nursing has to take into account different organizational levels, ranging form the hospital as a whole, the departments, the wards to the individual work tasks. The analysis of the latter represents the starting point for the design or the reintegration of complete work tasks. Results of work analyses, which were based on observations and interviews, have shown that work tasks in nursing on hospital wards are often 'partialized', i.e., that the division of labor has left these tasks 'incomplete' (Glaser, 1997). Tasks which require planning are often assigned to other occupations (e.g., the physicians in the case of ward rounds or admissions) or to other hierarchical positions (i.e., the nurses in charge or the shift supervisors in the case of care planning). This tayloristic principle of division of labour decreases the proportion of mentally challenging elements with higher cognitive regulation demands. Results are nursing tasks, which do not conform to the criteria of complete and therefore humane work. But the results of the observations and interviews also indicate that the characteristics of work tasks on different hospitals wards vary considerably, even if the wards have the same function and a similar structural situation (e.g., surgical wards in general hospitals with a similar number of beds and staff). A more fine-grained differentiation on the level of individual work tasks yielded the same result: Some jobs where organized to be 'complete' on some wards, while they were 'partialized' on others.

To describe such differences in the work organization on hospital wards we developed a systematization of nursing work (Glaser & Büssing, 1996a) with two dimensions. The dimension 'nursing organization' refers to the area of responsibility of the nurses, which can be individual patients, certain rooms, a section of the ward, certain groups of patients or the whole ward. The other dimension of the systematization is the so-called 'nursing principle', which is relatively independent of the first dimension. The 'nursing principle' describes the degree to which nursing is predominantly oriented on the execution of work functions or rather on the patients' individual needs. Holistic nursing can be defined as a combination of full responsibility of nurses for a certain number of patients and a high degree of patient-orientation in a complete sequential process of planning, executing, and controlling nursing work. The concept of holistic nursing thus integrates concepts from work psychology and nursing science.

The development and the test of such a holistic nursing system was conducted, documented, and evaluated in a research project in a general hospital, which was already mentioned in a previous section. One goal of the project was to restructure the work organization on designated model wards from a tayloristic system of function-oriented nursing in large patient groups to a system of holistic nursing within rather small nursing domains, which should result in a higher degree of task 'completeness', more autonomy and responsibility for the nurses, a reduction of work stressors, and – last but not least – an improvement of the quality and the economy of care. By choosing a participative bottom-up approach, the nurses were involved in the process of organizational development. Appropriate measures for work design were developed in task forces and workshops. Discussions, seminars, and measures for training on- and off-the-job were initiated to prepare the nurses for the new working situation. A special feature of this longitudinal project was the formative evaluation of the organizational development, which was conducted with the TAA-KH-S and other questionnaires on four points of measurement during a three-year period. The intermediary results were used to create a feedback-loop for the respective task forces to facilitate a continuous improvement of the reorganization effort.

The results of this evaluation have shown that regulation problems and their consequences, i.e., time pressure, interruptions, informational and motor impediments, additional effort, and risky action, which initially were among the most relevant stressors in nursing on hospital wards, could be reduced significantly by a reorganization of the nursing system. Additionally, mentally more demanding jobs with more responsibility for the nurses were created. As an unintended side-effect of the reorganization, however, stressors connected with the social interaction at work had increased and had resulted in some of the nurses withdrawing from certain patients. This phenomenon, already described above, has lead us to more strongly integrate the patients' perspective into our research by developing and testing instruments for patient surveys, which assess aspects of holistic nursing, characteristics of the social interaction, and the role of the patients.

Our approach of 'employee- and patient orientation' (MPO-approach[2]), which represents a design concept not limited to nursing but referring to health care in general, expands and rounds out our research program. The MPO-approach integrates findings of work psychology and nursing science with the goal of a complete health care service. It incorporates methodological and contentual findings from the analysis of demands, stressors, and resources in nursing, from the investigation of facets of the social interaction, as well as from the concept of holistic nursing, while at the same time expanding our perspective to include the perceptions of other occupational groups in hospitals and especially also the patients and their relatives (Büssing & Glaser, 2003).

Employee orientation refers to the creation of 'complete' work tasks in nursing, which are characterized by adequate psychological demands, low work stressors, and a high availability of work-related resources. These conditions can be assessed in an economic, reliable, and valid way with the screening version of the TAA-KH-S. The results of these analyses can be used directly as an input for work design projects.

Patient orientation complements employee orientation by focussing on the interaction between nurses and patients. For the measurement of the degree of patient orientation and of the completeness of the health care service form the perspective of the patients we developed the 'Munich Instrument for Patient Surveys' (MIP[3]; Büssing & Glaser, 2003). The MIP is a condition-oriented instrument with different comparable versions for patients and their relatives, which incorporates the conceptualization of patients as interactive co-producers of the health care service and not as mere 'consumers'. The assessed aspects of the interaction and the relationship between professionals and patients as well as of the quality and the completeness of the health care service allow for a joint optimization of employee- and patient orientation.

Several projects of work design in the context of quality management in hospitals have been conducted with the MPO-approach. For example, in a hospital for psychosomatic medicine for children and adolescents an assessment of the perspectives of the employees, the patients, and their relatives was used to initiate an improvement process in the course of a quality certification program.

---

[2] *The abbreviation 'MPO' refers to the German expression 'Mitarbeiter- und Patientenorientierung'.*

[3] *The abbreviation 'MIP' refers to the German name 'Münchener Instrument zur Patientenbefragung'.*

An important advantage of work design with the MPO-approach is that it corresponds with the postulates of total quality managements systems (e.g., EFQM) and therefore is met with positive response from practitioners. Not only does it provide abstract concepts but also concrete methods for evaluation, the condition-oriented operationalization of which prevents biases stemming from the use of attitudinal measures (e.g., the disproportionately high number of 'satisfied' employees and patients, which represent a problem well-known from the research on work satisfaction). Further advantages of this approach are its theoretical basis and the possibility to reconcile the perspectives of employees and patients in a common conceptual and methodological framework. By taking into account the perspectives of different groups of actors the MPO-approach makes a contribution to the generalization of previous results. Other aspects concerning generalizability are dealt within the next section.

Generalization and outlook

In this article I introduced a research program for the analysis, the evaluation, and the design of work, which was initiated by André Büssing in the mid 1980s in the context of psychiatric hospitals (Büssing, 1992). Together, we began with the development of the 'Work Analysis Instrument for Hospitals' (TAA-KH) and conducted several studies on the effects and consequences of working conditions in nursing. Current research projects have shown that the concepts and especially the instruments are generalizable to other fields of nursing. In a project funded by the Federal Institute For Occupational Safety and Health (FIOSH) the screening version of the TAA-KH-S was adapted to the context of home care. The psychometric properties of the adapted instrument are comparable to those obtained from the analysis of nursing in hospitals. The working situation in the field of home care, which has increasingly gained importance since the German nursing care insurance law was passed, shows some similarities to but also distinctive differences from the situation of nursing in hospitals. Working in the patients' homes brings about new demands and stressors, which are often related to inadequate material and spatial resources. Additionally, the nature of cooperation at work changes. Contacts to colleagues are often restricted to team meetings, while the patients' relatives tend to play a key role in daily work. Furthermore, home care also seems to be characterized by more responsibility and higher activity latitudes for the nurses.

In the cooperation project on interaction work in person-related services, which is funded by the Federal Ministry for Education and Research and was outlined in a previous section of this article, we thoroughly investigate nursing work in nursing homes for the elderly. The working situation, including the structural and legal conditions in nursing homes for the elderly, is examined and documented in a series of project reports. Besides the mentioned development of concepts and methods on interaction work, the introduction of a holistic nursing system, in which patients are assigned to nurses, who are responsible for their entire care, on three model wards of a nursing home for the elderly is a particularly interesting part of this project. The results of the evaluation, which was conducted on three points of measurement, indicate that this form of work organization is appropriate to support interaction work between nurses for the elderly and residents. The MPO-approach was also successfully modified for this new context, with the results of the survey for the patients' relatives being of special relevance in this project, because of a high proportion of demented patients.

In addition to general hospitals, the MPO-approach was also tested in hospitals for psychosomatic and psychiatric medicine. Currently it is employed in the quality management of state-run psychiatric hospitals. The collection of survey data from 3,889 employees, including nurses as well as other occupations, and from 1,612 patients was completed recently. The results show that the MPO-approach can be modified for psychiatric nursing and other professions. Such a generalization to different fields of nursing, which includes comparisons of conditions and effects of nursing work as well as the test of concepts for work design, seems important in the light of efforts to establish an integrated health care system (e.g., to improve the transfer between institutions for in- and out-patient care).

Beyond the generalization of concepts and instruments to different fields of nursing, research on the work of other occupational groups in the health care sector, which have been largely neglected by psychological research so far, is needed. First steps in this direction have been undertaken by adapting both the TAA-KH-S and the MIP for medical and therapeutic professions. Further work, e.g., on comparisons between different occupational groups in the health care sector, is in progress. Nursing is an important source of innovations – not only in hospitals but in all organizations of the health care sector. A generalization of our research program from nursing in hospitals to the broader field of health care therefore will contribute to improvements for an even larger number of employees and patients.

Overall, the research program presented here can be taken as a proof that nursing is not at all a 'simple job', but a complex, dialogical service task. It is possible to analyze nursing from the perspective of work psychology in a theory-based, reliable, valid, and economic way, which makes it possible to consolidate und serve the interests of both science and practice. It has also been shown that established concepts and models in work psychology can be adapted to the field of nursing. However, as a person-related service, nursing work has a dialogical character, which is due to the fact that – unlike industrial work – its main focus is not a 'work object' but a 'subject', i.e., another person. The model of goal-oriented action therefore needs to be expanded by taking into account facets of the interaction between nurse and patient. The concept of interaction work seems appropriate to close or at least to reduce this gap between the analysis of non-dialogical and dialogical work. As an applied discipline work psychology not only has to provide concepts and methods, but also evidence for their implementation in and their impact on the field. The reported projects of work design and organizational development show that this idea of an applied science is an integral part of the presented research program. Further developments of the research program, e.g., with regard to its generalization to other fields of health care, have been indicated. These and other issues represent work in progress, which are dealt with in currently running, third-party funded research projects.

References

Antonovsky, A. (1987). *Unraveling the mystery of health. How people manage stress and stay well*. San Francisco: Jossey-Bass.

Badura, B. (1995). Gesundheitsdienstleistungen im Wandel. In H.-J. Bullinger (Hrsg.), *Dienstleistung der Zukunft. Märkte, Unternehmen und Infrastruktur im Wandel* (S. 183-190). Wiesbaden: Gabler.

Becker, W. & Meifort, B. (1997). *Altenpflege: Eine Arbeit wie jede andere? Ein Beruf fürs Leben?* Bielefeld: Bertelsmann.

Böhle, F. (1999). Nicht nur mehr Qualität, sondern auch höhere Effizienz – Subjektivierendes Handeln in der Altenpflege. *Zeitschrift für Arbeitswissenschaft, 53,* 174-181.

Büssing, A. (1992). *Organisationsstruktur, Tätigkeit und Individuum*. Bern: Huber.

Büssing, A. & Glaser, J. (1991). Zusammenhänge zwischen Tätigkeitsspielräumen und Persönlichkeitsförderung in der Arbeitstätigkeit. *Zeitschrift für Arbeits- und Organisationspsychologie, 35,* 122-136.

Büssing, A. & Glaser, J. (1993). Qualifikationserfordernisse und -möglichkeiten als gesundheits- und persönlichkeitsförderliche Merkmale in der Arbeitstätigkeit. *Zeitschrift für Arbeits- und Organisationspsychologie, 37,* 154-162.

Büssing, A. & Glaser, J. (1999). Work stressors in nursing in the course of redesign: Implications for burnout and interactional stress. *European Journal of Work and Organizational Psychology, 8,* 401-426.

Büssing, A. & Glaser, J. (2000). The „four-stage process model of core factors of burnout". The role of work stressors and work-related resources. *Work & Stress, 14,* 329-346.

Büssing, A. & Glaser, J. (2001). Interaction work: Concept, measurement, and results from nursing. In J. de Jonge, P. Vlerick, A. Büssing & W. B. Schaufeli (Eds.), *Organizational Psychology and Health Care at the Start of a New Millenium* (pp. 175-196). München: Hampp.

Büssing, A. & Glaser, J. (2002). *Das Tätigkeits- und Arbeitsanalyseverfahren für das Krankenhaus – Selbstbeobachtungsversion (TAA-KH-S)*. Göttingen: Hogrefe.

Büssing, A. & Glaser, J. (2003). Employee and client orientation. Concept and evaluation of quality in health care. In J. Hellgren, K. Näswall, M. Sverke & M. Söderfeldt (Eds.), *New organizational challenges for human service work* (pp. 115-136) München: Hampp.

Büssing, A., Giesenbauer, B. & Glaser, J. (2003). Gefühlsarbeit. Beeinflussung der Gefühle von Bewohnern und Patienten in der stationären und ambulanten Altenpflege. *Pflege, 16,* 357-365.

Büssing, A., Glaser, J. & Herbig, B. (2000). Organizational interfaces, risk potentials and quality losses in nursing: A multi-level approach. In C. Vincent & B. DeMol (Eds.), *Safety in Medicine* (pp. 155-174). Amsterdam: Pergamon.

Büssing, A., Glaser, J. & Höge, T. (2001). Screening psychischer Belastungen in der stationären Krankenpflege (Belastungsscreening TAA-KH-S). *Diagnostica, 47,* 77-87.

Corcoran, S. A. (1986). Task complexity and nursing expertise as factors in decision making. *Nursing Research, 35,* 107-112.

Deutsches Institut für Angewandte Pflegeforschung (2002). *Pflege-Thermometer 2002. Frühjahrsbefragung zur Lage und Entwicklung des Pflegepersonalwesens in Deutschland.* Köln: Autor.

Giddens, A. (1991). *Modernity and self identity. Self and society in late modern age.* Stanford: University Press.

Glaser, J. (1997). *Aufgabenanalysen in der Krankenpflege. Eine arbeitspsychologische Analyse und Bewertung pflegerischer Aufgaben.* Münster: Waxmann.

Glaser, J. & Büssing, A. (1996a). Ganzheitliche Pflege: Präzisierung und Umsetzungschancen. *Pflege, 9,* 221-232.

Glaser, J. & Büssing, A. (1996b). Widersprüchliche Anforderungen in der Arbeitstätigkeit, Zusatzaufwand und psychischer Streß. Konzepte und Überprüfung eines Vermittlungsmodells. *Zeitschrift für Arbeits- und Organisationspsychologie, 40* (2), 87-91.

Greiner, B. A., Ragland, D. R., Krause, N., Syme, S. L. & Fisher, J. M. (1997). Objective measurement of occupational stress factors – An example with San Francisco urban transit operators. *Journal of Occupational Health Psychology, 2,* 325-342.

Hacker, W. (1998). *Allgemeine Arbeitspsychologie. Psychische Regulation von Arbeitstätigkeiten.* Bern: Huber.

Hochschild, A. R. (1983). *The managed heart: Commercialisation of human feeling.* Berkeley: University of California Press.

Hofmann, F. (1994). *Arbeitsbedingte Belastungen des Pflegepersonals.* Landsberg: Ecomed.

Kasl, S. V. (1987). Methodologies in stress and health: Past difficulties, present dilemmas, future directions. In S. V. Kasl & C. L. Cooper (Eds.), *Stress and Health: Issues in Research Methodology* (pp. 307-318). New York: Wiley.

Lazarus, R. S. & Launier, R. (1978). Stress-related transactions between persons and environment. In L. A. Pervin & M. Lewis (Eds.), *Perspectives in interactional psychology* (pp. 287-327). New York: Plenum.

Morris, J. A. & Feldman, D. C. (1996). The dimensions, antecedents, and consequences of emotional labor. *Academy of Management Review, 21,* 986-1010.

Rafaeli, A. & Sutton, R. I. (1987). Expression of emotion as part of the work role. *Academy of Management Review*, *12*, 23-37.

Schlüter, G. (1992). *Berufliche Belastungen in der Krankenpflege – Eine empirische Untersuchung.* Melsungen: Bibliomed.

Statistisches Bundesamt (2003a). *Gesundheitswesen* (abrufbar als www-Dokument unter URL http://www.destatis.de/themen/d/thm_gesundheit.htm [26.01.2004])

Statistisches Bundesamt (2003b). *Gesundheitsausgaben und Gesundheitspersonal 2001.* Wiesbaden: Autor.

Strauss, A., Fagerhaugh, S., Suczek, B. & Wiener, C. (1985). *Social organization of medical work.* Chicago: University Press.

Improving health care work environments: The need for evidence-based management

Denise M. Rousseau*

Heinz School of Public Policy and Tepper School of Business, Carnegie Mellon University, USA

There is a serious gap between the evidence of how to effectively manage complex organizations and the way in which contemporary healthcare workers, particularly nurses, are managed. I will focus on two key issues. First, nurses are key integrators and coordinators of patient care, but the way nurses in contemporary healthcare organizations are managed is largely ineffective and dysfunctional. Second, healthcare organizations have failed to practice evidence-based management, despite the existence of a substantial research base to guide more effective organizing and management of healthcare work. This paper outlines the evidence-based features of effective healthcare work environments.

Nurses as integrators and coordinators of patient care

Nurses are the primary deliverers of healthcare in contemporary hospitals. In the United States, for example, on average every fourth person working in a hospital is a licensed nurse. In addition to providing core health services, nurses are also the essential protectors of patients from medication errors, risk of infection, adverse drug interactions, and other threats to patient safety. The critical role that nurses play in providing patient care is evident in research on hospital management practices. Research has found that quality of patient care in the most nursing-intensive hospital settings, that is, critical care units, is directly tied to the unit's *nursing* culture and leadership (however, no parallel effect has been found for physician culture, Shortell, et al., 1994) The criticality of nurses to patient care quality is underscored in recent report by Barens (2000) finding that 1,720 hospital patient deaths and 9,584 injuries resulted from actions or inactions of registered nurses in the United States over 5 year period. A key question is why nurses, who are critical to protecting patient safety, account for these adverse outcomes.

The answer identified in a recent Institute of Medicine (IOM) report (Page, 2004) is linked to the high turnover rates among nurses, turnover, not only

---

* *Correspondence: Denise M. Rousseau, rousseau@andrew.cmu.edu*

from the hospitals that employ them but from the nursing profession itself (see table 1 for statistical information). Registered nurses are leaving nursing in record numbers (18.3% according to NSSRN data). Even among nurses remaining in the profession, 1 in 2 registered nurses leaves an employer annually, making many acute care hospitals in the United States veritable revolving doors. Nursing administrators, including nurse managers supervising those nurses with direct patient care responsibilities, also demonstrate increasingly high rates of turnover, adding to a degree of personnel instability that challenges healthcare organizations to manage effectively. This turnover rate corresponds to lower job satisfaction levels among nurses in comparison to workers generally.

Table 1

Facts about nurses (USA)
1 out of 4 acute care hospital employees is a licensed nurse
Registered nurses are leaving nursing in record numbers – 18.3% (NSSRN data)
• Turnover: in 2000 21% of acute care hospital nurses left their position.
• 2001 American Healthcare Association study indicated:
56% turnover rate among registered nurses,
45% for nurse administrators
78% for nursing assistants (non-licensed)
Only about 2% are contingent workers, often filling vacancies (Year 2000).
Nurses report satisfaction with current job (69% NSSRN in contrast with 85% workers in general and 90% professional workers, Spratley et al, 2000)
Registered nurses are older than workforce generally (Average age = 45.2 years) female 94.6%
1,720 deaths and 9,584 injuries of hospital patients from actions or inactions of RNs over 5 year period.

(Chicago Tribune Report by Berens, 2000 based on U.S. Department of Health and Human Services data)

The basis for this dissatisfaction is the increasingly stressful work environment nurses face (Table 2). Patients in acute care hospitals are sicker on admission, as a function of more home-based treatment of many clinical cases and an aging patient population. Sicker patients are particularly vulnerable to deviations in care quality. Patient turnover is greater, ranging from 1 in 4 to 1 in 2 patients turning over in an 8 hour period. Shorter stays give nurses less time to become familiar with patient needs. This movement of patients in and out of units creates its own problems because patient transfers increase the nursing workload, requiring greater coordination, information gathering and sharing, room preparation etc. More patient transfers translate into more gaps in the chain of care as each movement of a patient from one locale to another means that critical information regarding the patient's condition and prior treatment may be lost. Transfers also mean that more people, including nurses, aides, and orderlies, come in contact with the patient, increasing the probability of infection by making infection protection more difficult to sustain. Paperwork, often amounting to as much as 28% of nursing work time, is exacerbated by transfers, and in itself takes time away from direct patient care. Paperwork is a common cause of overtime among nurses. Sicker patients and fewer nurses to care for them means longer work hours for nurses, not uncommonly 12 or more hours in a 24 hour period.

Table 2

Nurses do more with less

Nurses face:

- ever sicker patients – especially vulnerable to deviations in care quality

- shorter stays – patient turnover ranges from 25 to 50 % in 8 hour period – means less time to become familiar with patient needs

- more transfers of patients in and out of work units increases work demands and slippage in chain of care

- longer work hours (12 or more in 24 hour period)

- paperwork that takes from 13 to 28% of time on job (away from patient care) –

    documentation is twice as high in home care nursing

    paperwork is common cause of overtime for nurses

The problems are exacerbated in patient care outside of hospitals, in settings characterized by even higher patient to nurse ratios. Nursing attrition has led to increasing use of temporaries (Anderson, Maloney, Knight & Jennings, 1996), higher patient to nurse ratios, and a decrease in the level of nursing experience (Narumi, Miyazawa, Miyata, Suzuki, Kohsaka & Kosuji, 1999). In nursing homes for example there is often only a single licensed nurse supervising non-licensed assistants. An IOM report concluded that high turnover among nurses was a major hazard to patient safety (Page, 2004). It further concluded that the root cause of this turnover was the chaotic and over-tasked work environment of nurses.

Healthcare settings lag in management practice

A recent IOM report concludes that the contemporary nursing work environment is a threat to patient safety (Page, 2004). How did it get this way? Healthcare organizations manage work and workers in a fashion more reminiscent of the 1950s than of well-managed 21st century firms. They are out of step with practices in well-managed organizations in other industries from manufacturing to other sectors focused upon human services. It is common for manufacturing firms to adopt effective practices from the service sector such as problem-solving approaches to customer service and vice versa as manifest in the widespread diffusion of Total Quality Management and related practices first developed in manufacturing. In contrast, healthcare organizations evince little uptake in management innovations. Modern management practices are effectively absent in the majority of healthcare organizations. Thus, we observed relatively little use of team building, electronic communication with employees, or real-time availability of performance metrics (Page, 2004). Moreover, there is persistent use of practices that have been demonstrated to be ineffective such as the continued use of punitive approaches to error reporting (IOM, 2000) and downsizing as a means of achieving efficiency (Cascio, Young & Morris, 1997; Cascio, 2002).

21st century management practice in leading edge organizations is based on pervasive evidence that professionals and other knowledge workers can produce high performance along multiple indicators of quality, efficiency, and member satisfaction. The conditions promoting this high performance represent a 'bundle' or set of mutually supportive management practices reflecting optimal use of worker skill in settings where management trusts workers to use their skills and discretion appropriately, and where information technology supports ('informates') optimum use of worker knowledge, skill and ability. Features of high performance work environments (Table 3) include information technology that enables workers, acting as effective decision supports and quality checks to reduce errors and eliminate administrative burdens. High performance environments offer on-going opportunity for worker development, becoming increasingly expert in their practice, and generating learning and innovation that can be captured, disseminated, and retained in the organization. This emphasis on learning reflects conscious efforts at knowledge management to continually identify and implement effective organizational processes. This learning orientation inclines organizations toward a problem focus by encouraging reporting of errors and potential operational problems. To support such practices organizational leaders themselves need to continually inform themselves regarding evidence-based management practice, to promote more effective ways of organizing, motivating staff, and managing knowledge.

Table 3

Healthcare organizations are out of step with contemporary management practice

21st Century Organizations	Healthcare Organizations
Information Technology enables work	Paper and non-linked data bases
Invest in worker development	Poor education and training
Non-punitive reporting systems	Punitive error reporting systems
Leaders educated in management practices	Leaders educated in technical processes
Emphasis on organizational learning and knowledge management	Little learning from daily errors and problem solving

Healthcare organizations in contrast are characterized by a host of disconnected and often mutually opposing management practices. Nursing turnover has diminished the availability of competent nurses in appropriate numbers to accomplish the complex tasks of providing quality clinical care while keeping patients safe. Nursing education and training are limited as shortages have reduced emphasis on up-skilling nurses. What limited use of information technology there is often involves isolated systems that are not themselves linked. Information technology in health care has not kept up with changes in contemporary work settings. It is rarely used to replace time-consuming non-clinical nursing activities with informated work practices. Charting and other communications are often paper-based. More serious still, the crush of work leaves little time for attention to learning from daily errors which thus often are repeated. Little on-going problem solving and solution sharing occur, which in turn are exacerbated by typically punitive responses to error reporting. Leaders in healthcare organizations tend to be educated in technical processes with little exposure to contemporary management practices or knowledge. In essence, healthcare managers typically are not trained to manage the complex work environments they confront.

Barriers to evidence-based management

Failure to train healthcare managers to manage leads to the neglect of evidence-based management in contemporary healthcare. Despite the key role of evidence in the adoption and implementation of patient care processes, healthcare managers generally make decisions regarding how to motivate healthcare workers and structure their work settings with no attention to contemporary management research. Moreover, in contrast to other industries where adoption of more flexible and developmental approaches to the workforce have heightened innovation and adaptability, healthcare management practices demonstrate limited innovation in the face of massive environmental and organizational challenge. Instead they remain rooted in largely authoritarian and inflexible work systems.

The persistence of management practices known to be ineffective is symptomatic of a larger problem in healthcare. Healthcare settings have expanded their use of temporary workers in critical roles (e.g., agency nurses) despite evidence that the presence of contingent workers elevates risk of accidents and errors and creates problems in effective coordination of work (Rousseau & Libuser, 1997). Downsizing is used as a means of achieving efficiency in healthcare, despite evidence that it erodes coordination and performance capabilities and does not typically reduce costs (Cascio, 2002). Persistent use of ineffective management practice is compounded by failure to employ practices of proven effectiveness where professionals and knowledge workers are concerned. For example, substantial organizational research exists on ways to balance the tension between efficiency and reliability (e.g., Roberts & Bea, 2001). Nonetheless, healthcare managers continue to view these performance metrics as trade-offs instead of goals to be managed simultaneously. Thus, healthcare organizations have failed to implement the existing evidence base regarding effective management practices. This failure occurs despite the emphasis on contemporary healthcare on evidence-based *clinical* practice.

A key issue is why management practices in healthcare are not subject to the same evidentiary requirements that clinical and policy innovations are. As well-articulated by Walshe and Rundell (2001), one reason may be that healthcare managers are a diverse group from different disciplinary backgrounds, lacking a shared language or terminology to describe what they do. As such there is no formal body of knowledge shared by all members of a 'healthcare management profession'. In consequence, personal experience and self-generated knowledge play a much larger part in determining how managers in healthcare approach their jobs than shared professional knowledge. Unlike practicing clinicians, healthcare managers often show little appreciation for the scientific method and seldom gather systematic information on the effectiveness of their practices (indeed this neglect of the scientific method is in contrast to contemporary approaches to manufacturing and other work systems where high performance is demanded). In contrast to management approaches embodied in TQM or Toyota Production System methods, healthcare managers often rely on armchair judgments and conjecture in making decisions affecting workers and the workplace. There is some degree of suspicion of the value and motives of researchers, perhaps because evidence generated externally is viewed as a threat to managerial control. Synthesizing, generalizing and transferring research findings from one setting to another are contested conceptually and methodologically, with a common discount being that the manager's organization is 'unique' or not 'comparable' to other settings where evidence regarding more effective practices exist.

Managerial scholarship compounds the problem of non-use of evidence in that there is no easy access to management information, outside of formal training programs. While clinical research is disseminated through healthcare bibliographic services that healthcare professionals can access and understand, there is no comparable bibliographic service for management professionals. Lastly, clinical decisions are often individual decisions, while managerial ones often involve others and may require compromise. Thus political criteria rather than professional standards of practice play a larger role in shaping management decisions.

Where do we go from here?

To protect patients while providing care in an efficient manner requires a radical shift in the way clinical care giving is organized. Evidence regarding effective management practices in promoting high quality and efficiency points directly to the need for a transformation in the way that clinical care and in particular nursing care is delivered.

A radical shift in the way work is organized worldwide and across many industries has resulted in greatly heightened organizational performance, in virtually all industries with the gaping exception of health care. Since the 1980s, for example, we have observed worldwide an evolution in organizing principles in manufacturing as the mass production system (which itself replaced the old 'craft' system in the early 20th century), morphed at the end of that century into 'flexible production' (Macduffie & Pil, 1996). This flexible production system reinforced by two related forces, the ever greater reliance on workers as the basis of organizational success and expanded trust managers have in their workers (Miles & Creed, 1995). The essence of this transformation of work is embodied in the high involvement work system (HIWS; Macduffie & Pil, 1996; Page, 2004). Such work systems promote greater contributions on the part of workers to the organization by releasing underutilized worker competence.

Features of HIWS include more decisions pushed down the organization's hierarchy, increasing worker responsibility for quality control (monitoring safety and taking action to prevent risks to safety or quality), and broadening the knowledge that workers possess regarding the activities of other work groups (e.g., through cross-functional teams, etc.). Members, managers, and executives all have changed roles in organizations based upon HIWS. All come to have new expectations for one another at odds with those associated with their traditional roles. Without a common understanding, it is difficult to establish new patterns of performance (Mohrman & Mohrman, 1997).

In effect, HIWS entails a new logic in health care management. A certain degree of unlearning is required for those who have worked in the traditional hierarchical health care organizations. Shifts from traditional hierarchical management to HIWS require time and flexible adaptation to local conditions and needs. The process of change is often gradual and cumulative. People 'not in the room' when initial changes are launched ultimately also have to change the way they think and as people and work units participate their competence and aspirations for what they can accomplish via HIWS will increase (Mohrman & Mohrman, 1997).

Core features of HIWS include:

- team structure as the basic organizational unit

- depth and expansion of competencies among workers and managers

- broader tasks performed at unit levels and by individual workers

- commitment to working collaborative among managers

- unit-level goals and rewards

- use of information technology and capital investment to support improved coordination of work, and release underutilized worker competence

- continuous feedback and redesign within and across teams to improve safety and quality

Teams

HIWS places authority and responsibility in appropriately composed teams. Many decisions typically the domain of the management hierarchies are moved into appropriate teams. To avoid confusion, responsibility and authority must be clearly delineated and communicated. Authority often cannot be neatly packaged. Teams can make some decisions only with information and input from others. They may make decisions that involve organizational resources and need approval from the management team or teams in other departments or specialties. Multiple teams may have to make a decision jointly. There needs to be a clear escalation point when teams cannot agree.

Deeper and expanded competencies

Competence on the part of workers and managers is a necessary condition of high involvement work, and skills typically broaden over the course of a career in a HIWS. Thus these work systems tend to emphasize retention and long term employment. The expanded set of worker skills involves clinical capabilities in the case of health care workers as well as group process and organizational skills. The latter skills are endemic in any HIWS. Group process skills include interpersonal skills in conflict management, negotiation, problem solving, and in representing work group concerns to others. Organizational skills include interpreting and responding to unit and organization-based performance indicators. As described below members are likely both within their groups and in cross-functional collaborations to monitor performance indicators and make performance improvements based on this feedback. These new skills and activities require greater training and more flexible work structures, often supported by greater technological supports for workers increasingly engaged in work that taps more of their knowledge and creativity and less of their physical strength or stamina (Carayon, Alvarado & Hundt, 2003).

Broader tasks

Broader tasks mean that HIWS members are responsible for a larger whole (referred to as a 'module') of the work. Patient care in the context of HIWS entails assigning responsibility to the level of the unit or team. Responsibility could include monitoring regarding use of normative practice for care giving (e.g., handwashing, use of gowns and masks when appropriate) and feedback regarding deviations form practice to promote overall patient safety within the unit.

Member authority is expanded in HIWS legitimating and supporting those workers who take responsibility to correct mistakes of others and employ their own solution to a problem when existing practices are unsuccessful. Team authority is extended to establish conditions under which the team determines its readiness to admit new patients. This extension of authority means that nurses would have the responsibility of deciding when to close a patient care unit based upon the adequacy of staffing and acuity of current patients. In such circumstances, nurses would collaborate with medical and administrative staff to determine the conditions associated with the unit's state of readiness to admit new patients. Team members would also take responsibility to interview new hires or transfers to their unit, with the goal of recruiting members whose values and skills coincide with the requirements of HIWS. Members also regularly conduct peer appraisals providing feedback aimed at developing the competencies of team members and promoting achievement of unit goals.

Greater attention to the continuum of care, rather than the explicit tasks of one's own job or unit is an important consequence of the HIWS's module approach. The team works together to complete a whole product (e.g., an automobile in manufacturing or a healthy resident in a long-term care home). Participants take responsibility to improve the quality of the whole product rather than being concerned only with quality problems that arise from their own tasks (Bailey & Sandy, 1999, p. 52). This more holistic view of the care giving process is expected to lead to greater interactions on the part of care giving team members with individuals outside the facility.

It is important to note that this expansion of the tasks clinical care givers perform under HIWS is not expected to lead to increased work load. Rather because of the streamlining of coordination and greater staff involvement in redesigning their own work efficiencies have been realized that reduce workers' experience of their workload and increase their satisfaction. Morey, Simon, Jay, Wears, Salisbury, Dukes and Berns (2002) studied a redesign of an emergency department in which physicians, nurses, and technicians participated. Following training in team structure, problem solving, communication, planning and workload management, a team structure led to reduced clinical errors in comparison with a control group of emergency departments and increased staff satisfaction, without change in the level of workload staff experienced.

Higher commitment from managers and workers

Management must make a commitment to institute a HIWS, such that investments workers and organization make in building such systems are sustained even when managers change. This commitment is most credible when based on discussions with workers regarding likely responses to conditions such as economic downturns. The vast majority of HIWS's are implemented with an explicit agreement, often taking the form of a memorandum of understanding signed by workers and managers (e.g., Weisman, Gordon, Cassard, Bergner & Wong, 1993). For example, Weisman and her colleagues report that the registered nurses at Johns Hopkins Hospital entered into a formal arrangement with the hospital to assume responsibility as a group for provision of 24 hour nursing care on the unit for a period of a year in exchange for gainsharing and the right to manage themselves as salaried rather than hourly personnel (p. 382).

Human resource practices need to be formulated to promote high commitment on the part of managers and workers to HIWS environments. Units participate in their own recruiting processes, interviewing applicants and screening in those workers seeking HIWS environments. Training and socialization processes (e.g., precepting) promote skills required to be effective at high involvement, including capabilities for taking responsibility, working with others, and collaborative problem solving. Since no selection and training system is perfect, there also must be meaningful accountabilities such that those who do not perform well in high involvement environment receive feedback and support to change, prior to possible termination.

Unit-level goals and rewards

Getting effective collaboration among different groups and levels in a traditional hierarchical organization requires that rewards and goals be aligned among workers within a unit and as well as across units. In a study of self-managing nursing units, an organizing committee of registered nurses and a nurse manager staffed units themselves, without recourse to agency or float pool personnel to improve patient care continuity and unit cost savings (Weisman et al., 1993). These shared goals were reinforced by a compensation system where nurses salaries were upgraded 10% over base pay to compensate for foregone overtime earnings. Gain sharing based on unit cost sharing were paid out yearly, with hospital-nurse shares negotiated yearly as part of an agreement, and the within unit-allocation determined by the nurses themselves (p. 382). Nurse satisfaction and retention were improved by this system. Similarly, unit-level agreement on the importance of monitoring and reporting medication errors and near misses has been found to be critical in encouraging error reporting such that unit members can learn from their mistakes (Edmondson, 1996). In particular, units where members share the belief that it is necessary to detect errors to promote patient safety are more likely to have members willing to report themselves as well as others when errors occur.

Note that effective motivation systems promoting patient safety within and across work units entail a set or combination of mutually reinforcing goals, metrics, incentives, and feedback, promoting shared expectations across all units and levels. Moreover, these goals would tend to combine performance associated with an individual's own job, the team or unit in which this person belongs, and also the larger organization. Edmondson (1996) reports that health care environments with tacit boundaries imposed by profession or rank are likely to reduce the amount of information shared, including feedback regarding performance problems. Typical HIWS team goals are multilevel, creating shared expectations not only within the unit but across units and to the larger organization as well. Such environments make it more likely that members of different work groups (e.g., pharmacists, nurses, doctors) will candidly share information regarding performance problems they have observed, because each recognizes the role that others play in promoting patient safety.

Information technology and capital equipment investment

Information technology promotes HIWS when designed to support new multidirectional communication links and information needs. HIWSs are characterized by greater use of electronic data interchange, particularly regarding incoming and outgoing orders placed by computer links. By systematizing how information is shared, teams can make the most of valuable face-to-face time – for deliberating, solving problems, and making decisions (Mohrman & Mohrman, 1997). Information technology can also make information accessible so that people identify important information quickly and share information in advance of meetings. Information needs to be widely distributed to that a big picture perspective is available to all, whether regarding the status of an individual patient or demands units are facing, so that people understand the system they are a part of. Promoting this big picture perspective gives people the understanding required to work together effectively and permits integration of the various parts of the care giving process (Roberts & Rousseau, 1989). Performance information is particularly important, especially ongoing feedback about results and plans for accomplishing goals.

Broader use of capital equipment, accompanies this expanded use of information technology, to get greatest value from labor contributions. HIWSs often use more capital equipment per worker to capitalize on the benefits of sophisticated technology when enabled by highly skilled workers (Applebaum, Bailey, Berg & Kalleberg, 1994). Moreover, it is typical for workers to have input into the tasks, the selection of equipment and technology, as well as the use and adaptation of equipment.

Feedback and redesign

Essential to the process of building a HIWS is team review of its performance against multiple metrics provided by unit stakeholders (patients). This process requires assessing agreed to performance indicators and periodic unit performance indicators and providing periodic feedback to the team. Of course, no review in itself can improve performance. Rather it is how work groups respond to feedback that matters. Improved performance results when feedback is used as a basis for problem solving and identifying more effective approaches to work.

Counter indicators

Note that HIWSs are less likely to be used and more difficult to implement where there is high use of immigrant labor, due to the lower quality of communication between management and workers, and the lower trust levels use of immigrant labor frequently accompanies. Typically organizations that rely on immigrant labor employ more hierarchical forms of controls (Bailey & Sandy, 1999). Similarly, firms that rely upon on temporary staff (e.g., registry nurses) and those experiencing high levels of turnover among key staff are less likely to have high involvement work practices because shared information and common experience are less likely (Wells, Kochan & Smith, 1991; Rousseau & Libuser, 1997).

Conclusion

Changing the work environment of nurses is an on-going process. A considerable body of evidence exists regarding how to effectively implement change that creates greater worker involvement in both day-to-day operational decisions and the decisions that shape their work environments in which they work. Healthcare organizations are challenged to learn from the considerable experience that exists in other industries. The stakeholders of healthcare organizations have reason to expect that this industry of all others would attend to the evidence base available in making decisions affecting the welfare of so many.

References

Anderson, F., Maloney, J., Knight, C. & Jennings, B. (1996). Utilization of supplemental agency nurses in an army medical center. *Military Medicine, 161*(1), 48-53.

Applebaum, E., Bailey, T., Berg, T. & Kalleberg, A. (1994). *Cross industry employer/Employee survey. Report of a pilot project.* Washington: Economic Policy Institute.

Bailey, T. & Sandy, C. (1999). The characteristics and determinants of organizational innovation in the apparel industry. In P. Cappelli (Ed.), *Employment practices and business strategy* (pp. 43-80). New York: Oxford.

Berens, M. (2000). Nursing mistakes kill, injure thousands annually. *Chicago Tribune, September 10*, p. 201.

Carayon, P., Alvarado, C. & Hundt, C. (2003) Reducing workload and increasing patient safety through work and workspace design. Paper commissioned by the Institute of Medicine Committee on the Work Environment for Nurses and Patient Safety.

Cascio, W. F. (2002). *Responsible restructuring: creative and profitable alternatives to layoffs.* San Francisco: Berrett-Koehler.

Cascio, W. F., Young, C. & E., Morris, J. R. (1997). Financial consequences of employment-changedecisions in major US corporations. *Academy of Management Journal, 40*, 1175-189.

Edmonson, A. C. (1996). Learning from mistakes is easier said than done: group and organizational influences on the detection and correction of human error. *Journal of Applied Behavioral Science, 32,* 5-28.

Harmon, J., Scott, D. J., Behson, S., Farias, G., Petzel, R., Neuman, J. H. & Keashly, L. (2002). Effects of high involvement work practices on employee satisfaction and service costs in the Veterans Health Administration. Unpublished manuscript, Farleigh Dickinson University, Madison, N.J.

Institute of Medicine (2000). *To err is human: Building a safer health system.* Washington DC: National Academy Press.

Macduffie, J. P. & Pil, F. K. (1996). 'High involvement' work practices and human resource policies: An international overview. In T. A. Kochan, R. Lansbury & J. P. Macduffie (Eds.), *Evolving employment practices in the world auto industry.* New York: Oxford.

Miles, R. E. & Creed, W. E. D. (1995). Organizational Forms and Managerial Philosophies: A Descriptive and Analytical Review. In B. M. Staw & L. L. Cummings (Eds.), *Research in Organizational Behavior* (Vol. 17). Greenwich, CT: JAI Press.

Mohrman, S. A. & Mohrman, A. M. (1997). *Designing and leading team-based organizations: a workbook for organizational self-design.* San Francisco: Jossey-Bass.

Morey, J. C., Simon, R., Jay, G. D., Wears, R. L., Salisbury, M., Dukes, K. A. & Berns, S. D. (2002). Error reduction and performance improvement in the emergency department thorugh formal teamwork training: Evaluation results of the MedTeams project. *Human Service Research, 37,* 1553-1581.

Narumi, J., Miyazawa, S., Miyata, H., Suzuki, A., Kohsaka, S. & Kosuji, H. (1999). Analysis of human error in nursing care. *Accident Analysis and Prevention, 31,* 625-629.

Page, A. (2004). *Keeping patients safe: Transforming the work environment of nurses.* Washington, DC: National Academy Press.

Roberts, K. H. & Bea, R. (2001). Must accidents happen? Lessons from high reliability organizations. *Academy of Management Executive, 15*(3), 70-78.

Roberts, K. H. & Rousseau, D. M. (1989). Research in nearly failure free high systems: Having the bubble. *IEEE Transactions on Engineering Management, 36,* 132-139.

Rousseau, D. M. & Libuser, C. (1997). Contingent workers in high-risk environments, *California Management Review, 39*(2), 103-123.

Shortell, S. M., Zimmerman, J., Rousseau, D. M., Gillies, R., Wagner, D., Draper, E., Knaus, W. & Duffy, J. (1994). The performance of intensive care units: Does good management make a difference? *Medical Care, 32,* 508-525.

Spratley, E., Johnson, A., Sochalski, J. F. M. & Spencer, W. (2000) *The registered nurse population findings from the national sample survey of registered nurses.* Washington, DC: U.S. Department of Health and Human Services.

Walshe, K. & Rundall, T. G. (2001). Evidence-based management: From theory to practice in health care. *The Millbank Quarterly, 79, 429-457.*

Weisman, C. S., Gordon, D. L., Cassard, S. D, Bergner, M. & Wong, R. (1993). The effects of unit self-management on hospital nurses' work process, satisfaction, and retention. *Medical Care, 31,* 381-393.

Wells, J. C., Kochan, T. A. & Smith, M. (1991), *Managing workforce safety and health: The case of contract labor in the U.S. petrochemical industry.* John Gray Institute.

Physicians' work climate at three hospitals under different types of ownership

Johnny Hellgren[*], *Magnus Sverke, Helena Falkenberg & Stephan Baraldi*
Deparment of Psychology, Stockholm University, Sweden

One of the most important and distinguishing features of Western economies can be observed in the tensions and differences that exist between the private and public sectors. The interrelationship and combining of a market-driven approach with one that is politically driven has been a central issue for a number of states in recent decades (Perry & Rainey, 1988). This trend has resulted in many of the traditionally public organizations becoming gradually privatized in order to be competitive in a market that is led by economic principles rather than political decisions. The prime motivator behind these changes in ownership has been the wish to minimize costs and increase the efficiency and productivity of the organization (Ferlie, Ashburner, Fitzgerald & Pettigrew, 1996; Hood, 1995). The gradual transforming of the public sector into private companies has been carried out in a number of different areas and branches, including public transportation, telecommunications, power production, electricity supplying, the maintenance of public areas, care for the elderly, and healthcare. These changes have also led to many organizations being forced out of the market, while others have been obliged to downsize their personnel or sell off portions of their business in order to survive. For the individual it has meant less secure employment and employment conditions, as well as less certain career paths and more unpredictability in regard to salary advancement (Burke & Cooper, 2000; Hellgren, Näswall, Sverke & Söderfeldt, 2003).

Changes in ownership such as the privatization of public enterprises are undertaken in an attempt to secure cost efficiency and high quality by exposing the business to a competitive environment. Within the area of healthcare in Sweden, as in many other industrialized countries, there have been efforts to create a market where various types of healthcare providers (private, public, co-operative) compete with each other over patients as well as healthcare personnel (Öhrming & Sverke, 2003). One possible benefit with this system could be that hospitals would become more autonomous by virtue of the fact that they will be making their own decisions and structuring the business

[*] *Correspondence: Johnny Hellgren, jhn@psychology.su.se*

The research reported here was supported by grants from the Swedish Council for Working Life and Social Research (FAS) and the Stockholm County Council (SLL).

according to their own wishes, as opposed to organizations that are more politically ruled and thereby subject to the decisions of the political majority (Lachman, 1985). In contrast to this, it could happen that a certain degree of tension or even outright antagonism may arise between the ownership and personnel in regard to the maximizing of business profits. There is even a good possibility that the transition from a public to a private service-production carries with it consequences that affect the work of the individual as well as the basic conditions underlying how work is carried out (Cunha, 2000). It is, for example, not at all unlikely that a newfound profit interest could bring about an increase in the workload and work pace for an organization's personnel.

It has also been suggested that work attitudes and motivations differ between individuals employed in private organizations and those who work for public organizations (Bozeman, 1987; Bozeman & Bretschneider, 1994). The majority of studies have however focused on managers and their attitudes and motivations. It has been found, for example, that managers in private organizations tend to report having more positive attitudes towards the organization in comparison to managers in public organizations (Buchanan, 1975). Studies have also shown that publicly employed managers report lower levels of job satisfaction and job security than their privately employed counterparts (Solomon, 1986). One of the few studies investigating the development towards privatization (Nelson, Cooper & Jackson, 1995) examined the effects of privatization on employees and found that job satisfaction and general well-being decreased for personnel in a British public organization that had been privatized. Today, there are still few studies, besides those mentioned above, that have attempted to investigate how experiences in the work environment differ between privately employed individuals and those who work for public organizations.

There are various models for an individual's motivation, behavior, and health (e.g., Hackman & Oldham, 1976; James & Sells, 1981). They all postulate, however, that an individual's experience of the immediate work environment – the psychological work climate – is of central importance to his or her motivation, behavior, and well-being at work. Therefore, an examination of whether these work environment experiences vary amongst individuals who work in organizations with different ownership types would be of interest. This is especially the case if we consider the fact that the privatization of emergency care has been the subject of a great deal of political debate over the past decade (Sverke, Hellgren & Öhrming, 1999). An important occupational group in healthcare is comprised of physicians who work across several departments and have both operational patient-related responsibilities and administrative duties. The present study therefore aims to investigate if and how environmental factors differ amongst physicians working at three hospitals that are run according to different operational types: one traditional public administration organization, one non-profit publicly-owned stock company, and one for-profit private stock company.

Work climate

The commitment and performance levels of individuals are believed to be associated with experiences of the work environment and those qualities of the work environment that the individual regards as being important or of particular personal significance (Brown & Leigh, 1996; Parker, Baltes, Young, Huff, Altmann, Lacost & Roberts, 2003). One cluster of theories that aids in the understanding of the connection between experiences of the work environment and the development of an individual's attitudes focuses on the psychological work climate. Psychological climate theories postulate that the motivation to perform work duties is a function of cognitive processes (James & Sells, 1981). These processes are assumed to reflect impressions from both situationally-based and individually-based domains. James and Sells define the psychological climate as the individual's cognitive representation of relatively immediate phenomena, expressed in terms that reflect psychological meaning and its significance for the individual. A main premise of psychological work climate theories is that individuals tend to interpret situations in psychological terms; they, in other words, assign psychological significance to attributes and happenings of their surroundings. Also of importance is the notion that the psychological climate refers to an individual's nearest environment, which can be more precisely defined as the immediate surroundings that an individual interacts with on a daily basis (James & Sells, 1981). There exists, accordingly, a difference between an individual's perception of the work situation, on one hand, and his/her perception of the organization as a whole and the organization's status in society, on the other. The latter aspects relate more directly to the concept of organizational culture and are governed by significantly stricter norms and values. The study of the psychological work climate, in contrast, is more concerned with the investigation of which attitudes are shaped by the work situation and what types of behavior these attitudes engender (James, Hater, Gent & Bruni, 1978).

More concretely, this implies that individuals create their own subjective representations of their work according to how they mentally perceive their work and its significance. According to James et al. (1978), these mental representations constitute different dimensions of the work and can interact to form more comprehensive or general conceptions of the work. The psychological climate is understood to consist of five central dimensions: role stress, job characteristics, leadership, work-group characteristics, and organizational climate (James & Sells, 1981). All of these areas will be investigated in the present study, with the exception of work-group characteristics. The reason for the exclusion of work-groups is primarily due to the fact that this study has physicians as its focus. The way in which physicians' work is organized makes it difficult for them to identify themselves with any specific work-group since they work across many departments and in a number of various work constellations.

For the purposes of this study, the dimension of role stress is represented by role overload, role conflict, and role ambiguity. Role overload is defined as the experience of having too much to do within the allotted work time (Beehr, Walsh & Taber, 1976). Role conflict reflects the degree to which individuals perceive that they are subject to contradictory demands from management or the degree to which they feel compelled to perform tasks that are in violation of the rules and policies (Rizzo, House & Lirtzman, 1970). Role ambiguity concerns the extent to which individuals feel that the goals, and degree of accountability, involved in their work is unclear and diffuse (Rizzo, House & Lirtzman, 1970). Earlier studies have shown that these types of stressors are important for an individual's conception of the work environment, and especially in the case of organizational changes (Hellgren & Sverke, 2001). Tombaugh and White (1990), for example, found that a personnel's experiences of role overload, role conflict, and role ambiguity increased after a reorganization that, among other things, involved reductions in personnel and a realignment of the spheres of accountability. An investigation done by Burke and Greenglass (2000) also found organizational restructuring to be related to a rise in the experiences of role stressors, such as workload. Previous research also suggests that experiences of role stress have a negative relation to job satisfaction in the case of hospital personnel (Pozner & Randolph, 1980). These results indicate the importance of examining what effects the different ownership types can have on physicians' experiences of role stress at work.

The job characteristics investigated in this study are job autonomy, job challenge, and knowledge of results. Autonomy reflects an individual's experiences pertaining to influence and control over the work. Job challenge relates to an individual's perceptions of work challenges and educational opportunities at work. And lastly, the factor of knowledge of results, as the name suggests, accounts for the amount of perceived feedback and criticism an individual receives regarding the work carried out. These central characteristics of work are derived from Hackman and Oldham's (1976) job facet theory and quality of worklife theory and have, in various investigations (e.g., Brown & Leigh, 1996) as well as in a meta-analysis (Parker et al., 2003), been shown to be of importance for an individual's levels of motivation and commitment at work. Previous research has found that reorganizations, which aim to enrich and advance the nature of an individual's work and job duties, are positively related to job characteristics such as autonomy, job challenge, and knowledge of results (Griffin, 1991). This could be an indication that physicians, for instance, might be amenable to privatization if there is a chance that it could lead to improved work content.

Individuals' perceptions of their most immediate managers are in the present study investigated through the consideration of three different types of leadership styles: production-oriented, employee-oriented, and change-oriented (Ekvall & Arvonen, 1994). Earlier studies have emphasized the importance of leadership when it comes to an individual's level of motivation and behavior in the organization (Yukl, 1999). The fact that previous research has identified the existence of differences in the motivations and attitudes of managers in private and public organizations (Bozeman, 1987; Solomon, 1986) testifies to leadership being an essential aspect in this connection. A question that remains, however, is whether human service employees in organizations with different types of ownership perceive their managers' behavior differently.

The perceptions of the physicians concerning differences in organizational climate are also investigated. Included among the organization-related factors investigated are justice and trust, which reflect individuals' perceptions of whether their organization's treatment is fair and how much confidence they have in management (Robinson, 1996). Justice and trust have been shown to be important for an individual's conception and evaluation of an organization, which is particularly true in regard to theories on the psychological contract (Robinson, 1996).

In contexts where the debate over the privatization of emergency medical care is at question, individuals' overall attitudes towards privatization of healthcare should be of central importance. Therefore the present study also investigates if differences exist between physicians employed in private care organizations and those in public when it comes to their attitudes towards private healthcare. Other factors such as participation in decision-making, job security, and employability are also important aspects of an individual's work experiences, and are of particular relevance in times that are characterized by reorganizations and turbulence in the labor market. Earlier studies have shown that participation in decision-making has a positive effect on an individual's conception of and attitude towards the organization (Heller, Pusić, Strauss & Wilpert, 1998). Today's working life is characterized by an uncertainty over future employment and research has shown the negative consequences of experiencing job insecurity (Sverke, Hellgren & Näswall, 2002). Previous research has also brought attention to the fact that managers in private and public organizations experience different levels of job insecurity, such that those publicly employed tend to report a higher degree of insecurity (Bozeman, 1987). Another important factor in the increasingly flexible working life concerns employability, which reflects an individual's estimation of his or her position in the labor market and how easily he or she could acquire a new job that is comparable to the present employment (Rajan, 1997).

An individual's perception of the psychological work climate is therefore believed to be an indicator of the general experiences of the work situation. It is also quite possible that the differences in the prevailing conditions of public and private organizations have an effect on the terms and conditions of the work itself – and thereby the perceptions of the climate. These climate perceptions are thus considered to be determining factors for an individual's level of motivation and behavior, and will end up having an effect on how well the various organizations succeed in their operations. Given the above argument, the aim of this study is to investigate whether there are differences in the four dimensions of the psychological work climate (role stress, job characteristics, leadership, and organizational climate) amongst physicians employed in three organizations that have different types of ownership.

Method

The focus of the present study concerns physicians' experiences of their work situation at three Swedish acute care hospitals with different types of ownership. The first hospital is run as a non-profit public administration unit, which means that the County Council, i.e., the local authority responsible for public service in the region, is in charge of the operations and activities at the hospital. The second hospital was transformed in 2000 from having been a non-profit public administration unit to a non-profit public stock company owned by the County Council. The third hospital was the first Swedish emergency hospital to be transformed into a public stock company in 1994, and was subsequently sold to a for-profit private stock company in 1999. Hence, the physicians compared in the present study worked at one publicly administrated hospital, one public stock company, and one privatized hospital. All three hospitals are located in the Stockholm region.

There are similarities in the development of the hospitals made into public stock companies in 2000 and 1994. There was a board of directors and an executive manager instated at each hospital. The transformation into a public stock company brought about a more distinct division of responsibilities, both between the County Council and the hospitals, as well as within the hospitals. The division of responsibilities and the increased autonomy in relation to the County Council facilitated the management of the hospitals as well as the outlining of goals and strategies for the operations. Along with the transformations, the staff was transferred from being employed by the County Council to being employees of the hospital. The staff felt that they achieved a stronger sense of commitment to the hospital after the transformation to a public stock company (Öhrming & Sverke, 2001). When one of the hospitals was sold to a private organization, an even greater degree of autonomy from the County Council was established, but it also meant that operations were to become profit-driven with a real demand for better earnings coming from the owners.

The three hospitals operate in the same region. They are all acute care hospitals and have rather similar specialties, while other factors, such as area of admissions, care taking capacity, and case-mix, vary to some extent amongst them. The public administration hospital, with its 292 beds, provides care chiefly in the areas of surgery, medicine, and obstetrics/gynecology, as well as in psychiatry and geriatrics. The public stock company, having 541 beds, offers services mainly in the areas of surgery, medicine, orthopedics, and obstetrics/gynecology. The privatized hospital has 287 beds and provides care mainly in the areas of surgery, medicine, orthopedics, and anesthetics.

The data collection was conducted during 2001 and 2002. Questionnaires were sent to the homes of all physicians at the three hospitals along with a letter explaining the purpose of the study. The letter also expressed that the responses would be treated with confidentiality and explained that participation in the study was voluntary. A second letter, in which management at each hospital expressed their support for the study, was also included. A pre-stamped envelope addressed to the research team was also part of the packet. In the publicly administrated hospital the questionnaire packet was sent to 149 physicians. A total of 91 physicians filled out and returned the questionnaire, which yielded a response rate of 61 percent. In the public stock company, 351 physicians were sent the packet, from which 239 questionnaires were filled out and sent back. This resulted in a response rate of 68 percent. In the privatized hospital, 207 questionnaires were sent out and 124 returned, which yielded a response rate of 60 percent.

The present study is based on those physicians who, after list-wise deletion of missing data, had complete data in all variables of the study. Hence, there were 78 physicians from the public administration unit, where the average age was 45 (SD = 11), 44 percent were women and the average length of employment at the hospital was 6 years (SD = 8). There were 217 physicians from the public stock company. The average age among them was 44 (SD = 10), 48 percent were women, and the mean organizational tenure was 8 years (SD = 9). Finally, there were 114 physicians from the privatized hospital displaying complete data in all variables. The mean age among these physicians was 45 years (SD = 10) and 33 percent were women; the average organizational tenure was 6 years (SD = 7). There were no differences between the physicians at the three hospitals in terms of age (F [2,453] = 0.27, $p>.05$), tenure (F [2,450] = 2.67, $p>.05$), or gender (a [2] = 0.06, $p>.05$). However, there were some differences between the effective sample and the internal attrition. The internal attrition group (n = 45) had shorter tenure (F [1,449] =

6.04, $p<05$), and were younger (F [1,452] = 4.55, $p<.05$) compared with the group with complete data on all study variables, but there were no gender differences (χ^2[1] = 3.57, $p>.05$).

The questionnaires that were directed to all physicians at the three hospitals focused on several different aspects of the work climate – role stress, job characteristics, leadership, and organizational climate – each of which consisted of several variables. Role stress comprised role overload, role conflict, and role ambiguity, and among the job characteristics were autonomy, job challenge, and knowledge of results. Leadership was measured using three dimensions: production-oriented, employee-oriented, and change-oriented leadership. The factors of organizational climate that were measured included perceptions of fair treatment by the hospital, trust in management, attitudes towards privatization, participation in decision-making, job insecurity, and employability. For most variables, respondents indicated their degree of agreement to the various statements by marking their answers on Likert-type scales ranging from 1 (strongly disagree) to 5 (strongly agree). An exception to this was leadership, where participants indicated how frequently their superiors engaged in various behaviors on a four-point scale (1 = seldom or never; 4 = almost all the time). After reversing negatively phrased statements, index variables were created by computing the mean values of answers to statements belonging to a particular variable. Table 1 shows basic information on each variable, namely its source and the number of items as well as the reliability estimates (Cronbach's α) for each hospital. All study variables were normally distributed, except employee-oriented leadership, job insecurity and tenure.

Table 1: Sources and number of items for all variables and reliability estimates for the three hospitals

| Variable | Number of items | Reliability | | | Source |
		Public admini- stration	Public stock company	Private company	
Role stress					
Role overload	3	.75	.77	.77	Beehr et al. (1976)
Role conflict	5	.74	.72	.74	Rizzo et al. (1970)
Role ambiguity	4	.77	.75	.75	Rizzo et al. (1970)
Job characteris- tics					
Autonomy	4	.77	.77	.77	Sverke & Sjöberg (1994)

Job challenge	3	.67	.66	.60	Hellgren et al. (1997)
Knowledge of results	3	.77	.79	.82	Hackman & Oldham (1975)
Leadership					
Production-oriented	3	.86	.84	.83	Ekvall & Arvonen (1994)
Employee-oriented	3	.88	.85	.86	Ekvall & Arvonen (1994)
Change-oriented	3	.87	.88	.87	Ekvall & Arvonen (1994)
Organizational climate					
Justice	3	.84	.88	.89	Brockner et al. (1992); Hellgren & Sverke (2001)
Trust	5	.61	.93	.94	Robinson (1996)
Attitude towards privatization	6	.63	.88	.87	Developed for the present study
Participation in decision-making	3	.77	.80	.80	Hellgren & Sverke (2001), based on Mellor et al. (1994)
Job insecurity	10	.80	.76	.80	Ashford et al. (1989)
Employability	4	.71	.70	.75	Developed for the present study

Results

In order to investigate whether the physicians from the three hospitals differed in terms of experiences of psychological work climate, a multivariate analysis of variance was carried out (MANOVA). All variables in the four categories of psychological climate (role stress, job characteristics, leadership, and organizational climate) were dependent variables in the analysis, while type of hospital (public administration unit, public stock company, and private stock company) was the independent variable. The results of this analysis showed that there was a multivariate difference between the physicians from the three hospitals (Multivariate F [30,786] = 2.71, $p<.001$). To further investigate where these differences could be found, follow-up univariate F-tests were conducted, which were complemented by post-hoc tests (Bonferroni) in order to identify exactly which hospitals differed from one another. Table 2 reports the results of these tests as well as the mean levels of all climate variables.

Table 2: Test for mean differences between hospitals

Variable	Public administration (1)	Public stock company (2)	Private stock company (3)	Univariate F	Post-hoc test (Bonferroni)
Role stress					
Role overload	3.77	3.95	3.89	0.99	–
Role conflict	2.47	2.52	2.37	1.22	–
Role ambiguity	2.20	2.14	2.10	0.29	–
Job characteristics					
Autonomy	3.10	3.15	3.21	0.38	–
Job challenge	3.98	4.31	4.24	7.54***	2>1, 3>1
Knowledge of results	3.04	3.09	3.04	0.11	–
Leadership					
Production-oriented	2.65	2.82	3.04	6.18**	3>1
Employee-oriented	2.97	3.37	3.33	8.63***	2>1, 3>1
Change-oriented	2.68	2.95	3.19	9.40***	3>2>1
Organizational climate					
Justice	2.96	3.39	3.34	8.74***	2>1, 3>1
Trust	2.83	3.16	3.34	6.85***	3>2>1
Attitude towards privatization	2.95	3.20	3.41	5.18**	3>1
Participation in decision-making	3.09	3.40	3.30	2.79	–
Job insecurity	1.53	1.59	1.49	1.17	–
Employability	4.41	4.51	4.48	0.70	–

** $p<.01$, *** $p<.001$
– Not applicable
Scale range: 1–5, except leadership variables (1-4)
Degrees of freedom for univariate F-tests: 2,406

There were no significant differences between the hospitals concerning the levels of role stress. This implies that the physicians' workload, despite being at a generally high level, does not seem to differ between hospitals with different types of ownership. Nor were there any differences in the physicians' experiences of role conflict or role ambiguity that could be explained by the ownership type of the hospitals. The levels of role conflict and role ambiguity were generally low at all three hospitals, while role overload was rather high.

Among the job characteristics there were significant differences on one variable. The levels of perceived job challenge were markedly higher at the two hospitals run as stock companies compared to the publicly administrated, but there was no difference between the public stock company and the privatized hospital. The levels of autonomy and knowledge of results were rather similar according to the physicians at the three hospitals. We may thus note that physicians at hospitals that are run as stock companies seem to have more variation in tasks and better opportunities for growth at work, while influence over work and feedback regarding work already done do not appear to depend on the type of ownership the hospital has.

The area of leadership displayed considerable differences between the hospitals, which was confirmed by the statistical significance found in all three leadership variables investigated. Our results show that the physicians at the privatized hospital generally perceived that their supervisors were practicing a more clear type of leadership. The degree of production-oriented leadership was significantly higher in the privatized hospital than in the publicly administrated, but there were no differences compared to the public stock company. When it comes to employee-oriented leadership, the physicians at both the privatized hospital and the public stock company scored higher on this variable as compared to their counterparts at the publicly administrated hospital. Concerning change-oriented leadership, there were differences that pointed in the same direction; the physicians at the privatized hospital had mean levels significantly higher than the physicians at the public stock company, who in turn reported higher levels of change-oriented leadership than the physicians at the public administration unit. These results indicate that hospitals that are run as stock companies appear to be better at creating the conditions necessary for a stronger leadership – when it comes to providing work structure as well as caring about the staff and working toward change. There is also a small indication that the leadership seems to be clearer in private for-profit organizations than in public non-profit stock companies.

The type of ownership of the hospital also appears to affect physicians' perceptions of organizational climate. There were significant differences for three of the aspects of organizational climate under study. The organizational justice perceptions were significantly stronger at both the privatized hospital and the public stock company as compared to the publicly administrated hospital. The trust in management also differed between the hospitals. The physicians at the privatized hospital showed greater trust compared to the physicians at the public stock company, who reported greater trust than the physicians at the public administration unit. There was also a statistically significant difference between the hospitals in terms of the attitude towards privatization. Not surprisingly, the physicians at the privatized hospital were more positively disposed to privately run acute healthcare than the physicians at the publicly administrated hospital, but no significant differences could be found concerning the public stock company. There were no differences between the hospitals in the levels of participation in decision-making, job insecurity, or employability. Based on the mean levels, the physicians in general had some degree of participation in the decision-making at their hospitals. Moreover the physicians at all three hospitals perceived their employment to be very secure and they had a strong confidence in their possibilities of acquiring new employment if desired.

Discussion

Given the gradual reorientation from public to private management characterizing the public sector in Sweden as well as in other countries over the last decade, the purpose of this study has been to investigate how different types of management, within the emergency healthcare sector, stand in connection with perceptions of the work environment. We have investigated how physicians employed at three Swedish acute care hospitals, run under different types of ownership (one public administration unit, one non-profit publicly owned stock company, and one for-profit private stock company), differ regard their immediate work environment in terms of their perceived psychological work climate. The psychological climate has been divided into four distinct categories: role stress, job characteristics, leadership, and organizational climate (James & Sells, 1981).

The results chiefly indicate that the transformation of hospitals into public or private companies was beneficial for physicians' perceptions of the work climate. In those cases where the differences between hospitals could be observed, the physicians at the private hospital and the public stock company reported more positive experiences of their work environment as compared with their colleagues at the public administration hospital. These results confirm, to a certain degree, previous research which has found that individuals employed in private organizations tend to have a more positive estimation of factors of the work environment and the organizational climate in comparison to those who work in public organizations (e.g., Buchanan, 1975; Solomon, 1986). One explanation for these differences amongst the physicians at the three hospitals could be that both the private hospital and the public stock company, to a greater degree, act autonomously and can therefore more easily carry through changes at the local level. It can also be said that certain aspects of the work climate appear to be unrelated to the type of ownership a hospital has.

The aspect of the work climate that most clearly emerges as important when considering the differences between the hospitals concerns physicians' perceptions of management. For all three dimensions of leadership behavior (production, employee, and change-oriented leadership), the management of the private as well as the public company was rated as being the most clear. This finding, that management plays an important role when comparing private and public organizations, has also been observed in previous research (e.g., Solomon, 1986). One explanation for our results could be that the management of the hospitals run as companies (public or private) gives a better impression of being clear than their counterparts at the public administration unit. Both the private and the public stock companies have undergone changes and made a transformation from public administration to their current organizational type. During such a process, management has the opportunity to play an important and prominent role as a promoter and agent of change. This can create the impression that the management of such organizations is clearer and more noticeable (Heller et al., 1998). In line with this, earlier studies have also found that employees' satisfaction with their closest supervisors tend to increase after a reorganization (e.g., Olson & Tetrick, 1988).

In terms of organizational climate, the results also show that physicians in the stock companies (public and private) rated aspects like justice and trust more highly than physicians in the public administration unit. One explanation for this may be that such aspects are associated with perceptions of clearer leadership, which would indicate that factors like trust in management and perceptions of justice in the organization are related to clarity of leadership. As previously discussed, it may be the degree of independence and autonomy accompanying the transformation into a stock company that contributes to a feeling of confidence and trust in management and in its ability to run the organization in a responsible and fair manner, which may not be the case at the public administration hospital which is more exposed to the policies of the County Council and its politicians. A related aspect of this involves the clarity of and proximity to the employer; in the stock companies, the employers and the hospitals are one in the same, whereas the workplace (the hospital) and the formal employer (the County Council) are separate for the employees in the public administration unit. Given the fact that physicians are an important part of hospital operations, it is reasonable to assume that the physicians in the stock companies have functioned as agents of change and that they, to some extent, have been active in transforming the hospital from a public administration unit to a stock company. This could account for their perceptions of justice and trust in the organization.

The results also show that the overall attitude towards privatization of healthcare was more positive in the privatized hospital than in the public administration unit. This could be attributed to feelings of uncertainty and skepticism

over the unknown, which would imply that the physicians in the public administration unit experience greater worry and anxiety about privatization
and, because of this, react more negatively towards the change then their
counterparts who already work in a private stock company (cf. Lazarus &
Folkman, 1984). A second plausible explanation is that those physicians who
welcome a private alternative in acute healthcare have already sought out
such organizations, which would imply that physicians working in the public
administration unit are more reserved and skeptical to the process of privatization.

It was also found that job insecurity and employability were unrelated to
ownership type. All of the physicians, regardless of hospital type, reported
relatively low levels of job insecurity and high levels of employability. This
can be explained, in part, by the existence of a favorable labor market for
physicians at the time of data collection.

An examination of job characteristics also revealed no substantial differences
between the physicians of the different hospitals. The physicians' perceptions
of autonomy were found to be unrelated to type of organizational ownership,
and there were no differences between the physicians of the organizations
regarding their perceptions of feedback from colleagues and patients. This
could be attributed to the fact that the occupation of physician, by definition,
is rather autonomous, and that this is not notably affected by organizational
ownership. The same can be said about the degree to which physicians have
knowledge of the results of their work. It is likely that physicians will,
through their patient services, receive feedback on their work, regardless of
the ownership of the hospital. When it comes to the perception of job challenge, however, the results showed that the physicians employed for the stock
companies experienced a higher degree of challenge in their work than the
physicians in the public administration unit.

Regarding the variables related to role stress, the results do not show any
differences between the physicians at the three hospitals. This contradicts the
assumption that privatization and the optimization of profits associated with it
would increase the workload and the perception of contradictory demands in
the organization. Rather, the results indicate that ownership type is not associated with the experiencing of role stress. These results are in agreement
with previous studies reporting that variables related to role stress were not
associated with organizational change (Olson & Tetrick, 1988; Shaw, Fields,
Thacker & Fisher, 1993). In a previous study investigating the differences
between a public administration hospital and a public stock company, it was
also found that there were no differences between the hospitals in regard to
the perceptions of role stress (Sverke, Hellgren & Öhrming, 1999). One explanation for these results may be that physicians' work situation as such is
characterized by high tempo and stress, regardless of organizational change or

ownership. However, there is research to suggest that different types of stress reactions take different amounts of time to develop and manifest themselves in the consciousness of the individual (Zapf, Dorman & Frese, 1996). There is, therefore, a possibility that it takes a longer time for stressors associated with a privatization to appear, which might explain why they were not identified in the present study.

Despite this study's finding that there are differences in psychological work climate between physicians at a publicly administrated, a non-profit public company, and a private company, we cannot be certain that the differences we identified were due to ownership type. It is possible that the various admission areas of the hospitals have an effect on physicians' perceptions of the work environment, even if all three of the hospitals are operating in the same metropolitan area. Another conceivable reason for the differences found between the organizations could be that the hospitals have partly different areas of specialty. These different areas of medical specialty can quite possibly generate different perceptions of the work climate (Öhrming & Sverke, 2001). Lastly, the possibility cannot be ruled out that the differing organizational cultures of the hospitals have had an influence on physicians' climate perceptions, since previous studies have found that the cultural aspects of an organization can constitute a determining factor in an individual's perceptions of the psychological climate (O'Driscoll & Evans, 1988).

Another possible source of error could stem from the special attention that the privatized hospital has received from the media, which was especially manifest since the privatized hospital studied here was the first Swedish hospital that was transformed into a public stock company and one of the first to be privatized (Öhrming & Sverke, 2003). This could have resulted in the personnel at the private hospital feeling that a great deal of attention was being centered on them, which could have led them to perceive their work environment more positively (cf. the Hawthorne studies; Roethlissberger & Dickson, 1939/1967). As was mentioned earlier, a certain degree of personal selection could come into play if we consider that those who are positive to the idea of privatized healthcare and wish to work within such a system who seek employment at the private and the public stock company, just as those who are negatively disposed choose to seek employment at public administration units.

Another limitation is that the results presented in this study are based on cross-sectional data and therefore should be interpreted with a reasonable degree of caution. This means that we did not utilize a baseline measure that would have allowed us to control for potential differences in initial levels between the hospitals under study. The reasons for this are that we wanted to compare all three ownership types with each other and were missing longitudinal data for the non-profit public stock company. Earlier studies from our project have however shown that there are only minor differences between the public administration unit and the private company in regard to initial levels of the work climate (Öhrming & Sverke, 2001; Sverke, Hellgren & Öhrming, 1999). It should also be noted that all of the data reported here have been collected through the use of questionnaires, which entails a risk of mono-method bias (Campbell & Fiske, 1959). The consequence of this is that a systematic error could be built into the method itself, which can have the effect of slanting the results in a particular direction. A replication of the results through other methods would therefore be desirable in order to increase the plausibility of our conclusions. Yet another issue that may affect the external validity of the present findings is the fact that those physicians who have responded to all study variables tended to have a longer tenure with the hospital as well as being older compared to those who were excluded due to internal attrition.

Despite these limitations, the results of this study do indicate that physicians working at the private hospital and public stock company tend to have a more positive perception of their immediate work environment. This can be seen as an indication that privatization of healthcare can have positive implications for a personnel's work environment. In the long run, this ought to also have positive effects on the attitudes and behavior of the employees, and thereby, eventually, lead to better efficiency and care quality for the entire hospital. These results, however, should be interpreted with a certain degree of caution since this study examined only physicians and their perceptions of the work climate. Therefore, to generalize and apply these results to other occupational groups within healthcare, and especially to other groups within public organizations that lie outside the healthcare sector, could be a problematic and unfeasible undertaking. In light of this, we would welcome future replication studies that could encompass a multitude of occupational groups, in a number of public organizations, across several different countries. The importance of this becomes all the more evident when all indications seem to be that the trend of increased privatization of healthcare, and the public sector on the whole, is here to stay for the foreseeable future.

References

Ashford, S. J., Lee, C. & Bobko, P. (1989). Content, causes, and consequences of job insecurity: A theory-based measure and substantive test. *Academy of Management Journal, 4*, 803-829.

Beehr, T. A., Walsh, J. T. & Taber, T. D. (1976). Relationships of stress to individually and organizationally valued states: Higher order needs as a moderator. *Journal of Applied Psychology, 61*, 41-47.

Bozeman, B. (1987). *All organizations are public: Bridging public and private organizational theories.* San Francisco: Jossey-Bass.

Bozeman, B. & Bretschneider, S. (1994). The 'Publicness Puzzle' in organization theory: A test of alternative explanations of differences between public and private organizations. *Journal of Public Administration Reseach and Theory, 4,* 197-223.

Brockner, J., Tyler, T. R. & Cooper-Schneider, R. (1992). The influence of prior commitment to an institution on reactions to perceived unfairness: The higher they are, the harder they fall. *Administrative Science Quarterly, 37,* 241-261.

Brown, S. P. & Leigh, T. W. (1996). A new look at psychological climate and its relationship to job involvement, effort, and performance. *Journal of Applied Psychology, 4,* 358-368.

Buchanan, B. (1975). Red-tape and the service ethic: Some unexpected differences between public and private managers. *Administration and Society, 6,* 423-438.

Burke, R. J. & Cooper, C. L. (2000). *The organization in crisis: Downsizing, restructuring, and privatization.* Oxford: Blackwell.

Burke, R. J. & Greenglass, E. R. (2000). Organizational restructuring: Identifying effective hospital downsizing processes. In R. J. Burke & C. L. Cooper (Eds.), *The organization in crisis: Downsizing, restructuring, and privatization* (pp. 284-303). Oxford: Blackwell.

Campbell, D. T. & Fiske, D. M. (1959). Convergent and discriminant validation by the multitrait-multimethod matrix. *Psychological Bulletin, 56,* 81-105.

Cunha, R. C. (2000). Impact of privatization in Portugal. In R. J. Burke & C. L. Cooper (Eds.), *The organization in crisis: Downsizing, restructuring, and privatization* (pp. 44-57). Oxford: Blackwell.

Ekvall, G. & Arvonen, J. (1994). Leadership profiles, situation and effectiveness. *Creativity and Innovation Management, 3,* 139-161.

Ferlie, E., Ashburner, L., Fitzgerald, L. & Pettigrew, A. (1996). *The new public management in action.* Oxford: Oxford University Press.

Griffin, R. W. (1991). Effects of work redesign on employee perceptions, attitudes, and behaviors: A long-term investigation. *Academy of Management Journal, 34,* 425-435.

Hackman, J. R. & Oldham, G. R. (1975). Development of the job diagnostic survey. *Journal of Applied Psychology, 60,* 159-170.

Hackman, J. R. & Oldham, G. R. (1976). Motivation through the design of work: Test of a theory. *Organizational Behavior and Human Performance, 16,* 250-279.

Heller, F., Pusić, E., Strauss, G. & Wilpert, B. (1998). *Organizational participation: Myth and reality.* Oxford: University Press.

Hellgren, J. & Sverke, M. (2001). Unionized employees' perceptions of role stress and fairness during organizational downsizing: Consequences for job satisfaction, union satisfaction and well-being. *Economic and Industrial Democracy, 4,* 543-567.

Hellgren, J., Sjöberg, A. & Sverke, M. (1997). Intention to quit: Effects of job satisfaction and job perceptions. In F. Avallone, J. Arnold & H. De Witte (Eds.), *Feelings work in Europe* (pp. 415-423). Milano: Guerini.

Hellgren, J., Näswall, K., Sverke, M. & Söderfeldt, M. (2003) Introduction. In J. Hellgren, K. Näswall, M. Sverke & M. Söderfeldt (Eds.), *New organizational challenges for human service work* (pp. 9-24). Munich: Rainer Hampp Verlag.

Hood, C. (1995). The new public management in the 1980s. *Accounting, Organizations and Society, 20*, 93-109.

James, L. R. & Sells, S. B. (1981). Psychological climate: Theoretical perspectives and empirical research. In D. Magnusson (Ed.), *Toward a psychology of situations: An interactional perspective* (pp. 275-295). Hillsdale, NJ: Lawrence Erlbaum.

James, L. R., Hater, J. J., Gent, M. J. & Bruni, J. R. (1978). Psychological climate: Implications from cognitive social learning theory and interactional psychology. *Personnel Psychology, 31*, 783-813.

Lachman, R. (1985). Public and private sector differences: CEOs' perceptions of their role environments. *Academy of Management Journal, 28*, 671-680.

Lazarus, R. S. & Folkman, S. (1984). *Stress, appraisal, and coping.* New York: Springer.

Mellor, S., Mathieu, J. E. & Swim, J. K. (1994). Cross-level analysis of the influence of local union structure on women's and men's union commitment. *Journal of Applied Psychology, 79*, 203-210.

Nelson, A., Cooper, C. L. & Jackson, P. R. (1995). Uncertainty amidst change: The impact of privatization on employee job satisfaction and well-being. *Journal of Occupational & Organizational Psychology, 68*, 57-71.

O'Driscoll, M. P. & Evans, R. (1988). Organizational factors and perceptions of climate in three psychiatric units. *Human Relations, 41*, 371-388.

Öhrming, J. & Sverke, M. (2001). *Bolagiseringen av S:t Görans sjukhus: En proaktiv organisering* [The corporatization of S:t Göran hospital: Proactive organizing]. Lund: Studentlitteratur.

Öhrming, J. & Sverke, M. (2003). Transition towards privatization: Uncertainty and sensemaking in two Swedish emergency hospitals. In J. Hellgren, K. Näswall, M. Sverke & M. Söderfeldt (Eds.), *New organizational challenges for human service work* (pp. 75-93). München: Rainer Hampp Verlag.

Olson, D. A. & Tetrick, L. E. (1988). Organizational restructuring: The impact on role perceptions, work relationships, and satisfaction. *Group & Organization Studies, 13*, 374-388.

Parker, C. P., Baltes, B. B., Young, S. A., Huff, J. W., Altmann, R. A., Lacost, H. A. & Roberts, J. E. (2003). Relationships between psychological climate perceptions and work outcomes: A meta-analytic review. *Journal of Organizational Behavior, 24*, 389-416.

Perry, J. L. & Rainey, H. G. (1988). The public-private distinction in organization theory: A critique and research strategy. *Academy of Management Review, 13*, 182-201.

Pozner, B. Z. & Randolph, W. A. (1980). Moderators of role stress among hospital personnel. *Journal of Psychology, 105*, 215-224.

Rajan, A. (1997). Employability in the finance sector: Rhetoric vs. reality. *Human Resource Management Journal, 7*, 67-78.

Rizzo, J. R., House, R. J. & Lirtzman, S. I. (1970). Role conflict and ambiguity in complex organizations. *Administrative Science Quarterly, 15*, 150-163.

Robinson, S. L. (1996). Trust and breach of the psychological contract. *Administrative Science Quarterly, 41*, 574-599.

Roethlisberger, F. J. & Dickson, W. J. (1939/1967). *Management and the worker*. Cambridge: Harvard University Press.

Shaw, J. B., Fields, M. W., Thacker, J. W. & Fisher, C. D. (1993). The availability of external coping resources: Their impact on job stress and employee attitudes during organizational restructuring. *Work & Stress, 7*, 229-246.

Solomon, E. E. (1986). Private and public sector managers: An empirical investigation of job characteristics and organizational climate. *Journal of Applied Psychology, 71*, 247-259.

Sverke, M. & Sjöberg, A. (1994). Dual commitment to company and union in Sweden: An examination of predictors and taxonomic split methods. *Economic and Industrial Democracy, 15*, 531-564.

Sverke, M., Hellgren, J. & Näswall, K. (2002). No security: A meta-analysis and review of job insecurity and its consequences. *Journal of Occupational Health Psychology, 7*, 242-264.

Sverke, M., Hellgren, J. & Öhrming, J. (1999). Organizational restructuring and health care work: A quasi-experimental study. In P. M. le Blanc, M. C. W. Peeters, A. Büssing & W. B. Schaufeli (Eds.), *Organizational psychology and health care: European contributions* (pp. 15-32). München: Rainer Hampp Verlag.

Tombaugh, J. R. & White, L. P. (1990). Downsizing: An empirical assessment of survivors' perceptions in a postlayoff environment. *Organization Development Journal, 8*, 32-43.

Yukl, G. (1999). An evaluative essay on current conceptions of effective leadership. *European Journal of Work and Organizational Psychology, 8*, 33-48.

Zapf, D., Dormann, C. & Frese, M. (1996). Longitudinal studies in organizational stress research: A review of the literature with reference to methodological issues. *Journal of Occupational Health Psychology, 1*, 145-169.

Attitudes toward individualized pay among human service workers in the public sector

Teresia Andersson-Stråberg[*], Magnus Sverke, Johnny Hellgren and Katharina Näswall
Department of Psychology, Stockholm University, Sweden

In order to keep up in a changing world, work organizations in Europe have been forced to adjust (Ferlie, Ashburner, Fitzgerald & Pettigrew, 1996). Among other things, industrial reformation, economic recessions, technical advancements, and intensified global competition have increased the pressure on organizations to be more cost-efficient, and improve the quality of services or products produced. The public sector has, in many ways, followed practices that characterize the private sector through what is known as the New Public Management (NPM) movement, which has influenced Europe as well as other industrialized countries over the world (Ferlie et al., 1996; Pfeffer, 1997). These working life changes have also involved a partial replacement of traditional wage systems in order to make way for individualized, performance-based pay. By focusing more strongly on individualized wages, i.e., pay raises based on performance (or skill), rather than factors such as education and seniority, employers hope to increase organizational efficiency and productivity (Eriksson, Sverke, Hellgren & Wallenberg, 2002; Pfeffer, 1997).

A report from the OECD (1995) reveals that the increased use of individualized pay in the public sector is a current trend within all OECD countries. Sweden, along with countries such as Denmark and Great Britain, is one of the OECD countries where performance-based pay has had a vast breakthrough (Hood, 1995). In the early 1990s, public sector organizations in Sweden began a process to, at least in part, replace traditional wage systems and make way for systems that include pay raises based on performance. The principles behind this emerging method of wage distribution were influenced by a system that had been used in the private sector since the 1950s. These pay-related adjustments affect human service employees in a number of ways, especially in service-oriented occupations, where the nature of work tasks may be vague and the performance results problematic to assess. Using a sample of assistant nurses from the Swedish public sector, this chapter fo-

[*] *Correspondence to: Teresia Andersson-Stråberg, tag@psychology.su.se*

Acknowledgement: The research reported here was financed by the Swedish Council for Working Life and Social Research (FAS).

cuses on employee attitudes toward individualized pay and investigates some of the factors that might predict such attitudes.

Performance-based pay

There are several reasons for the current trend towards individualized, performance-based pay in the public sector. One is that today's society is becoming increasingly more centered on individualistic values (Ferlie et al., 1996). Organizations – and even unions – seem to be all the more convinced that individualized pay is something that employees desire (Wallenberg, 2002). The second reason is rooted in the ambition to increase mobility between the private and public sectors, and lessen the pay differences between these sectors (Ferlie et al., 1996). Thirdly, in organizational research, pay is often seen as a motivational factor, a means of getting employees to enjoy their work more and exert themselves towards the achievement of organizational goals (Lawler, 1991). Accordingly, employers expect that individualized pay will lead to certain outcomes such as higher organizational productivity and greater effectiveness among the employees. However, in order for individualized pay to have such effects, employees need to be positively disposed to the idea of individualized pay and believe that their work efforts are truly reflected in their pay.

Earlier studies have shown that employees might have quite positive feelings toward individualized pay (Wallenberg, 2000). They may see it as an opportunity to exert a greater influence over their salary and a way to affect their salary through their performance. The greatest difficulty with individualized wages concerns how the underlying 'objective' criteria for performance evaluation should be determined. Some professions as well as certain work tasks will inevitably be harder to assess than others. Should, for example, the nurse with a great deal of empathy, who often sits and converses at the bedsides of patients, or the nurse who does the medicine round more effectively receive the highest salary? In view of this, individualized pay could present new challenges for organizations when it comes to deciding how they are to evaluate different types of work tasks, or when determining what sort of criteria should be used in assessing the employees' work performances in order to settle wages. Since individuals hold different views on the fairness of their pay, are more or less satisfied with their salaries, and also differ in their attitudes toward factors such as how their pay and pay raises are decided, it is imperative to study human service workers' pay-related attitudes from a broad perspective. In our opinion, it is not enough just to study a single pay attitude, since attitudes can vary depending on whether they concern the pay level itself (e.g., pay equity and pay satisfaction) or more specific aspects of pay (such as attitudes toward individualized pay and preferences for local wage settling).

Employees' attitudes toward their pay can be manifested in various ways. Perhaps one of the most essential attitudes concerns pay equity, which refers to the way employees evaluate their relationships with co-workers by assessing their ratios of rewards (i.e., pay) to contributions (i.e., work performance) in comparison to the corresponding ratios of the other employees (Bing & Burroughs, 2001). Inevitably, individuals compare themselves to others – both within and outside their organization – as a way of deciding if the compensation, in terms of pay or pay raises, reflects the work effort that they feel they put in. It could be expected that employees with high estimations of their own performance would regard their pay as being more unfair since they might not consider it to be a reflection of their work effort. This is often explained by the fact that individuals' perceptions of their own work performance tend to differ from that of the person who establishes the salary (Motowidlo, 1982). Another attitude central to pay is that of pay satisfaction. One way of explaining the concept is to say that if employees feel that they receive a reasonable amount of compensation, they also tend to feel satisfied. Accordingly, individuals' level of pay satisfaction reflects how content they generally are with the financial compensation that the job provides (Judge & Welbourne, 1994).

Both pay equity and pay satisfaction represent rather general attitudes toward pay as a whole. But, in the context of individualized pay, it is also important to take more specific attitudes into consideration, such as how employees feel about individualized pay as a concept (Eriksson et al., 2002). In general, views on individualized pay are shaped by how employees react to the whole procedure of receiving pay based on their performance. According to several researchers, employees' attitudes toward individualized pay are related to factors such as motivation, engagement, and work performance (e.g., Mamman, 1997). This, in turn, underscores the importance of positive attitudes for enhanced employee productivity and work effort in the organization.

The traditional, and more collectivistic, industrial society has slowly moved towards being more individualistic, post-industrial, and knowledge-based (Ester, Halman & de Moor, 1994). This development has resulted in collective agreements, on a central level, becoming less specific in regard to general pay raises, and wages, to an increasingly greater extent, being set at the local workplace level (Andersen, 1997). This has also lead to an increased desire from the employees' side to negotiate their salaries personally with their closest manager (Wallenberg, 2000). This development touches the very core of the concept of individualized pay since it concerns how strong employee preferences are when it comes to their choice of whether pay raises are to be negotiated at the local or the central level (Cable & Judge, 1994). Hence, local preferences in terms of wage determination represent an important aspect of employees' attitudes toward wage systems (Wagner & Moch, 1986).

Predicting pay attitudes

The present study concentrates on three categories of predictors of pay attitudes – demographics, performance-related factors, and characteristics of the work environment. In terms of demographics, research suggests that pay satisfaction tends to increase with age, which could be explained by the fact that seniority usually leads to pay raises (Kacmar & Ferris, 1989). However, it appears that older workers are less likely to believe that an enhanced work effort would produce desired benefits; consequently, older employees might be less inclined to embrace individualized pay since they do not see it as something they could benefit from (Arvey & Neel, 1976; Davis, Matthews & Wong, 1991). In contrast, younger employees, who do not benefit from a system where general pay raises are based on seniority, could be expected to prefer individualized pay and regard it as an opportunity to advance financially. Organizational tenure is another factor that must be taken into consideration. The same rationale that applied to age can be used here – if employees have long organizational tenure, then they probably have already been receiving pay raises automatically, which might have an impact on their pay attitudes (Pfeffer, 1997). Another factor of potential relevance to pay attitudes is gender. Various studies have indicated that gender differences and discrimination can affect pay levels and pay negotiations (Pfeffer, 1997). However, since the present study almost exclusively involves women as participants, gender differences in pay attitudes were impossible to examine empirically.

Performance-related factors (e.g., experiences of pay-for-performance and perceived performance differences) represent an additional set of potential predictors of pay attitudes. Individuals are typically inclined to feel more positive toward things that they already have experiences of and are familiar with (Muchinsky, 1993; Wallenberg, 2000). Hence, employees who have had previous experiences of individualized pay may be more in favor of individualized pay than those who lack such experiences. Another performance-related factor concerns subjectively perceived performance differences in the work group. Employees who compare themselves to their co-workers, and conclude that they themselves perform at a higher capacity, would probably feel more positive towards individualized pay since they might assume that such a pay system would benefit them (Daly & Geyer, 1994). Accordingly, perceptions of performance differences are more likely to be negatively associated with attitudes concerning pay level (pay satisfaction and pay equity) and positively related to attitudes toward individualized pay and local preferences in wage determination.

A third set of factors that may affect pay attitudes concerns perceptions of the work environment (e.g., role overload, autonomy, feedback, and job challenge). Role overload reflects the balance between the magnitude of the workload and the time given to carry it out (Kahn, Wolfe, Quinn, Snoek & Rosenthal, 1964). Employees who feel that they have too much to do within the time available could be expected to be more positively disposed to the option of individualized pay, and see it as a way of obtaining a salary that better reflects the perceived work effort (Daly & Geyer, 1994). Autonomy refers to the amount of control an employee perceives she has when it comes to choosing among work assignments, deciding how work tasks should be carried out, and setting the work pace (Hackman & Oldham, 1976). This factor could have an effect on employees' attitudes toward individualized pay, in the sense that the more control and freedom employees perceive they have, the better able they are to influence their work situation – and hence the pay level, as long as it is based on performance. Feedback essentially reflects the extent to which there is correct and precise information available about how effectively a worker is performing (Hackman & Oldham, 1976). Since feedback gives employees an insight into what adjustments are wanted in order to increase their performance, it could be expected that employees who are given sufficient feedback may feel more positive towards individualized pay. Job challenge reflects the extent to which a job entails a range of job skills that challenges employees intellectually and offers a variety of assignments (Brown & Leigh, 1996). When employees regard their work as challenging, positive outcomes such as increased motivation and higher-quality performance can occur (Hackman & Oldham, 1976). This might suggest that the more employees are challenged at work, the more positively disposed they will be to individualized pay.

Another key aspect of the work environment concerns job satisfaction. According to a widely known definition, job satisfaction can be described as the pleasurable emotional state that may result from the positive appraisal of one's job or job experiences (Locke, 1976). Research suggests that job satisfaction involves a fairly stable evaluative judgment on how well one's job fulfills one's needs, wishes, and expectations. Employees who are satisfied with their jobs in general, may also be more content with their financial outcomes in terms of pay (Quarstein, McAfee & Glassman, 1992). There for it is possible that the more positively disposed they might be to individualized pay.

Present study

The aim of this study was to investigate some of the factors that may influence attitudes towards individualized pay among human service workers in the public sector. We chose to differentiate between a number of pay attitudes – pay equity, pay satisfaction, attitudes toward individualized pay, and local preferences in pay determination. Predictors such as demographics, performance-related factors, and characteristics of the work environment were investigated to find out whether they might explain the variations in pay attitudes.

Method

Sample

The study was based on data collected among Swedish assistant nurses affiliated with the Swedish Municipal Workers' Union (Kommunal). This union, which is the largest union in the Swedish Trade Union Confederation (LO), organizes service and human service workers with low levels of education, primarily in the public sector, and its unionization rate is around 90 percent (Kjellberg, 2002). Questionnaires were mailed to the home addresses of a sample of 800 assistant nurses, randomly selected from the national membership roster of the union. A total of 581 usable questionnaires were returned in pre-stamped envelopes, which provided a response rate of 74.5 percent. Listwise correction for internal attrition resulted in an effective sample of 491 individuals with complete data on all study variables. The respondents' mean age was 45 years (SD = 11), their average tenure 14 years (SD = 7), and the proportion of women was 96 percent.

Measures

Unless otherwise stated, responses to the study variables were obtained using a five-point Likert scale, ranging from 1 (strongly disagree) to 5 (strongly agree). Negatively phrased items were reverse coded prior to analysis, and variable indices were constructed using mean values of the items comprised by the respective measures. For descriptive purposes, Table 1 presents correlations, means, standard deviations, and reliability estimates (Cronbach's α), for all study variables. In general, the coefficient α reliabilities were satisfactory.

Table 1: Correlation matrix and descriptive statistics for all variables in the study

Variables	1	2	3	4	5	6	7	8	9	10	11	12	13	M	SD	α
Demographics																
1 Age	1.00													45.40	11.19	–
2 Organizational tenure	.51	1.00												14.23	7.68	–
Performance-related factors																
3 Pay-for-performance	-.02	.02	1.00											1.92	1.51	–
4 Performance differences	-.08	-.09	.02	1.00										3.12	1.23	–
Work environment																
5 Role overload	.02	.07	-.06	.12	1.00									3.61	1.01	0.76
6 Autonomy	.08	-.01	.04	-.03	-.18	1.00								3.26	0.80	0.70
7 Job challenge	.14	.01	.06	-.06	.08	.42	1.00							3.22	0.91	0.61
8 Feedback	.11	-.00	.10	-.07	-.07	.33	.33	1.00						2.50	1.16	0.87
9 Job satisfaction	.25	.09	.02	-.19	-.18	.52	.46	.35	1.00					3.77	0.99	0.84
Pay attitudes																
10 Pay equity	.07	.03	.16	-.07	-.16	.08	.07	.21	.15	1.00				1.89	0.91	0.73
11 Pay satisfaction	.12	.03	.24	-.06	-.17	.13	.12	.17	.20	.80	1.00			1.70	0.98	0.92
12 Attitude towards individualized pay	-.14	-.16	.11	.35	-.04	.08	.04	.08	-.07	.19	.19	1.00		2.68	0.91	0.82
13 Local preference	-.24	-.17	.07	.17	-.04	.05	-.00	.02	-.00	.04	-.01	.38	1.00	3.23	1.54	–

For $r > .09$, $p < .05$
– = not applicable
Scale range 1-5 for all variables except age and tenure (years)

The first set of predictor variables – *demographics* – consisted of age and organizational tenure, both measured in years. The second category was *performance-related variables*. Pay-for-performance was measured with a single item ("Do you feel that your pay depends on how well you perform?"), with response alternatives ranging from 1 (not at all) to 5 (most definitely). Performance differences were also assessed using a single item ("Do you feel that your co-workers with similar work tasks are performing differently?"), with response alternatives ranging from 1 (there are very small differences) to 5 (there are very large differences). The set of *work environment* factors included five variables. Role overload (e.g., "It happens fairly often that I have to work under heavy time pressure") was measured using the four-item scale developed by Beehr, Walsh and Taber (1976). Autonomy (e.g., "It is possible for me to decide how to organize my work assignments") was assessed with Sverke and Sjöberg's (1994) four-item scale. Job challenge (e.g., "I am constantly learning new things in my job") was measured with Hellgren, Sjöberg and Sverke's (1997) three-item scale. Feedback (e.g., "I frequently get feedback on whether I am doing a good job or not") was measured with four items developed by Hackman and Oldham (1975). Job satisfaction (e.g., "I am satisfied with my job") was measured with a three-item scale developed by Hellgren et al. (1997).

Four *pay attitudes* were focused on in this study. Pay equity (e.g., "I consider my pay to be fair in comparison with that of others within my organization") was measured using Sverke and Sjöberg's (1994) three-item scale. Pay satisfaction (e.g., "I am satisfied with the amount of pay I get") was captured by four items derived from Seashore, Lawler, Mirvis and Camman (1982). Attitude towards individualized pay (e.g., "I think it is a good idea to connect performance with pay") was assessed using a five-item scale by Eriksson et al. (2002). Local preference was measured using a single item ("How do you think your pay should be determined?") that was developed and designed for the purpose of this study. The response alternatives ranged from 1 ("I prefer my salary determined at a central level between the employer federation and the union") to 5 ("I prefer my salary settled between myself and my closest supervisor").

Results

We examined the effects of all predictor variables on the four pay attitudes using multiple regression analysis. Table 2 presents the results of these analyses.

Table 2: Results of multiple regressions predicting pay attitudes (standard-ized regression coefficients)

Predictors	Pay equity	Pay satisfaction	Attitude towards individual-ized pay	Local preference
Demographics				
Age	.05**	.08	-.05	-.21**
Organizational tenure	.02	-.03	-.10*	-.06
Performance-related factors				
Pay-for-performance	.19**	.23**	.10*	.07
Performance differences	-.07**	-.03	.33**	.17**
Work environ-ment				
Role overload	-.14**	-.13**	-.07	-.02
Autonomy	.01	.00	.05	.03
Job challenge	-.06**	.03	.04	-.02
Feedback	.13**	.06	.08	.02
Job satisfaction	.09**	.10	-.07	.06
Adjusted R^2	.12**	.11**	.15**	.08**

* $p<.05$, ** $p<.01$

Seven variables emerged as significant predictors of pay equity. Age, pay-for-performance, feedback, and job satisfaction showed a positive relationship with pay equity, while performance differences, role overload, and job challenge evidenced a negative relationship. The only two independent variables that did not predict pay equity were organizational tenure and autonomy. The results indicate that employees who view their pay level as being fair are comparably older, regard their pay as depending on their work performance, receive sufficient feedback from their supervisors, and are quite satisfied with their jobs. Furthermore, they tend to experience only minor performance differences between their co-workers, have a workload that is not too high, and perceive their job as less challenging in comparison with those assistant nurses who find their pay less equitable. Altogether, the predictors accounted for 12 percent of the variance in pay equity.

Pay satisfaction was predicted by two variables. Pay-for-performance displayed a rather strong positive relationship with pay satisfaction, while role overload was negatively related to the criterion. Neither of the remaining predictor variables reached significance. The results suggest that those employees who are satisfied with their pay believe that pay is contingent on their work performance and do not regard their workload as too high. In total, 11 percent of the variance in pay satisfaction was explained by the predictor variables.

Attitude towards individualized pay was predicted by organizational tenure, pay-for-performance, and performance differences. Organizational tenure demonstrated a negative association with attitude towards individualized pay, whereas pay-for-performance and performance differences showed a positive relationship with the criterion. None of the other predictors had significant impact. The results indicate that employees who are positively disposed towards individualized pay tend to have relatively short organizational tenure, regard their pay as depending on their work performance, and consider the performance differences between co-workers with similar work tasks as substantial. Altogether, the predictors accounted for 15 percent of the variance in attitude towards individualized pay.

The two variables that significantly predicted local preference were age, which demonstrated a negative relationship with the criterion, and performance differences, which evidenced a positive relationship. None of the other variables reached significance. This result suggests that employees who prefer their pay bargained at a more local level are comparably younger and regard performance differences between co-workers with similar work tasks to be sizable. As a whole, the model explained 8 percent of the variance in local preference.

Discussion

The purpose of this study was to investigate some of the factors underlying the attitudes human service workers have toward individualized pay. The predictor variables included were divided into three areas: demographics, performance-related factors, and characteristics of the work environment. Demographics and performance-related factors generally predicted attitudes toward individualized pay, whereas work environment variables, in contrast, were more strongly related to pay level attitudes (pay satisfaction and pay equity). The results indicate that an individual could feel positively toward individualized pay as a concept, but at the same time be dissatisfied with his or her actual pay level.

The effects of the demographics included in this study formed a somewhat mixed pattern. As expected, comparatively older employees regarded their pay as being more fair, and were more opposed to having pay negotiations at a local level, whereas employees with shorter tenure were found to be more in favor of individualized pay. These results concur with previous research indicating that younger individuals are quicker to embrace organizational novelties, as they may benefit from individualized pay rather than wages based on factors like seniority (Arvey & Neel, 1976; Kacmar & Ferris, 1989). Older employees have been shown to express more loyalty towards traditional work values, which could be explained by the fact that traditional wage systems, to a higher degree, support the financial advancement of older employees (Mamman, Sulaiman & Fadel, 1996; Pfeffer, 1997). Along with the increasing individualism in society, younger employees might prefer wage forms such as individualized pay (Ester et al., 1994).

The pay-for-performance variable showed a positive relation with three of the pay attitudes (the non-significant association with local preference being the exception). As in previous research, this finding suggests that individuals with prior experiences of individualized pay tend to be more satisfied with their pay, regard it as being more fair, and hold more positive attitudes toward individualized pay as a wage system (Quarstein, McAfee & Glassman, 1992; Wallenberg, 2000). This indicates that having experiences of individualized pay not only may promote positive pay attitudes as a whole, but also that individualized pay may be an effective management practice in human service organizations (Muchinsky, 1993). However, in contrast to pay-for-performance, which primarily predicted attitudes concerning the actual pay level (pay satisfaction and pay equity), perceived performance differences mainly predicted attitudes toward individualized pay and local preferences. This finding indicates, as in previous research, that individuals who view their own performance as being better than that of others may consider their pay to be unfair and believe that an individualized pay system could be of personal benefit to them (Lawler & Jenkins, 1992).

Work environment variables predicted attitudes concerning the current level of pay and, in particular, pay equity, which in part supports earlier research (e.g., Mamman, 1992). The results indicate that the more individuals perceive their workload as being too high, and the more they consider their job to be challenging, the less fair they seem to regard their pay to be. Autonomy was the only predictor not to show a significant relation with any of the pay attitudes. The fact that job challenge was negatively related to pay equity was unexpected, based on the previous literature (e.g., Lawler & Jenkins, 1992). This might be a consequence of employees with high degrees of job challenge viewing their performances as being better in comparison with those of their co-workers and, in turn, feeling that they deserve a higher salary. The results also suggest that the more feedback employees receive, and the more satisfied they are with their jobs, the more equitable they perceive their pay to be. All in all, our results indicate that factors of the work environment are of some importance for individuals' pay-related attitudes concerning pay level (especially pay equity) and not so critical for their attitudes toward individualized pay and local preference.

One important finding of the present study concerns the fact that those human service employees who already have experiences of individualized, performance-based pay tend to be quite satisfied with this type of wage system. However, even with this finding, the important question of how wages are to be settled still remains. Individualized wage criteria do more than just motivate effort; they also let people know specifically what is valued and regarded as being of importance in the context of the organization. In this sense, incentives or wage criteria are similar to goal setting, which also can have a powerful effect on performance (Locke & Latham, 1990; Pfeffer, 1997).

It is unquestionably a difficult task to try to decide what constitutes a good work performance. Pay incentives are effective only to the extent that the assessment systems underlying them measure the 'right criteria'. If the indices used to evaluate employees' performance are inappropriate, either because they do not measure the right aspects of performance or because they do not properly identify individual contributions, the reward systems can be grossly inefficient or even counterproductive (Pfeffer, 1997). It has been suggested that pay-for-performance is more successful when productivity can be assessed less ambiguously, that is, when employees are aware of – and accept – the underlying criteria (Konrad & Pfeffer, 1990).

There are some issues connected with individualized pay that call for further investigation. It is important for future studies to try to illustrate the possible fears and misgivings that may arise in connection with individualized pay and the wage settling process. It is also imperative to investigate the evaluation criteria and how the perception of the applied wage criteria may affect employees' attitudes, motivation and performance. Our study points out certain factors that are related to pay attitudes. Performance-related factors were shown to have the most influence when it came to attitudes toward individualized pay, whereas work characteristics were more predictive of attitudes concerning the pay level itself. This indicates the importance of focusing on different types of pay attitudes, since they tend to be predicted, at least in part, by different variables. In a similar vein, different pay attitudes may relate to various outcomes differently. Nevertheless, one cannot ignore the fact that our model explained approximately 10-15 percent of the variation in pay attitudes, which, on one hand, is comparable to earlier studies of pay attitudes (e.g., Swiercz, Icenogle, Bryan & Renn, 1993), but, on the other, leaves room for additional explanatory factors. Variables that might be of interest in future studies are personality, goal-setting, gender, and socio-economic status. Other potential limitations concern the cross-sectional nature of the study, as well as the use of only self-report measures to assess the central variables (Campbell & Fiske, 1959). However, although mono-method bias may represent a problem, self-reports are probably the best alternative available for dealing with the types of variables included in the present study (cf. Perrewé & Zellars, 1999). Replications of this study, using a longitudinal design, a more even gender distribution, and including non-unionized as well as unionized participants from other professions and countries, would contribute to a clearer picture of the determinants of pay attitudes.

To summarize, the findings of the present study imply that the issue of having fair performance evaluation criteria is especially important in human service organizations, which sometimes have goals that are hard to define. Thus, a proper evaluation process requires that both supervisors and employees not only accept the criteria that are to be used, but also have a similar understanding of which criteria are to be used in the evaluation process. A shared view on how work goals can be accomplished in order for the work criteria and performance evaluations to be regarded as fair is also necessary. The results of this study could be of use for organizations that are planning to introduce an individualized pay system. By identifying factors that are associated with pay-related attitudes, it is possible for organizations to take action in order to minimize undesired attitudes. This could be accomplished, for example, through the use of preventive measures that aim to increase the level of employee participation in the pay settling and evaluation process. Not only has this study shown that it is indeed important to study pay attitudes from a wide variety of perspectives, it has also pointed out that although we have captured some of the factors that predict human service workers' attitudes toward individualized pay, there are additional predictors that need to be investigated.

References

Andersen, T. (1997). Decentralization in the Danish public sector: The emergence of local pay bargaining strategies. In M. Sverke (Ed.), *The future of trade unionism* (pp. 161-175). Aldershot, UK: Ashgate.

Arvey, R. D. & Neel, C. W. (1976). Motivation and obsolescence in engineers. *Industrial Gerontology, 3*, 113-120.

Beehr, T. A., Walsh, J. T. & Taber, T. D. (1976). Relationship of stress to individually and organizationally valued states: Higher order needs as a moderator. *Journal of Applied Psychology, 35*, 41-47.

Bing, M. N. & Burroughs, S. M. (2001). The predictive and interactive effects of equity sensitivity in teamwork-oriented organizations. *Journal of Organizational Behavior, 22*, 271-290.

Brown, S. R. & Leigh, T. W. (1996). A new look at psychological climate and its relationship to job involvement, effort, and performance. *Journal of Applied Psychology, 81,* 358-368.

Cable, D. M. & Judge, T. A. (1994). Pay preferences and job search decisions: A person-organization fit perspective. *Personnel Psychology, 47*, 317-348.

Campbell, D. T. & Fiske, D. W. (1959). Convergent and discriminant validation by the multitrait-multimethod matrix. *Psychological Bulletin, 56,* 81-105.

Daly, J. P. & Geyer, P. D. (1994). The role of fairness in implementing large-scale change: Employee evaluations of process and outcome in seven facility relocations. *Journal of Organizational Behavior, 15,* 623-638

Davis, D. R., Matthews, G. & Wong, C. S. K. (1991). Ageing and work. In C. L. Cooper and I. T. Robertson (Eds.), *International review of industrial and organizational psychology* (pp. 149-211). Chichester: Wiley.

Eriksson, A., Sverke, M., Hellgren, J. & Wallenberg, J. (2002). Lön som styrmedel. Konsekvenser för kommunanställdas attityder och prestation. [Pay as an instrument of control: Consequences for attitudes and performance of public sector employees]. *Arbetsmarknad & Arbetsliv, 3,* 205-216.

Ester, P., Halman, L. & de Moor, R. (Eds.) (1994*). The individualizing society: Value change in Europe and North America.* Tilburg: Tilburg University Press.

Ferlie, E., Ashburner, L., Fitzgerald, L. & Pettigrew, A. (1996). *The new public management in action.* Oxford: Oxford University Press.

Hackman, J. R. & Oldham, G. R. (1975). Development of the job diagnostic survey. *Journal of Applied Psychology, 60,* 159-170.

Hackman, J. R. & Oldham, G. R. (1976). Motivation through the design of work: Test of a theory. *Organizational Behavior and Human Decision Processes, 16,* 250-279.

Hellgren, J., Sjöberg, A. & Sverke, M. (1997). Intention to quit: Effects of job satisfaction and job perceptions. In F. Avallone, J. Arnold & K. de Witte (Eds.), *Feelings work in Europe* (pp. 415-423). Milano: Guerini.

Hood, C. (1995). The new public management in the 1980's: Variations on a theme. *Accounting, Organizations and Society, 20,* 93-109.

Judge, T. A. & Welbourne, T. M. (1994). A confirmatory investigation of the dimensionality of the pay satisfaction questionnaire. *Journal of Applied Psychology, 79,* 461-466.

Kacmar, K. M. & Ferris, G. R. (1989). Theoretical and methodological considerations in the age-job satisfaction relationship. *Journal of Applied Psychology, 74,* 201-207.

Kahn, R. L., Wolfe, D. M., Quinn, R. P., Snoek, J. D. & Rosenthal, R. A. (1964). *Organizational stress: Studies in role conflict and ambiguity.* New York: Wiley.

Kjellberg, A. (2002). Ett nytt fackligt landskap – I Sverige och utomlands. [Unionism's new landscape – In Sweden and abroad]. *Arkiv, No 86/87,* 44-95.

Konrad, A. M. & Pfeffer, J. (1990). Do you get what you deserve? Factors affecting the relationship between productivity and pay. *Administrative Science Quarterly, 35,* 258-285.

Lawler, E. E. III (1991). Reward systems in organizations. In R. M. Steers & L. W. Porter (Eds.), *Motivation and work behaviour* (pp. 1009-1055). New York: McGraw-Hill.

Lawler, E. E. III & Jenkins, G. D. Jr. (1992). Strategic reward systems. In M. D. Dunette & L. M. Hough (Eds), *Handbook of industrial and organizational psychology* (pp. 1009-1055). Palo Alto, CA, US: Consulting Psychologists Press.

Locke, E. A. (1976). The nature and causes of job satisfaction. In M. D. Dunnette (Ed.), *The Handbook of industrial and organizational psychology.* Chicago: Rand McNally.

Locke, E. A. & Latham, G. P. (1990). *A theory of goal-setting and task performance.* Englewood Cliffs, N.J.: Prentice Hall.

Mamman, A. (1992). Employees' preferences for payment systems: Theoretical approaches and an empirical test. *International Journal of Human Resource Management, 3,* 329-341.

Mamman, A. (1997). Employees' attitudes toward criteria for pay systems. *Journal of Social Psychology, 137,* 33-41.

Mamman, A., Sulaiman, M. & Fadel, A. (1996). Attitudes to pay systems: An exploratory study within and across cultures. *International Journal of Human Resource Management, 7,* 101-121.

Motowidlo, S. J. (1982). Relationship between self-rated performance and pay satisfaction among sales representatives. *Journal of Applied Psychology, 67,* 209-213.

Muchinsky, P. M. (1993). *Psychology applied to work.* Pacific Grove, CA: Brooks/Cole.

OECD (1995). *Trends in public sector pay in OECD countries.* Paris: OECD.

Perrewé, P. L. & Zellars, K. L. (1999). An examination of attributions and emotions in the transactional approach to the organizational stress process. *Journal of Organizational Behavior, 20,* 739-752.

Pfeffer, J. (1997). *New directions for organizational theory: Problems and prospects.* New York: Oxford University Press.

Quarstein, V., McAfee, R. & Glassman, M. (1992). The situational occurrences theory of job satisfaction. *Human Relations, 45,* 859-873.

Seashore, S. E., Lawler, E. E., Mirvis, P. & Camman, C. (Eds.) (1982). *Observing and measuring organizational change: A guide to field practice.* New York: Wiley.

Sverke, M. & Sjöberg, A. (1994). Dual commitment to company and union in Sweden: An examination of predictors and taxonomic split methods. *Economic and Industrial Democracy, 15,* 531-564.

Swiercz, P. M., Icenogle, M. L., Bryan N. B. & Renn, R. W. (1993). Do perceptions of performance appraisal fairness predict employee attitudes and performance? *Academy of Management Proceedings, 1,* 304-309.

Wagner, J. A. & Moch, M. K. (1986). Individualism-collectivism: Concept and measure. *Group and Organization Studies, 11,* 280-303.

Wallenberg, J. (2000). *Löner och arbetsplatsförhållanden för Kommunals medlemmar.* [Wages and working conditions among members of the Swedish Municipal Workers' Union]. Stockholm: Svenska kommunalarbetareförbundet.

Wallenberg, J. (2002). Kommunals lönepolitik och medlemsopinionen. [The wage policy of the Swedish municipal workers' union and membership opinion] In M. Sverke and J. Hellgren (Eds.), *Medlemmen, facket och flexibiliteten: Svensk fackföreningsrörelse i det moderna arbetslivet* [Members, unions, and flexibility: Swedish unionism in the modern working life] (pp. 161-173). Lund: Arkiv förlag.

From structures to attitudes: A process model of empowerment, job satisfaction and affective commitment

Pádraig Mac Neela[1]*, Anne Scott[2], Anne Matthews[2], Melissa Corbally[2], Anne Walsh-Daneshmandi[2] & Pamela Gallagher[2]

[1] *Department of Psychology, NUI Galway, Ireland*
[2] *School of Nursing, Dublin City University, Ireland*

In Ireland, as elsewhere, healthcare systems are undergoing extensive structural changes as a result of new health policies (e.g., Department of Health and Children, 2001) and the changing demands of the public. Nurses comprise over 40% of health service employees in Ireland and, as in other European countries, comprise the single most extensive human resource. Nurses perform key roles, both formal and informal, in health care provision, and their effectiveness is mediated by organisational factors such as staffing levels, autonomy and resourcing (see Page, 2004).

Internationally, organisational re-structuring has sometimes had the effect of reducing nurses' job satisfaction, with possible implications for the retention of nurses, and ultimately for the quality of patient care (e.g., Aiken et al., 2001). In the current climate of changing sociotechnical systems, it is therefore important to examine possible consequences for work attitudes of nurses. An increased critical awareness of complex health care systems is required to understand the factors that empower professionals to make decisions and act on them for the benefit of patients.

A national survey of nurses was carried out in 2002 as part of a study funded by the Irish Department of Health and Children, to investigate the nursing workforce's understanding and experience of empowerment (Scott, Matthews & Corbally, 2003). The study yielded a large dataset on the job satisfaction, affective commitment and empowerment of nurses, an evidence base to influence policy and organisational planning. The dataset permits important questions about work effectiveness to be addressed. For instance, while links between affective organisational commitment (Meyer & Allen, 1997) and job satisfaction (e.g., Warr, Cook & Wall, 1979) have been explored, possible relations with workplace empowerment (Laschinger, Finnegan, Shamian & Almost, 2001a) have not been considered. Understanding interactions be-

---

* *Correspondence: Pádraig Mac Neela, padraig.macneela@nuigalway.ie*

tween these factors benefits both organisations and employees in identifying how empowering (or dis-empowering) environmental conditions may lead to eventual outcomes such as commitment to stay or intent to leave.

Theoretical focus: Affective commitment, empowerment and job satisfaction

In the nursing literature, empowerment is "used with reference to a process and outcome that might lead to an individual's increased efficiency, perceived control and well-being" (Ellefsen & Hamilton, 2000, p. 108). An empowered work role is one in which employees feel supported in autonomous decision-making, and as such is largely a desirable attribute. Empowerment is particularly relevant in considering nurses' contribution to care, as the nursing profession stands in distinct power and status relations to other professional groups (e.g., Manias & Street, 2001).

Kanter (1993) devised a conceptual model to explain the empowerment process, arguing that work organisations enable the experience of empowerment through structural preconditions (access to information, resources and support, and the opportunity to learn). Kanter proposed that employees assess their opportunities rationally, resulting in a particular level of psychological empowerment. Developing this concept further, Spreitzer (1995) described four components of psychological empowerment – a sense of meaning, competence, self-determination and impact. Much of this literature recalls Hackman & Oldham's (1975) influential work on job characteristics and motivation. Drawing on previous work, Laschinger et al. (2000a) have devised a model of empowerment that is applied to nursing, and which is operationally assessed via questionnaire.

There is ample evidence that, in the healthcare work environment, empowering conditions are linked to outcomes such as work satisfaction, job tension, accountability, and levels of burnout (Spreitzer, Kizilos & Nasan, 1997; Laschinger & Havens, 1996; Laschinger, Wong, McMahon & Kaufmann, 1999; Hatcher & Laschinger, 1996). An indicative study is that of Laschinger et al. (2001a), who examined relationships between job strain, job content, empowerment, organisational commitment and global job satisfaction, among a random sample of 404 Canadian nurses. Nurses experiencing higher job strain experienced significantly lower levels of perceived structural empowerment, psychological empowerment, organisational commitment, and work satisfaction. While findings such as these allude to links between empowerment, commitment and satisfaction, empowerment has yet to be integrated with concepts such as organisational commitment and job satisfaction.

Organisational commitment

Organisational commitment has been defined as "a force that binds an individual to a course of action" (Meyer & Herscovitch, 2001, p. 301), a multidimensional construct (Meyer & Allen, 1991) with three hypothesised components – normative, continuance and affective commitment. Of these, affective commitment is the single most influential dimension of organisational commitment (e.g., Meyer & Allen, 1997). Affective commitment has been defined as "the employee's emotional attachment to, identification with, and involvement in the organisation" (Meyer & Allen, 1991, p. 67) – a psychological state in which the individual *wants* to pursue a course of action, as opposed to feeling obliged or lacking in choice (Mowday, Porter & Steers, 1982). Affective organisational commitment is related to key variables such as turnover, absenteeism and intent to leave (e.g., Tett & Meyer, 1993).

The study of affective commitment appears particularly relevant in a nursing context. Using a sample of nurses, Meyer, Allen and Smith (1993) established that affective commitment predicts outcomes such as organisational citizenship behaviour (OCB). Positive correlations were also noted between affective commitment and variables that are conceptually linked to empowerment – voice (willing to suggest improvements), loyalty (accepting things as they are), and neglect (withdrawing passively). Again, these implicit linkages have not been followed up to investigate how commitment relates to empowerment.

Job satisfaction

Job satisfaction is one of the most familiar constructs in the study of organisational behaviour, based on an evaluative attitude toward work ("… the degree to which people like their jobs", Spector, 1997, p. vii; "a pleasurable or positive emotional state resulting from the appraisal of one's job or job experiences", Locke, 1976, p. 1300), and which is associated with outcomes such as intent to leave and turnover (Clugston, 2000; Eby, Freeman, Rush & Lance, 1999). Given the conceptual breadth of the construct, and its intuitive appeal as a key element of the experience of work, there are many different measures and foci of job satisfaction (Becker & Billings, 1993).

Measures of job satisfaction reflect our feelings and thoughts about the jobs we do, and tend to reflect facet-based and global approaches to assessment. There is an ongoing debate on how best to conceptualise and measure job satisfaction. Whereas the construct is evaluative, many widely used measures are cognitively-based (Eagly & Chaiken, 1993). Due to their wording, global measures certainly tend to provoke a more generalised, affective response. Warr, Cook and Wall's (1979) job satisfaction scale is a typical example of a facet-based scale, addressing intrinsic and extrinsic elements of job satisfaction. Intrinsic satisfaction items include references to freedom in choosing work methods, recognition and responsibility, and task variety. Extrinsic items require evaluation of elements such as physical work conditions, colleagues and superiors, and rate of pay.

A process model of empowerment, satisfaction and affective commitment

A process model (Donebedian, 1966) sets out antecedents, experiences and consequences related to a given phenomenon. Process-based accounts help to clarify connections between concepts that originate from different theoretical positions. For instance, organisational commitment can be considered a consequence arising from earlier stages of an employee's organisational experience (e.g., Meyer & Allen, 1997; Eby et al., 1999). Some research evidence is available to map the path from empowerment into organisational commitment and onto outcomes such as absenteeism and turnover. Laschinger, Finegan, Shamian and Wilk (2001b) used a sample of nurses to test a process model comprising three stages: structural empowerment – psychological empowerment – job satisfaction. Structural equation modelling demonstrated that the model fit the data well and accounted for 58% of variance. While this model identifies the influence of structural conditions on job satisfaction, mediated by psychological empowerment, it did not incorporate commitment.

Eby et al.'s (1999) influential paper proposed that (a) structural factors, such as supportiveness and participation, give rise to (b) experiences such as empowerment. These in turn impact on (c) intrinsic motivation, (d) job satisfaction and (e) affective commitment, eventually mediating (f) outcomes such as deciding to leave a job. Eby et al. (1999) used meta-analytic techniques in conjunction with structural equation modelling to study relationships between structural factors (including empowerment), commitment and job satisfaction.

Empowerment was assessed through the use of two proxy variables, rather than using an operationalisation of a theory-based approach. The variables chosen were supervisory satisfaction (designed to capture perceptions of supportiveness and participation) and pay satisfaction (to capture perceptions of fairness). Support was obtained for a model in which intrinsic motivation partly mediates the relationship between job characteristics, work context and work attitudes (such as commitment and job satisfaction). Eby et al.'s (1999) proxy measures of empowerment contributed indirectly to general job satisfaction and affective commitment, while job satisfaction strongly predicted affective commitment.

Taking this body of research as a whole, there is evidence to suggest that empowerment, job satisfaction and affective commitment are related to one another. To date, this relationship has not been researched based on simultaneous consideration of the three factors using specifically designed measures.

Examining this question from a nursing perspective helps assess how this important health care resource is affected by organisational structures, at a time when policy and public opinion exert increasing pressure to re-structure the mechanisms through which health care is delivered.

Research questions

While key psychological states related to workplace experience, the interrelationship of empowerment, job satisfaction, and affective commitment has yet to be explored from a process perspective. This lack of clarity is reflected in contradictory or ambiguous findings. Affective commitment has been considered both a precursor to, and consequence of, empowerment-like constructs (Eby et al., 1999; Meyer, Allen & Smith, 1993), and empowerment has been operationalised using proxy measures (e.g., Eby et al., 1999). The present investigation uses Laschinger et al.'s (2000a) operationalisation of empowerment in nursing, based on Kanter's (1993) conceptual model, to represent empowering conditions and experiences.

No analysis to date has considered the relationship between satisfaction, commitment and empowerment within the same data set. These are conceptually separable constructs, and those structural conditions described by Kanter (1993) and Laschinger et al. (2001a) as representing empowerment, should logically precede and influence job satisfaction. There is less evidence to suggest a relationship between empowerment and affective commitment.

A conceptual model was developed using a process framework as a basis for model development, with empowerment as a precursor to job satisfaction, and job satisfaction a precursor to affective commitment. Empowerment was proposed to influence levels of job satisfaction directly. While job satisfaction was predicted to exert a direct influence on affective commitment, empowerment was proposed to influence commitment mediated through its impact on job satisfaction.

Methodology

Sampling

Six nursing disciplines were included in the survey (general, mental health, intellectual disability, public health, midwifery and paediatric nursing), with weighted sampling measures used to ensure a viable sample for several of the small disciplines. A total of 1,781 individuals responded to a survey package sent randomly to 3,854 nurses and midwives on the Live Register of An Bord Altranais (the Irish Nursing Board), a response rate of 46%. Of these respondents, 441 reported that they were not currently practising nurses and were therefore removed from the analysis, leaving a final sample of 1,340 respondents.

The gender profile of the sample was overwhelmingly female (92.6%), reflecting national figures. Respondents tended to possess more nursing qualifications and to be older than the nursing workforce as a whole. Ten per cent were aged 20-29 years, 28.1% 30-39, 38.8% 40-49, 20.8% 50-59, and 2.3% were over 60. The greatest inconsistencies with the national figures were in the age categories 20-29 (17.0% nationally) and 40-49 (27.0% nationally). The configuration of the sample is partly a result of weighted sampling used to ensure representation of all areas of practice, which necessitated two qualifications to be held in the case of midwives and three in the case of public health nurses.

Rating scales

Empowerment. Laschinger et al. (2000a) have developed and validated several self-report scales to assess empowering conditions and experiences, comprising 1-5 Likert scales. The Conditions of Workplace Effectiveness Questionnaire (CWEQ) measures four empowering structural factors: support, opportunity, information and resources, each measured using three items. Two other scales assess the subjective experience of power, the Job Activity Scale (JAS) (three items, to assess formal power), and the Organisational Relationship Scale (ORS) (three items, to assess informal power). The global empowerment scale is a two-item measure to provide a global overview of the experience of empowerment.

Affective commitment. Affective commitment was measured through the six-item 1-5 Likert sub-scale devised by Allen & Meyer (1996), which has been extensively validated. For the purposes of this analysis, the scale was divided into 2 parts, with Part 1 comprising the first 3 items and Part 2 comprising the remaining items.

Job satisfaction. The 15-item Job Satisfaction sub-scale of Warr, Cook and Wall's (1979) Work, Life and Attitudes Survey Scale was used. The scale has been used previously to study job satisfaction among nurses in Ireland. It includes intrinsic and extrinsic dimensions of job satisfaction, rated on a 7-point scale. Global job satisfaction was measured using two items piloted in a survey of stress among a sample of Irish nurses (Wynne, Clarkin & McNieve 1993).

Data analysis

Structural Equation Modelling was conducted using AMOS 5.0 to investigate the conceptual model proposed in the study, having replaced missing values with means. The four CWEQ sub-scales were compiled as a total workplace effectiveness score, and scores on the Job Activities and Organisational Relationships Scales were combined as a measure of the subjective experience of empowerment. A Maximum Likelihood estimation was used to evaluate the fit of the hypothesized model to the empirical data. Acceptable model fit is generally indicated by a goodness of fit index (GFI) and adjusted GFI (AGFI) greater than .90, and a root mean square error of approximation (RMSEA) not significantly greater than .05 (Rovniak, Anderson, Winett & Stephens, 2002).

Achieving parsimony in assessing model fit involves statistical goodness of fit and review of the number of estimated parameters (e.g., Walsh-Daneshmandi, 2002). The Bentler & Bonnet (1980) Normed Fit Index (NFI) has been widely adopted alongside the revised (Bentler, 1990) Comparative Fit Index (CFI). Both are given in AMOS output but Bentler asserts that the CFI should be the index of choice as it accounts for sample size. Values for both NFI and CFI range from zero to one and are a function of comparison between the null model and the hypothesised model. Each yields an indication of complete variation in the data, a value greater than 0.90 is synonymous with an acceptable fit to the data. The squared multiple correlation (R^2) associated with the latent variable of Affective Commitment was used to evaluate the effectiveness of the model in explaining the variance observed in Affective Commitment scores.

Results

Table 1 lists, for each of the measured variables, the means, standard deviations and inter-correlations. Measures of internal scale consistency (Cronbach's α) can be found on the diagonal of table 1. The mean item ratings on the components of empowerment were generally somewhat lower than previous European and American work has indicated (e.g., Ellefsen & Hamilton, 2000). The mean affective commitment score recorded by the sample was higher than in Laschinger et al.'s (2001a) study using Canadian nurses.

Table 1: *Cronbach's α, inter-correlations, means and standard deviations for model variables*

	Affective commitment part 1	Affective commitment part 2	Global job satisfaction	Job satisfaction subscale	Organisational relationships scale	Job activities scale	CWEQ	Global empowerment
Affective commitment part 1	.61							
Affective commitment part 2	.61	.63						
Global job satisfaction	-.40	-.47	.74					
Job satisfaction subscale	-.39	-.42	.67	.90				
Organisational relationships scale	-.26	-.22	.37	.35	.70			
Job activities scale	-.25	-.30	.44	.56	.33	.72		
CWEQ	-.30	-.33	.52	.58	.38	.59	.82	
Global empowerment	.38	.42	-.55	-.61	-.33	-.51	-.55	.87
M	2.69	2.78	5.02	4.50	3.32	2.67	11.29	2.82
SD	.81	.84	1.31	.93	.93	.87	2.39	.96

The measurement components of the model were evaluated to confirm the factor structure of the latent variables; Empowerment, Job satisfaction and Affective commitment. The measurement components of the model can be seen in figure 1 as arrows pointing from the latent variables (ellipses) to the measured variables (rectangles).

Results from the initial testing of the model indicated the following: χ^2 (17, n=1340) = 130.77, p = .00; GFI = .98; AGFI = .95; RMSEA = .07. Having reviewed the modification indices provided by AMOS, the two most striking changes suggested allowing a correlation between the errors (i.e., unique variance) associated with the Job Activities Scale and both the CWEQ (MI = 24.48) and the Global Job Satsifaction Scale (MI = 24.93). Given the ensuing reduction in χ^2 value alongside the absence of contraindications from a theoretical stance (i.e., significant correlation coefficients, see table 1), these changes were effected in the model. The subsequent fit indices (χ^2(15, n = 1340) = 73.56, p = .00; GFI = .99; AGFI = .97; RMSEA = .05) indicate that the model is a good fit to the data. Although the χ^2 probability is less than .05, this must be evaluated within the context of the large sample size (see Cochran, 1952). However, in keeping with Bentler, Bonnet and Douglas (1980), the NFI of 0.98 and the CFI of .99, were further indications that the hypothesised model represented an adequate fit to the data. In addition, the model explained 42% of the variance in affective commitment.

Figure 1: Measurement components of the proposed model

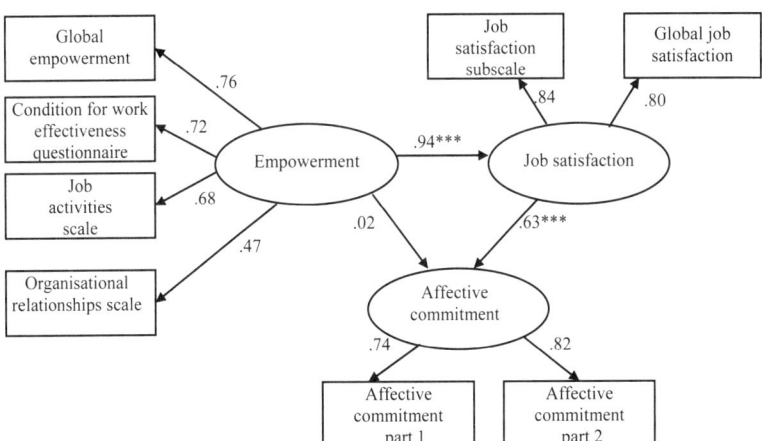

Within the structural element of the proposed model, the total effect is the sum of direct and indirect effects of empowerment and job satisfaction on affective commitment. Direct effects relate to the portion of total effects not explained by mediating variables. Here, this reflects the independent contribution of empowerment and job satisfaction on affective commitment. Indirect effects refer to the portion of total effect mediated by a latent variable in a model. The mediating variable in this case is job satisfaction.

The standardised total effect of empowerment on affective commitment was .65. The direct effect (.02) was considerably lower than the indirect effect (.63) demonstrating the important mediating role that job satisfaction plays on the relationship between empowerment and affective commitment.

Discussion

Empowerment, job satisfaction and affective commitment are integral to employees' experience of work, particularly in the case of highly qualified health care professionals such as experienced clinical nurses. Successful implementation of health care reforms is dependent on maintaining this critical human resource, and identifying how structural changes can increase its effectiveness. High quality patient care is predicated on a strongly motivated and capable professional workforce. This research proposed to link appraisals of organisational structure with both subjective evaluations of the work and nurses' relationship with the organisation.

This was operationalised through a process model comprising empowerment, job satisfaction and affective commitment, and tested with a dataset from a large-scale national survey of nurses in Ireland. Structural equation modelling found empowerment to be a strong predictor of job satisfaction, and job satisfaction to strongly predict affective commitment. There was no support for a direct link between empowerment and affective commitment, but a strong indirect link was found, mediated through job satisfaction. These findings are consistent with previous work (e.g., Clugston, 2000; Eby et al., 1999; Laschinger et al., 2001a/b), and extend our understanding by considering all three variables simultaneously, using measures devised specifically for the purpose, and indicating a strong indirect relationship between empowerment and affective commitment.

The findings provide support for a stage-based conceptualisation of the workplace experience beginning with the impact of organisational structure on feelings of empowerment, leading into evaluations of the job, and concluding with a degree of affective commitment toward continued involvement. This model helps to clarify the relationship between distal features of the organisation, subjective judgements of the work and of the organisation, with implications for decisions such as intentions to leave.

Considering the strength of direct and indirect links between empowerment and other constructs, it appears that the explanatory value of this variable has been overlooked to date. This is important to note in the Irish context, as elsewhere, where widespread amendments to health care planning, management and delivery are proposed. The findings of this research demonstrate the importance of assessing employees' views on key organisational structures and their perceptions of power. Health care systems depend on nurses to be proactive in crucial but largely informal nursing roles such as surveillance and monitoring of patients' health status. Changing organisational structures without due regard to empowerment and employee motivation may well have the effect of weakening this bulwark of the health care system.

Limitations of the research and future directions

The proposed process model indicates a role for empowerment in explaining levels of job satisfaction and affective commitment. While these are important outcomes in their own right, one of the reasons that researchers have focused on them is because of their relationship to eventual outcomes such as OCB, intent to leave, absenteeism and turnover. While the process model is supported in this research, it is not possible to draw a definitive link with distal outcomes such as turnover. Future research could consider this link directly, and further integrate empowerment with existing theory by examining links between empowerment, intentions and behaviours themselves (Ajzen, 1991). One strength of the research is the applicability of the findings to nurses working in clinical care, a key occupational group in a vital area of service provision. This work can be extended by considering the generalisability of the structural model of empowerment proposed by Kanter (1993) and Laschinger et al. (2000a) to other occupational groups, in health care and other industries.

References

Aiken, L., Clarke, S., Sloane, D., Sochalski, J., Busse, R., Clarke, H., Giovanetti, P., Hunt, J., Rafferty, A. & Shamian, J. (2001). Nurses' reports on hospital care in five countries. *Health Affairs, 20*, 43-53.

Ajzen, I. (1991). The theory of planned behaviour. *Organisational Behaviour and Human Decision Processes, 50*, 179-211.

Allen, N. J. & Meyer, J. P. (1996). Affective, continuance, and normative commitment to the organisation: An examination of construct validity. *Journal of Vocational Behaviour, 49*, 252-276.

Becker, T. E. & Billings, R. S. (1993). Profiles of commitment: An empirical test. *Journal of Organisational Behaviour, 14*, 177-190.

Bentler, P. M. (1990). Comparative fit indexes in structural models. *Psychological Bulletin, 107*, 238-246.

Bentler, P. M., Bonnet, D. G. & Douglas, G. (1980). Significance tests and goodness of fit in the analysis of covariance structures. *Psychological Bulletin, 88*, 588-606.

Clugston, M. (2000). The mediating effects of multidimensional commitment on job satisfaction and intent to leave. *Journal of Organisational Behaviour, 21*, 477-486.

Cochran, W. G. (1952). The χ^2 test of goodness of fit. *Annals of Mathematical Statistics, 23,* 315-345.

Department of Health and Children (2001). *Quality and fairness: A health system for you.* Dublin: The Stationery Office.

Donabedian, A. (1966). Evaluating the quality of medical care. *Milbank Memorial Fund Quarterly, 44*, 166-206.

Eagly, A. H. & Chaiken, S. (1993). *The psychology of attitudes*. San Deigo, CA: Harcourt Brace Jovanovich.

Eby, L. T., Freeman, D. M., Rush, M. C. & Lance, C. E. (1999). Motivational bases of affective organisational commitment: A partial test of an integrative theoretical model. *Journal of Occupational and Organisational Psychology, 72*, 463-483.

Ellefsen, B. & Hamilton, G. (2000). Empowered nurses? Nurses in Norway and the USA compared. *International Nursing Review, 47,* 106-120.

Hackman, J. R. & Oldham, G. R. (1975). Development of a Job Diagnostic Survey. *Journal of Applied Psychology, 60*, 159-170.

Hatcher, S. & Laschinger, H. K. (1996). Staff nurses' perceptions of power and opportunity and level of burnout: A test of Kanter's structural theory of organisational behaviour. *Canadian Journal of Nursing Administration, 9*, 2, 74-94.

Kanter, R. M. (1993). *Men and women of the corporation*. New York: Basic Books.

Laschinger, H. K. & Havens, D. S. (1996). Staff nurse empowerment and perceived control over nursing practice. *Journal of Nursing Administration, 26*(9), 27-35.

Laschinger, H. K., Finegan, J., Shamian, J. & Almost, J. (2001a). Testing Karasek's demands-control model in restructured health settings: Effects of job strain on staff nurses' quality of work life. *Journal of Nursing Administration, 31*(5), 233-243.

Laschinger, H. K., Finegan, J., Shamian, J. & Casier, S. (2000a). Organisational trust and restructured health care settings: Effect on staff nurse commitment. *Journal of Nursing Administration, 30*, 413-425.

Laschinger, H. K., Finegan, J., Shamian, J. & Wilk, P. (2001b). Impact of structural and psychological empowerment on job strain in nursing work settings. *Journal of Nursing Administration, 31*(5) 260-272.

Laschinger, H. K., Finegan, J., Wilk, P. & Shamian, J. (2000b). *A confirmatory factor analysis of the CWEQ, JAS, ORS, ITW and OCQ*. Working paper, University of Western Ontario.

Laschinger, H. K., Wong, C., McMahon, L. & Kaufmann, C. (1999). Leader behaviour impact on staff nurse empowerment, job tension and work effectiveness. *Journal of Nursing Administration, 29*(5) 28-39.

Locke, E. A. (1976). The nature and causes of job satisfaction. In M. D. Dunnette (Ed.), *Handbook of industrial and organisational psychology* (pp. 1297-1349). Chicago: Rand McNally.

Manias, E. & Street, A. (2001). The interplay of knowledge and decision-making between nurses and doctors in critical care. *International Journal of Nursing Studies, 38*, 129-140.

Meyer, J. P. & Allen, N. J. (1991). A three-component conceptualisation of organisational commitment. *Human Resource Management Review, 1*, 61-89.

Meyer, J. P. & Allen, N. J. (1997). *Commitment in the workplace: Theory, research, and application*. Thousand Oaks, CA: Sage.

Meyer, J. P. & Herscovitch, L. (2001). Commitment in the workplace: Toward a general model. *Human Resource Management Review, 11*, 299-326.

Meyer, J. P., Allen, N. J. & Smith, C. A. (1993). Commitment to organisations and occupations: Extension and test of a three-component conceptualisation. *Journal of Applied Psychology, 78*, 538-551.

Mowday, R. T., Porter, L. W. & Steers, R. (1982). *Organisational linkages: The psychology of commitment, absenteeism, and turnover*. San Diego: Academic Press.

Page, A. (2004). *Keeping patients safe: Transforming the work environment of nurses*. Washington: Institute of Medicine.

Rovniak, L. S., Anderson E. S., Winett, R. A. & Stephens, R. S. (2002). Social cognitive determinants of physical activity in young adults: A prospective structural equation analysis. *Annals of Behavioral Medicine, 24*, 149-156.

Scott, P. A., Matthews, A. & Corbally, M. (2003). *Nurses' and midwives' understanding and experience of empowerment in Ireland*. Dublin: Department of Health and Children.

Spector, P. E. (1997). *Job satisfaction: Application, assessment, causes, and consequences*. San Diego: Sage.

Spreitzer, G. (1995). Psychological empowerment in the workplace: Dimensions, measurement, and validation. *Academy of Management Journal, 38*(5) 1442-1462.

Spreitzer, G., Kizilos, M. A. & Nason, S. W. (1997). A dimensional analysis of the relations between psychological empowerment and effectiveness, satisfaction, and strain. *Journal of Management, 23*(5) 679-704.

Tett, R. P. & Meyer, J. P. (1993). Job satisfaction, organisational commitment, turnover intention, and turnover: Path analyses based on meta-analytic findings. *Personnel Psychology, 46*, 259-293.

Walsh-Daneshmandi, A. (2002). *Environmental philosophy, threat and well-being*. Unpublished PhD Thesis: Department of Psychology. Dublin, Trinity College.

Warr, P., Cook, J. & Wall, T. (1979). Scales for the measurement of some work attitudes and aspects of psychological well-being. *Journal of Occupational Psychology, 52*, 129-148.

Wynne, R., Clarkin, N. & McNieve, A. (1993). *The experience of stress among Irish nurses – a survey of Irish Nurses' Organisation members*. Dublin: Irish Nurses' Organisation.

The added value of innovative HRM and organisational practices for the quality of care and care work: An application in Flemish old age and nursing homes

Peggy De Prins, Erik Henderickx, Ria Janvier & Ingrid Willems*
Department of Management, University of Antwerp, Belgium

It is too readily accepted that HRM will automatically contribute to the quality and competitive position of the organisation and its staff. It forms one of the basic premises in many of the normative HRM subject libraries. There is actually very little sector-specific research on the subject to support this premise empirically. It is equally our most definite conviction that it is precisely this kind of (contextual) research which can provide a firm and solid basis for initiatives in policy optimalisation and innovation, rather than blindly following the normative HR discourse. HRM cannot be regarded as a universal and 'perfect' system of personnel management which can be applied equally within every modern organisation and its (changing) environment. Searching empirically and sector-specifically for effective (innovative) policy practices will make it clear in which way HRM can be implemented successfully within specific organisational contexts. In the paper an attempt has been made to undertake an empirical study as against the theoretical dynamics of HRM in the sector of Flemish old age and nursing homes. Performance output criteria were the quality of labour (indicators = stress and burnout) and the quality of care (indicator = individually tailored care).

Theoretical background and formation of hypotheses

The search for the best practices in relation to quality results takes place partly within the organisational and sociological tradition of conditional or risk-statement research in the area of 'quality of the work/the product(ion)'. Key variables within this tradition are usually the labour division, whether or not this is combined with the covering personnel policy or the employment relationship. According to advocates of the conditional approach, there is a need for models which establish the relationship between, for example, the reduction of the work fragmentation on the one side and the increase in individual welfare and efficiency on the other. A good example of such a model is that

---

* *Correspondence: Peggy De Prins, Peggy.deprins@ua.ac.be*

of Karasek (1979; Karasek & Theorell, 1990), which was later expanded into more integral quality and organisational models such as, for example, the socio-technical model (de Sitter, 1994). Karasek's model consists of two factors: job demands (problems encountered by the staff during or as a result of work) and job control (the autonomy, independence, or decision making scope which people have when they carry out their work). The combination of both these factors determines whether or not the work contains a risk of stress (several regulation problems combined with little opportunity to regulate), or opportunities to learn (several regulation problems combined with several opportunities to regulate). In the former case, the model suggests demoralising or tense work, in the latter it suggests active or challenging work.

Although this model has been widely known and advocated for many years, it has been subjected to critical discussion. The 'status quaestionis' which is deployed in various critical overview articles (e.g., Kristensen, 1996; De Jonge & Kompier, 1997; Van der Doef & Maes, 1999) shows that there are still scores of empirical and conceptual gaps and problems, despite the rich tradition in research. From an organisational-sociological (but also managerial) viewpoint, the most important conceptual gap can be identified: the lack of organisational support structures on which job demands and job control can be based. An expansion of this model is presented graphically in figure 1. The model can be read as a systematic and theoretical expansion of the socio-technical theory into the area of organisational sociology.

Figure 1: Conceptual framework

ORGANISATION

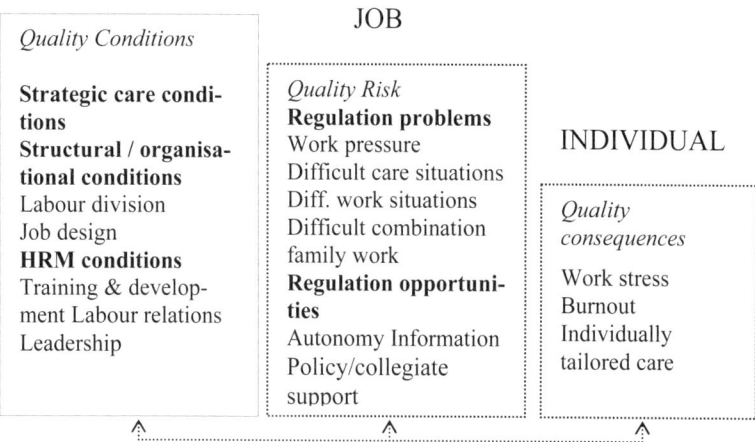

Within the organisational model the starting point is the system level of the care organisation. Most attention is given to the way in which care organisations affect and could affect quality sources. Care organisations will use strategic policy options to group, divide, and co-ordinate the work of professional groups. The organisational reasoning is also reflected by the way in which the personnel policy is implemented. The same work can be carried out under various forms of work allocation, leadership and labour relations. Together with the strategic and organizational conditions they make up the organisation oriented quality conditions under which care professionals practise their career.

Quality conditions can generate certain 'autonomous' quality dynamics, or at least several normative theories about (care) organisation and personnel policy would lead us to believe. The assumption is that the care institutions with innovative policies with regard to strategy, care content, organisation, and personnel are more successful in keeping work stress under control and making best use of individually tailored care. In addition, they largely condition the regulation problems and opportunities which care workers experience within their specific professional work.

We regard regulation problems as those problems which the staff experience during (or as a result of) their work within a certain organisational context and which call upon their 'regulating' capacities. Regulation problems are an indication of potential quality risks. Care work employees are confronted with all sorts of problems during their work. They face difficult care situations (for example, dealing with awkward or emotionally vulnerable old people), difficult work situations (for example, working under time pressure or dealing with disruptions as a result of having to wait for other services), and the difficult combination of work and family (for example, as a result of working irregular hours). Some of these problems can almost be completely eliminated (for example, disruptions as a result of having to wait for other services), but there is no real solution to others (for example, dealing with emotionally vulnerable old people or doing shift work). A workplace without regulation problems does not exist. It is, however, important that the first kind of problem is eliminated and that there is sufficient provision of regulation space for the second kind. Otherwise, there is the risk of a decrease in quality. We define regulation opportunities as the opportunities which the staff have to deal with regulation problems effectively. In the example of dealing with emotionally vulnerable old people, this could mean, for example, the provision of sufficient autonomy, collegiate and/or policy deliberation, and support. Whenever there are a lot of regulation problems and few regulation opportunities in workplaces (but also more generally within organisations), this is an indication of quality risks.

Finally, at the last mentioned individual level, quality is affected and it shows up specifically, for example, in terms of stress and individually tailored care. Signs of stress and perceptions of individually tailored care are examples of personal attributes which can be observed empirically at the individual level. The question is then whether and how these personal symptoms are affected or structured more broadly by symptoms from work or the job on the one hand, and characteristics of the organisation on the other.

In this context two basic hypotheses are formulated in accordance with the difference between quality conditions and quality risks. First of all, we suggest that few regulation problems in terms of the above mentioned difficult work and care situations, the pressure of work, the difficulty in combining work and family, and several regulation opportunities in terms of (e.g.) autonomy, involvement or support, will mean reduced stress and increased individually tailored care. Secondly, to repeat ourselves, our starting point is that innovative policies in terms of organisation and personnel increase the chance of lower stress rates and more individually tailored care.

Methodology

To test both hypotheses, we refer to the results of a related research survey carried out in Flemish old age and nursing homes at the beginning of the year 2000. A total of 91 institutional managers and 2426 nurses and care workers took part in the survey. Managers filled out the organisation survey, whilst employee nurses and care workers filled out the personnel survey. At the organisational level, only 10% refused to answer. At the personnel level, 78.2% took part. In accordance with our analogous conceptual model, the survey included questions about both quality conditions and quality risks as well as quality consequences. Quality conditions concerning characteristics of the organisation were surveyed almost entirely at this level by means of the organisation survey. Quality chances and risks were found at the lower level of the work situation and were surveyed entirely at personnel level. Quality consequences were surveyed by means of the personnel survey. This related to the symptoms of the individual.

To gain a quantitative impression, as regards stress and burnout we referred to two scientific funded research questionnaires which have been used for many years in social scientific and psycho-medical research. These are (1) the Dutch version of the General Health Questionnaire (Koeter, 1991) and (2) the Flemish edition of the Maslach Burnout Inventory (Vlerick, 1994). The General Health Questionnaire uses 12 questions to gauge the occurrence and severity of psychological complaints (Cronbach's $\alpha = 0.88$). Examples of their questions include: "Have you lost a lot of sleep recently on account of worry?" and "Have you felt recently that you are constantly under pressure?"

The Maslach Burnout Inventory uses 16 questions on a scale from 0 (= never) to 6 (= every day) to gauge the severity and measure of a person's burnout. Burnout thereby comes under three distinct dimensions: (1) the frequency of occurrence and the emotionally exhausted feelings (exhaustion) (Cronbach's α = 0.82); (2) the frequency of occurrence of dehumanising job behaviour (this is the extent to which the staff develop a hardened, cynical attitude with regard to the people with whom they work) (Cronbach's α = 0.55)[1] (avoidance); and (3) the frequency of occurrence of a low self-assessment of job skill (competence) (Cronbach's α = 0.73).

Certainly in comparison with the tradition which surrounds stress and burnout research, quantitative research regarding employee perceptions of quality of care is still in its early stages. Nevertheless, in both the subject literature and public opinion there is already a great deal of consensus on what a humane or qualitative good patient care and treatment can involve. In this regard one thing is sure: the global concept fields various dimensions or aspects, each of which contributes to a global qualitative patient treatment. Before recording these various dimensions we let existing foreign quantitative and qualitative research inspire us and we arrived at our own devised stock of questions. Two dimensions have been distinguished: (1) the emotional individually tailored care within one's own work (with questions presented: "Can you indicate which resident oriented activities may occur during the course of your work: stimulating physical self-help activities?/focussing involuntary attention on your work?/...") (Cronbach's α = 0.78); and (2) the individually tailored care culture within the institution; examples of questions include: To what extent do you agree with the following propositions: "In our institution attention given to residents and/or family members is not really seen as work?/In our institution the staff often have no time to give attention to the residents?" (Cronbach's α = 0.71). Even for the quantitative recording of quality risks (summarised as symptoms of the regulation problems and opportunities) and quality conditions (summarised as signs of strategic, work-organisatorial, and personnel areas), use has often been made of our own devised questions and scales (sometimes inspired by existing question stocks such as the Job Content Instrument (Karasek, 1985).

Within the framework of further reporting the results, we will first present some results of innovations or re-orientations in the areas of work organisation and HRM[2]. Later on we will deal with the results of the explanatory analyses. We will examine whether or not the innovations have actually had a

---

[1] Comparable with Vlerick (1994).

[2] Innovations at a strategic and care-content level are not included here.

positive effect upon the stress and individually tailored care situations of the nurses and care workers.

Innovations detected

Functional versus resident oriented care structuring

Since Mintzberg professional bureaucracies carried out research and recorded their findings, we know that those types of organisations base their co-ordination on the standardisation of skills, which are gained mainly via official training courses. Using what Mintzberg (1983, p. 176) indicates as 'pigeon holing' (the organisation tries to link a pre-determined case to a standard programme), professional bureaucracy can separate the various executed tasks from each other and give them to separate, relatively autonomous groups or solo (para) professionals. Departments and staff services endeavour to tackle the complexity by means of standard instructions and procedures. No account can be taken of the fact that everyone wants something different. The solutions which are supplied are then also 'mediated solutions'. These solutions are less than optimal for the one receiving care and they stand in stark contrast to the requirements of demand oriented care. In order to anticipate these and other (quality) malfunctions, the concept of customer oriented (resident oriented) team is becoming increasingly prominent. At the heart of this team concept is the idea of a minimum of functionalising. This means that the various professional groups and their qualifications will no longer be used as the major structuring principles, but rather the various clients with their specific care features and questions. An attempt will be made to link every client family to their own, fully equipped sub-systems.

What do the research results suggest about the actual penetration level of resident oriented structures? In the first instance the results indicate a triumphal procession for the resident oriented structures. The majority of the institutions (70.9%) state explicitly that they work with one or more forms of departmental operation. This would be a surprisingly high percentage. However, behind this percentage there lurks a hybrid reality. Institutions always have to take various selective steps to arrive finally at a definite plan for a practical structure. The initial selection concerns the choice of applying the grouping or departmental principle to all the residents or merely a limited number of them. Larger institutions will perhaps tend rather to divide the entire resident population into separate entities, while smaller institutions will design a separate section for a limited group (e.g., severe dementia profile). This latter option is dominant in our sample of institutions. A second and, for our purposes, more important selection which the organisation must make is whether or not to allocate (permanent) staff to entities. In order to speak in terms of integrated personnel work teams, we will employ the following two requirements: (1) all the care personal operates unit oriented; and (2) all the nursing personal operates unit oriented, except for any required night duties. At this point the data gives a less triumphant picture: about 25% of the institutions satisfy the two integrated work team requirements. This is not surprising. It could be assumed that the need to organise consciously according to target groups is a recent requirement so that many institutions find themselves in a kind of 'transitional phase'. The relative small scale of many old age and nursing homes also serves to make its implementation less urgent. Moreover, a re-organisation involves considerable extra cost. In order to keep costs to an absolute minimum, mixed forms prove very persuasive in practice.

The optimistic versus pessimistic scenarios in function enlargement

The past decade has had a lot to do with task enlargement and task splitting scenarios within care work. Mainly as a result of the threatening scarcity on the labour market, changes in the work itself, and the increasing work pressure, ways have been investigated to formulate an answer by means of function differentiation to all sorts of questions related to quality, organisation, and personnel. By and large, there are two visions which stand out: 'Some nurses fear the creation of a lower rank of less trained staff, while others believe that innovative practices require all nurses to be highly trained. In some ways this debate within nursing reflects the division between Pioire and Sabel's (1984) optimism about the extent of job upskilling and Atkinsons (1986) model of a division between core and peripheral workers. (Walby, Greenwell, Mackay & Soothill, 1994; pp. 176-177). In what follows, both visions are confronted with the empiric material.

Table 1: Present level of task enlargement (in %)

	Already carry out this task				
	Managers $n = 94$	Nurses $n = 150$	Nurse assistants $n = 529$	Care workers $n = 1,170$	χ^2 test Sign.
Quality tasks	76.6	30.7	23.1	15.7	.000
Palliative tasks	66.3	31.6	25.4	13.4	.000
Responsible person	56.0	40.0	36.1	36.3	.000
Training tasks	77.7	28.4	15.6	9.0	.000
Therapeutic tasks	16.1	10.6	5.3	8.5	.000
Accompanying students/new staff	91.8	60.9	43.6	40.3	.000
Purchase/supply control	64.2	20.3	12.6	9.7	.000

As table 1 makes clear, the pessimistic scenario can be supported. Where there is mention of function enlargement, this occurs mainly among the senior nursing staff. Alongside quality tasks, palliative tasks, consideration tasks, training tasks, accompanying tasks, supply control and purchasing tasks occur the most at this function level, relatively speaking. The lower the hierarchical position, the less mention of integrated functions. The function enlargement scenario manifests itself in Flemish old age and nursing homes as a one-sided scenario: mainly senior positioned staff and more highly trained staff benefit from it. Notice also that at present there is no significant link between the extent of task enlargement and the broader labour organisational principles. And so, institutions which operate with a maximum of integrated entities do not score significantly better on task integration. It could be expected that a structural establishment of an inter-disciplinary approach within the institution should also stimulate function flexibility. The results cannot (yet) confirm this premise.

Sham versus genuine occupational market segments

It is generally accepted that care institutions have little scope to implement a dynamic policy regarding the stream of semi-professionals. Traditionally, there has been talk of an influx and little or no circulation. In order to fill up jobs, one buys the necessary qualifications directly from the labour market. There is always a corresponding occupational market segment on which the required qualifications are ready for service. The concept of an occupational market segment has been acknowledged mainly in the classical labour market typology of Lutz and Sengenberger (1974) ('betriebsspezifische Qualifikationen'). Jobs within occupational market segments do not have a specific organisational character, but require professional qualifications which the organisation does not need to supply to those involved. Functions within these market segments lead to closed segments and strongly reduced function and salary classifications. Little or no mobility is possible between these segments. Concepts such as career policy, career planning, and mobility are not generally accepted in the care sector.

However, at the discourse level changes are being perceived. In accordance with the employability discourse within organisations other than social profit ones, there is an increasing call for horizontal career initiatives instead of vertical ones. A career within the organisation is then not a career linked to remuneration, but a career from novice to expert (Benner, 1984) within the profession. Research shows that suitable horizontal career policies are not yet being made available at present because of factors such as tight staffing levels. Institutions are 'forced' to devote their potential in a universal fashion during the career. The professional career sought within an occupational market segment seems unachievable in this way. Therefore, there is rather talk of what we would like to call sham occupational market segments. There is no place in the structure here for experience valorisation. The disappointing results in table 2 bear witness to this. Age conscious personnel policies are implemented in terms of limiting working hours and not, or hardly, in terms of limiting heavy tasks and/or valorisation of emotional or co-ordinate care tasks. Task flexibility in terms of career expertise is still meager. At present, discussion of this point deviates strongly from the specific personnel practices within care institutions.

Table 2: Indications of age conscious personnel policy and experience valori-sation (in %) (n = 89)

	Is applied as much as possible	Is some-times applied/ sometimes not	Is not applied/not feasible
Age conscious personnel policy			
Older staff are relieved of demanding physical work.	7.2	21.7	71.9
Older staff are given priority in choosing to work part-time.	41.7	11.9	46.4
Experience valorisation			
Experience is valued by offering them the oppor-tunity to carry out co-ordinating tasks	27.1	56.5	16.5
Experience is valued by giving them more opportunities to tend to the psychological and emotional care of the residents.	17.6	35.3	47.1

With regard to training a more optimistic picture can be presented, at least as far as the investment in quantitative training is concerned. It is noticeable that the majority of the institutions easily exceed the annual regulated limit of 8 hours training for each staff member of the nursing and caring corps: ex-tremes of between 40 and 50 hours training can be noted. These relatively favourable figures can only be welcomed. Within the framework of promot-ing expertise on the one hand and increasing regulation opportunities on the other, the development of a thorough in-service training policy is always of prime importance. It forms a supportive measure throughout the care profes-sion and it can be employed to anticipate changes in job demands. Initiatives in task enlargement also increase the importance of opportunities for profes-sional development.

So far we see a positive empiric image again. The same research shows however, that while obligatory training gives rise to a quantitative investment in staff training, the qualitative investment in training and developmental policies is rather minimal. In the best case scenario (Stewart, 1999), institutions are going from a so called training circuit; they start by signalling training problems or needs, and this is followed by an analysis and the establishing of training aims. After the training has been completed, the effectiveness and efficiency of the training can be assessed on the basis of evaluation criteria established in advance. Ideally, this is not limited to the response level and the learning level, but the work conduct level and the organisational level are also assessed. If it is desirable to stimulate inter-collegiate study, then the assessment involves not only the managers, but also colleagues. The confrontation between the ideal situation and actual practice reveals the following results: only one out of two institutions formally enquires about systematic training needs, and only one out of three institutions maintains an individual training file per staff member. It is evident that only 58 % of the institutions surveyed anticipate and provide replacements when some of the care staff follow training courses. For some institutions, investment in training is linked to a temporary increase in work pressure on others. Perhaps the lack of a systematic personnel buffer in most institutions lies at the bottom of this. The training items which score relatively worst of all are the assessments between colleagues and managers. It seems that training and assessment are not an established practice within the sector. This is regrettable since it hinders individual, organisational and collegiate learning.

Control versus involvement

Management systems contain an implicit summary concerning conduct, especially concerning staff motivation. Management systems can be typified according to the extent to which they are more or less geared to control and extrinsic stimulation or stimulating intrinsic involvement in the work and the organisation (Friedman, 1977). Control and involvement are not mutually exclusive strategic dimensions. They are often in line with each other and can be at odds. This tension is noticeable, for example, when the employee is expected to display both subordination and initiative at the same time. This is the case in care organisations because the quality of care is largely determined by direct interaction with the patient/client. At the same time it is assumed that the work is carried out as far as possible according to the guidelines and that it is sufficiently flexible to respond to the wishes and requirements of those requiring care. Whenever these things are out of balance, problems threaten, not only in the interactive balance between employee and client, but also in the attaining of broader organisational objectives, whether official or not (see Goffman, 1961; Lipsky, 1980).

The results in table 3 indicate the relatively critical relationship of care staff with their supervisors. Fewer than half of the respondents think that their immediate supervisor has a sufficient overview over the work to make accurate assessments (35.5 %), accurate estimations (37.2 %), effective plans (43.7 %), and to act as a representative for the staff (46.3 %). A considerable number of respondents are also of the opinion that their supervisors do not treat all staff equally and do not make it clear if their staff do their work well. Most of the respondents receive general appreciation from their immediate supervisors and, likewise, stimulation to work together with colleagues. 57.7 % are also of the opinion that their supervisor is capable of developing an effective care work vision. Relationships with colleagues are also given a positive assessment: in 71.4 % of the cases colleagues cover for each other. In addition, colleagues usually show sufficient appreciation for each other's work and take sufficient account of each other's feelings.

Table 3: The perceived quality of leadership and labour relations (in %)

	Agree	Not sure	Disagree
Perceived leadership qualities			
My supervisor has sufficient overview over the work to :			
1. plan it effectively	43.7	46.2	10.1
2. make accurate estimations	37.2	51.1	11.7
3. assess the staff accurately	35.5	51.7	12.8
4. develop an effective vision for residential care	57.7	35.7	6.6
5. act as representative for the staff	46.3	40.8	12.9
Relationship with immediate supervisor			
1. My supervisor shows appreciation of my work.	65.2	23.9	10.9
2. My supervisor treats all staff equally.	54.9	22.2	22.9
3. My supervisor encourages mutual co-operation in the department/in the institution.	65.9	21.4	12.7
4. My supervisor makes it clear if I do my work well.	48.7	28.7	22.5
Relationship with colleagues			
1. My colleagues show sufficient appreciation for my work.	68.1	26.7	5.2
2. My colleagues take my feelings into account.	67.4	27.4	5.2
My colleagues make it clear if I do my work well.	54.2	34.3	11.5

Innovations assessed

After examining the outlined results with regard to innovations, we now turn our attention to the results of the explanatory analyses. The explanatory analyses were carried out via the multi-level method (Goldstein 1995). This method allows findings to be recorded at various levels (organisational, individual) explicitly and simultaneously in the analysis. This benefits the impartiality of the observations and therefore the trustworthiness of the statistical tests (Snijders & Basker, 1999). In addition, analyses have been carried out on the basis of the difference between excellent institutions ($n = 20$), average institutions ($n = 50$), and risk institutions ($n = 21$). This division was obtained after the institutions had been positioned according to the aggregate scores on the consequences for quality (stress, burnout and individually tailored care). The (variance) analyses on the basis of this difference still show the findings of the multi-level regression analysis; moreover, these findings also give rise to a number of supplementary and/or more pronounced conclusions.

Innovations = best practices?

How do the excellent institutions fare in the sample? It appears from table 4 that excellent institutions do not vary in their scores on an innovative organisational structure. Excellent institutions do strive somewhat more for greater task enlargement. In other words, there is a greater chance that nurses and care workers in excellent institutions can also carry out palliative tasks, consideration tasks, training tasks, supportive tasks, and purchase tasks as well as their basic duties. The difference is not so significant. Excellent institutions do not differ significantly from risk or average institutions because of their (innovative) training and development policies. Where they do differ extremely is in the dimensions of labour relations and labour management. More specifically, the relatively positive relationship with the immediate supervisor and the perceived quality of the management is in view here. Despite the generally critical staff attitudes towards their immediate supervisors, the excellent quality practices reveal themselves in optimal mutual work relationships, adjoining well assessed management qualities. These practices generate a specific quality impact much more than other policy areas.

Table 4: *Risk, average, and excellent institutions typified by the quality of their conditions. Results from One-way Anova with Bonferroni-test/effect sizes.*

	Excellent institutions (1)	Average institutions (2)	Risk institutions (3)	p	Significant group differences	Partial Eta squared
Integrated work entities	20.0 % (n = 19)	38.0 % (n = 47)	14.3 % (n = 19)	.083	-	.020
Measure of task enlargement*	2.17 (n = 20)	1.90 (n = 50)	1.77 (n = 21)	.212	-	.035
Training conditions*	6.16 (n = 19)	5.77 (n = 47)	6.61 (n = 19)	.308	-	.028
Development conditions*	4.47 (n = 19)	4.13 (n = 46)	4.12 (n = 18)	.847	-	.004
Relationship with management*	7.46 (n = 20)	6.51 (n = 50)	6.13 (n = 21)	.000	1>2.3	.171
Relationship with colleagues*	7.21 (n = 20)	6.91 (n = 50)	6.69 (n = 21)	.050	1>3	.066
Management qualities*	7.91 (n = 20)	6.46 (n = 50)	6.20 (n = 21)	.000	1>2.3	.185

* scale from 0 to 10

Our basic hypothesis can only be partly confirmed. The data supplies little empirical evidence for forming hypotheses with a normative connotation. This means: hypotheses in which unintended positive quality effects are expected from innovative policy practices. Explanations for this have already been given. The tabled results still show that there are no, or hardly any, (mature) innovations in the area of labour allocation, and this means that direct quality effects can hardly be expected. In the area of organisation there are mainly 'crumbled' versions, which once again leave little scope for direct quality results. A question which arises directly from this is whether our search for 'best practices' then forms a measure for nothing. We do not think so. The reference framework for our search must be turned round. This can be done by no longer starting from the normative (practice) theory, but starting instead with the 'excellent' practice which can teach us important content and policy lessons. We will first examine the results of the regulation problems and opportunities.

Best Practices = ?

If we examine the regulation problems from the difference between 'excellent, risk, and average institutions' (see table 5), then it is immediately noticeable that excellent institutions always score significantly lower. It is mainly the work pressure and difficult working situations which generate relatively fewer complaints in excellent institutions. This is partly to be expected: difficult working situations (e.g., waiting for other services, problems of work means, …) and the pressure of work are profiled as organisatorial problems which can be tackled in contrast with, for example, difficult care situations (handling awkward, aggressive, terminally sick … residents). This means that regulation problems can be dealt with and reduced effectively. And so, as regards the regulation opportunities, the difference between opportunities for policy consultation and support is noticeable. On average, excellent institutions score 7.72 on this dimension (scale runs from 0 to 10) in comparison with 6.5 in average institutions, and 5.91 in risk institutions. The policy consultation and support dimension seem to be the most prominent factor in the profiling of excellent institutions. It can be assumed that the favourable scores on work pressure and difficult work situations are related to the proven merits of these (external) regulation opportunities in the past. Whenever work pressure problems and/or difficult work situations are discussed systematically and effectively with the supervisors and within the framework of a basic consultation structure, this produces results, even in the long term. They no longer function (merely) as a means of cure, but also as a means of prevention by offering regulation opportunities.

Table 5: *Risk, average, and excellent institutions typified according to regulation problems and opportunities. Results from One-way Anova with Bonferroni-test/effect sizes.*

	Excellent institutions (1)	Average institutions (2)	Risk institutions (3)	p	Significant group differences	Partial Eta squared
Regulation problems						
Work pressure*	4.58 (*n* = 20)	5.44 (*n* = 50)	6.26 (*n* = 21)	.000	1<2.3	.319
Difficult care situations*	5.11 (*n* = 20)	5.59 (*n* = 50)	5.87 (*n* = 21)	.016	1<3	.090
Difficult work situations*	2.92 (*n* = 20)	3.45 (*n* = 50)	4.06 (*n* = 21)	.000	1<2.3	.257
Difficulty in combining family and work*	2.70 (*n* = 20)	3.05 (*n* = 50)	3.76 (*n* = 21)	.000	1<3	.189
Regulation opportunities						
Autonomy*	7.80 (*n* = 20)	7.53 (*n* = 50)	6.77 (*n* = 21)	.001	1>3	.147
Information*	6.98 (*n* = 20)	5.87 (*n* = 50)	4.93 (*n* = 21)	.000	1>2.3	.208
Policy consultation and support*	7.72 (*n* = 20)	6.50 (*n* = 50)	5.91 (*n* = 21)	.000	1>2.3	.273
Collegiate consultation and support*	7.50 (*n* = 20)	7.14 (*n* = 50)	6.64 (*n* = 21)	.004	1>3	.116

* scale runs from 0 to 10

In line with the presented results, comparative multiple (multi-level) regression analyses show that models with regulation problems/opportunities as dependent variables always generate a higher model fit than those models with quality conditions as independent variables. This means that the effective presence of autonomy, information, support, and consultation better explains the variation between the institutions and the individuals than their accommodating quality contexts. Moreover, the policy consultation and support scores as dominant regulation opportunities confirm the already established importance of healthy human relations and a share in leadership within the institution. On the basis of these results it could be stated that the outlook of the Human Relations movement which is regarded by many as antiquated deserves fresh consideration: (much) more than innovative structuring and allocation principles, good management and healthy labour relations make up the outstanding quality conditions within the context of an intra-mural care setting.

Discussion

Economic and social developments are to a large extent decisive for approaching personnel and organisational issues. Movements in the social profit sector also reflect these developments. The increasing demands from the relevant stakeholders (the subsidising authority, the clientele, and the staff) necessitate a different and optimalised organisation and HR policy; a policy in which and whereby human skills and (semi-) professional talents can be used and developed to the fullest. The stated research results give an indication of the relevance, but also the difficulty/multi-dimensionality of implementing an HR policy to fit social profit care. The results show that in Flemish old age and nursing homes, innovative policy practices have very little effect on the realities of stress and individually tailored care. The exceptions to the rule are the labour relations and the quality of management on the work floor. More than innovative organisation and HR principles, good management and healthy mutual work relationships make up the foremost quality conditions within the context of an intra-mural care setting. Both of these must accommodate one another.

It should be emphasized that due to the cross-sectional character of the research, it is difficult to make any causal interferences. A second and related point that needs to be mentioned for discussion is that many of the measured HR-innovations are not at all mature. Therefore, the data supplies little empirical evidence for forming hypotheses with a normative connotation. Ideally, the research model should be retested using longitudinal data at the level of both individuals and organisations.

References

Atkinson, J. & Meager, N. (1986). *New Forms Of Work Organisation*. Brighton: Institute Of Manpower Studies.

Benner, P. (1984). *From novice to expert. Excellence and power in clinical nursing practice*. California: Addison-Wesley.

De Jonge, J. & Kompier, M. A. J (1997). A critical examination of the Demand-Control-Support Model from a work psychological perspective. *International Journal of Stress Management, 4*, 235-258.

De Sitter, L.U. (1994). *Synergetisch produceren*. Assen: Van Gorcum.

Friedman, A. (1977). *Industry and labour: class struggle at work and monopoly capitalism*. London: Macmillan.

Goffman, E. (1961). *Asylums. Essays on the social situation of mental patients and other inmates*. Garden City, New York: Doubleday Anchor Books.

Goldstein, H. (1995). *Multilevel statistical models*. London: Edward Arnold.

Karasek, R. (1979). Job Demands, Job Decision Latitude and Mental Strain: Implications for Job Design. *Administrative Science Quarterly, 24*, 285-308.

Karasek, R. (1985). *Job Content Instrument: Questionnaire and User's Guide*. Los Angeles: Department of Industrial and Systems Engineering, University of Southern California.

Karasek, R. & Theorell, T. (1990). *Healthy work. Stress, Productivity and the Reconstruction of Working Life*. New York: Basis Books.

Koeter, M. W. & Ormel, J. (1991). *General Health Questionnaire: Nederlandse bewerking en handleiding*. Lisse: Swets Test Services.

Kristensen, T. S. (1996). Job stress and cardiovascular disease: A theoretical critical review. *Journal of Occupational Health Psychology, 3*, 246-260.

Lipsky, M. (1980). *Street-level bureaucracy. Dilemmas of the individual in public services*. New York: Russel Sage Foundation.

Lutz, B. & Sengenberger, W. (1974). *Arbeitsmarktstrukturen und öffentliche Arbeitsmarktpolitik*. Göttingen: Otto Schwartz & Co.

Mintzberg, H. (1983). *Structures in fives. Designing effective organizations*. Englewood Cliffs, NJ: Prentice-Hall.

Piore, M. J. Sabel, S. J. (1984). *The Industrial Divide: Possibilities for Prosperity*. New York: Basic Books.

Snijders, T. A. B. & Bosker, R. J. (1999). *Multilevel Analysis. An introduction to basic and advanced multilevel modelling*. London/Thousands Oaks/New Delhi: SAGE publications

Stewart, J. (1999). *Employee development practice*. London: Pitman Publishing.

Van der Doef, M. P. & Maes, S. (1999). The Job Demand-Control(-Support) Model and psychological well-being: A review of 20 years of empirical research. *Work & Stress 13*(2), 87-114.

Vlerick, P. (1994). *Onderzoek naar de antecedenten en gevolgen van burnout bij verpleeg-kundigen in algemene ziekenhuizen*. Gent: Facultcit Psychologie en Pedagogische Wetenschappen.

Walby, S., Greenwell J., Mackay; L. & Soothill, K. (1994). *Medicine and nursing*. Professions in a changing Health Service. London: Sage Publications.

Employee well-being and customer satisfaction in the context of work environment changes

Ilse Cornelis* and Peter Vlerick
Department of Developmental, Personality and Social Psychology; Department of Personnel Management, Work and Organizational Psychology, Ghent University, Belgium

In recent years, for a variety of reasons, there have been a large number of organisations that have introduced some kind or organisational change, be it a merging operation, acquisition, downsizing or restructuring of some type. Although these are introduced to improve organisational performance, it is unclear to what degree they may possibly have adverse effects on customer satisfaction (CS), either by directly influencing customers' perceptions of organisational performance or through the impact these changes have on the well-being of employees confronted with these changes. Furthermore, it is still unclear in the literature to what degree there exist linkages between employee well-being or indicators of well-being and customer satisfaction. Although this linkage seems intuitively attractive, until now it has only been demonstrated with alternating success.

In the present study we will examine this relationship between job satisfaction and intention to leave the organisation with customer satisfaction ratings from three different sources, and we will explore whether we can find evidence for effects of work environment changes on CS.

Work environment changes

Numerous authors have outlined the possible negative consequences of downsizing, mergers or other large scale change operations for both employees that have been laid off as well as for the 'survivors' (Ashford, 1988; Kets De Vries & Balazs, 1997; Kozlowski, Chao, Smith & Hedlund, 1993). Other studies provided more mixed results: whereas in short term the desired effects are achieved, for instance improvements in productivity or risk taking, there might at the same time be considerable deterioration of employee morale,

* *Correspondence: Ilse Cornelis, ilse.cornelis@Ugent.be*

This research was sponsored by the Federal Services for Scientific Affairs, grant PS/02/31.

workplace climate or organisational commitment (Gilmore, Shea & Useem, 1997).

Most of these studies concentrate on investigating the effect of one or more major organisational changes on individuals' responses, which makes it difficult to know exactly *what* has changed for each individual employee. In the study reported here, rather than examining the effects of large scale organisational changes, we chose to obtain information on changes in the work environment that each individual employee was directly confronted with (changes in direct superior, tasks, co-workers, working hours and/or work rhythm).

Secondly, according to a transactional perspective (Lazarus & Folkman, 1984), the appraisal of an event or the way in which an individual evaluates a situation may be more important to employee well-being than the actual presence of stressors. This evaluation process results in a certain emotional response (positive or negative) which will in turn lead to certain coping responses. Following this line of reasoning, Payne and Morrison (1999) argued that it is important to distinguish possible 'stressful' or 'harmful' situations from the 'importance' or affective value of these situations for the individual. In a transactional perspective, the changes in the work environment of employees will have a differential impact on employee well-being according to the way they are evaluated and experienced. Here, we examined not only the 'objective' changes in employees' work environment, but also the degree to which employees perceived a certain control over changes and the degree to which they experienced these changes as stressful. These factors are partially derived from the conceptual framework provided by Karasek's Demand-Control model (Karasek, 1979), which characterizes the working environment in terms of psychological demands and control. An abundance of empirical studies have shown that these factors have indeed significant and important direct effects on employee well-being indicators such as burnout and job satisfaction (Van der Doef & Maes, 1999). It is hypothesised here that the perception of changes as uncontrollable and the experience of changes as stressful, demanding events will be more important in determining employee well-being than the number of work environment changes actually experienced.

Employee well-being and customer satisfaction

Nowadays, many organisations are searching for ways to measure, manage and ultimately improve customer satisfaction with their organisation – being forced to do so either by the highly competitive nature of certain markets or driven by societal concerns that result in governmental regulations.

Especially in the service sector, customer satisfaction will at least partly depend on customers' perceptions of employee behaviours such as friendliness and helpfulness (Dant, Lumpkin & Rawwas, 1998; Parasuraman, Zeithaml & Berry, 1985). It can be argued that these employees' behaviours will depend on their attitudes towards their work and the organisations they work for and their sense of well-being at work, and this line of reasoning has been integrated in popular models such as the 'service-profit chain' (Heskett, Sasser & Schlesinger, 1997). Based on this argument, the issue of improving customer satisfaction in services has resulted in recent years in a combination of two fields of research that traditionally have been separated, namely research on organisational behaviour and research in marketing. These two fields are combined in order to assess the effects of certain organisational aspects (either at higher levels, such as managerial practices, or at the level of individual employees, such as job satisfaction) on customer satisfaction. Research conducted in this particular field has yielded mixed results until now.

We chose here to include only a limited number of indicators of employee well-being, and we opted for a general level of job satisfaction and intention to leave. *Job satisfaction* is often conceived as a core measure of job related well-being (Van der Doef & Maes, 1999) and was included already in a number of studies examining the hypothesis that an individual's job satisfaction will have an impact on their performance and will ultimately influence customer satisfaction levels as well. *Intention to leave* the organisation is included here as another indicator of employee well-being, since it can be suspected that people who intend or wish to leave the organisation will tend to exhibit less positive customer-oriented behaviours and will thus tend to report and receive lower customer satisfaction.

Several studies have found direct relationships between employee job satisfaction and indicators of customer satisfaction in a variety of service employee settings (Atkins, Marshall & Javalgi, 1996; Hartline & Ferrell, 1996; Ryan, Schmit & Johnson, 1996). On the other hand, job satisfaction was included in a number of studies that did not yield direct effects of job satisfaction on CS indicators (Herrington & Lomax, 1999; Schneider, Parkington & Buxton, 1980; Todd, Robson & Lomax, 2000). A study from Griffith (2001) on the relationships between staff job satisfaction and parents' and students' satisfaction with school support services staff showed different results depending on the CS rating source (parents or students). It thus seems meaningful to distinguish in certain cases between different 'types' of customers or sources of CS ratings in order to allow meaningful interpretations. In the study reported here, we made a distinction between three separate sources of CS ratings for nursing homes, ratings that were given by either the residents of the nursing homes, family members of residents or members of staff. These can be considered as three fairly separate groups with different perspectives and expectations.

A final issue that merits our attention here is the question of the level of analysis when examining linkages between employees and customers. In this study, employees' perception of CS was related in a straightforward manner to the antecedent employee variables (both at the individual level). However, since the focus in this study was on the effects of changes in the working environment of individual employees' and their well-being at work on CS, these ratings were conceptual group level variables and were thus aggregated for both residents and family members within each organisation. The individual employee is the unit of analysis here, and aggregated scores for resident and family CS were assigned to each employee (see Wetzels, de Ruyter & Bloemer, 2000, for a similar procedure).

In this study we examined three main research questions dealing with the relationship between work environment changes, employee well-being and customer satisfaction. Firstly, can we find evidence for a relationship between employee well-being (job satisfaction and intention to leave) and CS ratings from three sources? Secondly, is there any evidence for a direct effect of work environment changes or the perception of these changes on CS, or are the effects mediated through employee well-being? In order to examine this latter question, we will compare two models, one being a direct effects model in which work environment changes and the perception of changes are allowed to have a direct effect on CS from three sources, and a mediated effects model in which changes have only an indirect effect on CS. Finally, if work environment changes and perception of changes only have an indirect impact, the final issue worth investigating is the hypothesis (according to a transactional perspective) that the number of work environment changes in itself will have a less important effect on employee well-being than the perceptions of these changes.

Method

Participants and procedure

The data were collected in a study on quality and satisfaction conducted in 39 nursing homes. Nursing homes participated on a voluntary basis to the study, which included standardised structured interviews of all residents that were mentally able to participate to such an interview. They could also participate to conduct a survey of family members or close acquaintances of residents, and a survey of all staff members.

In total we analysed data from 882 employees (88.5% females, mean age = 37 years), 2315 residents and 1481 family members of residents. CS data for residents and family were aggregated at the level of nursing homes and linked with individual employee data (average within group interrater reliability for family ratings was $r_{wg(j)}$ = .93 and for residents $r_{wg(j)}$ = .86; James, Demaree & Wolf, 1984). Aggregated data for resident CS ranged from 1.94 for the nursing home with the lowest satisfaction rating to 2.89 for the highest scoring nursing home (measured on a 4-point scale, M_{homes} = 2.39, SD = .22). Family CS ratings were scored on a 7-point scale and aggregated scores ranged from 4.75 to 6.46 (M_{homes} = 5.83, SD = .32, see table 1).

Measures

Staff questionnaires contained indicators of work environment changes (total number, control and stress associated with changes), well-being (job satisfaction and intention to leave) and perceived CS. Family members completed a similar questionnaire as staff members on perceived CS, and residents were asked four CS questions (see table 1).

Table 1: Indicators in staff, residents and family questionnaires

Staff questionnaire	Cronbach's α	M	SD
Work environment changes (during past 6 months) 1. Change of tasks 2. Change of working hours 3. Change of working rhythm (pace) 4. Change of direct superior 5. Change of co-workers = Total number of changes in working environment	NA	2.10	1.13
Perceived control over changes 1. I felt in control over these changes (from 1 = completely disagree to 5 = completely agree)	NA	1.98	1.18
Stress experienced when confronted with changes 1. Indicate on a scale from 0 to 100 the degree of stress you experienced when confronted with these changes (0 = no stress; 100 = enormous amount of stress).	NA	31.96	28.06
Job satisfaction (7-point scale) 1. How satisfied are you with your work in general? 2. How satisfied are you with the content of your work? 3. How satisfied are you with your job compared with jobs in other organisations?	.82	5.37	.99
Intention to leave (7-point scale) 1. I regularly consider leaving the organisation 2. It is unlikely I will be working here next year	.61	2.52	1.42
Perceived customer satisfaction (7-point scale) 1. How satisfied do you think residents are with the tangible aspects of the home (meals, attractiveness, comfort and cleanliness of bedroom, leisure rooms and buildings)?	.82	5.31	.78

2. How satisfied do you think residents are with empathy of staff?
3. How satisfied do you think residents are with helpfulness of staff?
4. How satisfied do you think residents are with the reliability of the institution (keeping files and administration, keeping appointments, ...)
5. How satisfied do you think residents are with courteousness of staff?

Resident questionaire	Cronbach's α	M homes	SD homes
Perceived customer satisfaction (4-point scale) 1. How satisfied are you with empathy of staff? 2. How satisfied are you with the atmosphere in the home? 3. To what degree do you feel at home in this institution? 4. To what degree would you recommend this home to others?	.83	2.39	.22

Family questionaire	Cronbach's α	M homes	SD homes
Perceived customer satisfaction (7-point scale) 1. How satisfied do you think residents are with the tangible aspects of the home (meals, attractiveness, comfort and cleanliness of bedroom, leisure rooms and buildings)? 2. How satisfied do you think residents are with empathy of staff? 3. How satisfied do you think residents are with helpfulness of staff? 4. How satisfied do you think residents are with the reliability of the institution (keeping files and administration, keeping appointments, ...) 5. How satisfied do you think residents are with courteousness of staff?	.88	5.83	.32

Results

The rank order correlations between the averaged CS ratings with nursing homes from the three different sources (Table 2) are moderately associated. The strongest association exists between ratings from staff and family, but this might be due to the use of an identical questionnaire for these ratings.

Table 2: Rank order correlations between customer satisfaction ratings from 3 sources (n = 882)

	Staff Perceived Satisfaction	**Resident Satisfaction**	**Family Perceived Satisfaction**
Staff perceived satisfaction	.82		
Resident satisfaction	.32**	.83	
Family perceived satisfaction.	.42**	.24**	.88

Note: Cronbach's α on diagonal

** $p < .01$

In order to see to what degree there exists a direct or indirect relationship between the number of work environment changes, the perception of changes and CS ratings, we compared two models for each of the three CS ratings (staff, residents and family). The first model shown each time is a mediated effects model, where work environment changes and the perceptions of changes are allowed to have an effect on CS through job satisfaction and intention to leave. The second model tested for direct effects of work environment changes on CS.

The first two models, for staff perceived CS, show that only employee job satisfaction is related directly to CS. The number of changes in employee work environment is significantly but weakly and negatively related to job satisfaction, but not to intention to leave. Perceived control over changes is positively related to employee job satisfaction and negatively to intention to leave, whereas stress associated with work environment changes is related positively to intention to leave and negatively to employee job satisfaction. Although the mediated effects model did not show a superior fit ($\chi^2 = 211.55$; $df = 55$; RMSEA = .057; NNFI = .95; CFI = .96; GFI = .96) than the direct effects model ($\chi^2 = 207.80$; $df = 52$; RMSEA = .058; NNFI = .94; CFI = .96; GFI = .97), it is clear from the path coefficients that there was no evidence to support direct effects from work environment changes on staff perceived CS.

Figure 1: Relationships between work environment changes, well-being and staff perceived satisfaction (mediated effects model, standardised coefficients, n = 882)

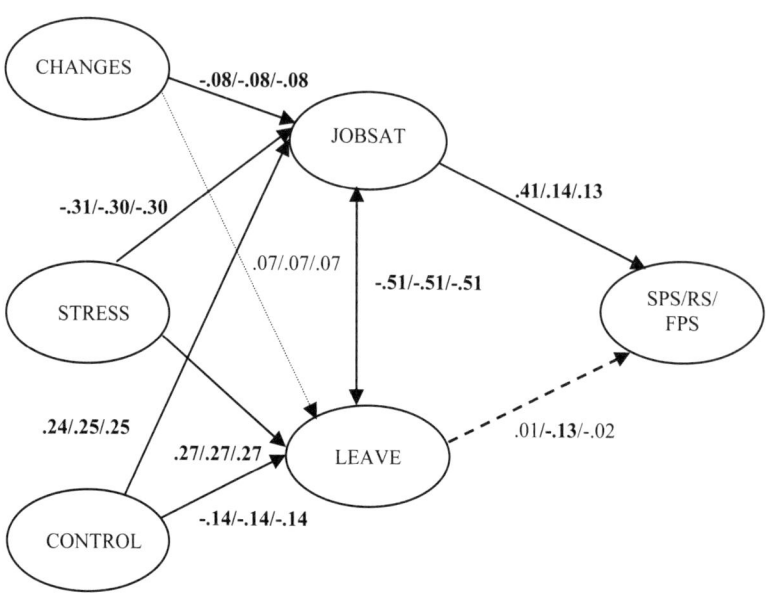

CHANGES = the number of work environment changes, STRESS = stress experienced due to the changes, CONTROL = the degree of perceived control over changes, JOBSAT = job satisfaction; LEAVE = intention to leave the organisation, SPS = staff perceived resident satisfaction, RS = resident satisfaction, FPS = family perceived satisfaction.

Figure 2: Relationships between work environment changes, well-being and staff perceived satisfaction (direct effects model, standardised coefficients, n = 882)

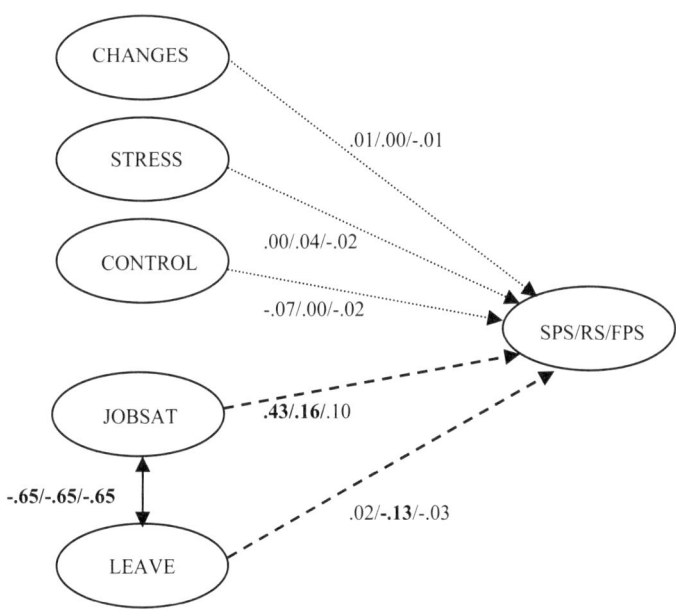

CHANGES = the number of work environment changes, STRESS = stress experienced due to the changes, CONTROL = the degree of perceived control over changes, JOBSAT = job satisfaction; LEAVE = intention to leave the organisation, SPS = staff perceived resident satisfaction, RS = resident satisfaction, FPS = family perceived satisfaction.

The third and fourth models indicate that both employee job satisfaction and employees' intention to leave are related to resident satisfaction (RCS), and there are no significant direct relationships between changes, the perception of changes and RCS. Again, the mediated effects model was not superior in fit (χ^2 = 122.87; df = 45; RMSEA = .04; NNFI = .96; CFI = .98; GFI = .98) when compared to the direct effects model (χ^2 = 121.67; df = 42; RMSEA = .046; NNFI = .96; CFI = .98; GFI = .98)

The two final models indicate again no direct links between changes, perceptions of changes and family perceived CS (FCS), and there is only a direct link between employee job satisfaction and FCS. Model fit for the mediated effects model ($\chi^2 = 219.97$; $df = 55$; RMSEA = .058; NNFI = .97; CFI = .97; GFI = .96) was not significantly better than for the direct effects model ($\chi^2 = 216.16$; $df = 52$; RMSEA = .06; NNFI = .96; CFI = .98; GFI = .96).

The proportion of the variance explained in the three different indicators for CS however was rather small and ranges from a mere 3% for FCS over 6% in RS to 17% in SPS.

Discussion

The aim of this study was to examine whether we could find evidence for direct detrimental effects of work environment changes on customer satisfaction, or whether changes within organisations might affect customer satisfaction indirectly through a decrease in employee well-being.

We did not find evidence for direct detrimental effects of the number of work environment changes, the perception of these changes as controllable events or the degree of stress associated with these changes on CS. Employee job satisfaction was strongly related to staff perceived CS, and to a lesser degree but still significantly related to resident CS and to family perceived CS. Intention to leave the organisation, another indicator of employee well-being, was negatively associated only to resident satisfaction ratings. Thus it seems that while higher employee job satisfaction is associated with higher levels of perceived CS in staff, residents as well as family of residents, stronger intentions to leave the organisation from employees are only associated with lower levels of resident CS.

Secondly, we found that the number of changes in employees' work environment is only weakly associated with job satisfaction. The degree of stress experienced when confronted to changes and to a lesser degree the perception of control over these changes seems to have had a far stronger effect on employee job satisfaction and intention to leave. These findings corroborate with the transactional perspective that stresses the importance of distinguishing between actual events and the appraisal of the event, in this case in terms of emotionally demandingness and controllability. In this context we would like to emphasise the importance of the manner in which certain changes are introduced and communicated to the employees. If an organisation can manage to introduce these changes in consultation with employees and ensuring a minimal level of stress, according to our findings, the impact on employee well-being will be considerably less negative.

Our finding that intention to leave the organisation is related to a far smaller and sometimes non-significant extent to CS might be explained by the fact that perhaps this indicator is not a reliable indicator of the degree to which an individual feels good in his or her job and organisation. Employees might have a variety of reasons to leave the organisation, including choosing a job closer to home, that are not directly related to employee well-being.

The explanation for the finding that intention to leave had an impact only on resident satisfaction ratings and not on employee or family CS is difficult to explain without further information. A possible but by no means final explanation might be that for employees who intend to leave the organisation, even though this might be for reasons not related to well-being and even though they themselves might have the impression of providing the services with the same care and thoroughness as before, a slight 'sloppiness' in services, engagement, ... somehow is perceived by residents who interact with these employees on a very regular basis. Family members of resident who have far less contact with employees can be expected not to notice this.

It is unclear however, to what degree intention to leave and job satisfaction are causally related to CS. It might be, that employees who feel less positive toward their job and the organisation they work for will tend to engage less in positive customer oriented behaviours that will results in higher levels of quality and CS. Or, alternatively, employees with more negative attitudes towards their work tend to display less positive emotions which influence customers' perceptions of service quality and satisfaction through an emotional contagion process (Pugh, 2001). Another explanation however might be that employees, working in an organisation with limited managerial concerns with maintaining a high level of service quality and resident satisfaction, might feel less satisfied, while at the same time this absence of 'a climate for service' might result in lower levels of CS. In order to clarify these relationships, similar research which includes more indicators, both on the organisational as well as on the employee level is needed.

Finally, the proportion of variance explained in CS by the variables included in this study was rather small. Although we found significant relationships between employee job satisfaction and customer satisfaction ratings from three sources, there is a large proportion of customer satisfaction that remains unexplained. Taking into account that job satisfaction is a fairly robust indicator of employee well-being, this study might provide additional evidence that the link between employee well-being and customer satisfaction is not as strong as is often assumed. Additional analyses that were conducted on these data have shown that one of the most important determinants of resident and family satisfaction was level of education, with respondents with higher education being more critical and less satisfied in general. The impact of such effects was obscured while aggregating the data from residents and family members within each nursing home in order to be able to link them with employee data.

Another limitation in this study is the very specific context in which the survey was conducted. In a nursing home context, the range of dissatisfaction might actually be larger than in other contexts since dissatisfied 'customers', in this case elderly people who are often in need of help for a number of daily activities, are highly unlikely to 'switch' homes.

Thirdly, we included in this study changes in the working environment and examined the effect of the number of changes, with no regard to the type of change reported. It might be that some work environment changes actually do have direct effects on CS, but that these effects were obscured by treating all changes equally and taking into account only the number of changes.

In concluding, we can say that at least in this study we could not demonstrate direct negative effects from work environment changes on CS, but there was evidence for a link between the perception of changes as controllable events and the degree to which the changes were rated as stressful and disruptive and job satisfaction which was in turn related to CS from three different sources.

This study was a first exploratory attempt to relate changes and the perception of changes in the working environment to employee well-being and customer satisfaction and as such should be considered a starting point for further research into the largely ignored domain of the effect of changes within organisations on organisational performance which would seem largely determined in the context of health care by employees' attitudes and behaviours.

References

Ashford, S. J. (1988). Individual strategies for coping with stress during organizational transitions. *Journal of Applied Behavioral Science, 24*, 19-36.

Atkins, P. M., Marshall, B. S. & Javalgi, R. G. (1996). Happy employees lead to loyal patients. *Journal of Health Care Marketing, winter*, 15-23.

Dant, R. P., Lumpkin, J. R .& Rawwas, M. Y. A. (1998). Sources of generalized versus issue specific dissatisfaction in service channels of distribution: a review and comparative investigation. *Journal of Business Research, 42*, 7-23.

Gilmore, T., Shea, G. & Useem, M. (1997). Side effects of corporate cultural transformation. *Journal of Applied Behavioral Science, 33*, 174-189.

Griffith, J. (2001). Do satisfied employees satisfy customers? Support services staff morale and satisfaction among public school administrators, students and parents. *Journal of Applied Social Psychology, 31*, 1627-1658.

Hartline, M. D., Ferrell, O. C. (1996). The management of customer-contact service employees: an empirical investigation. *Journal of Marketing, 60*, 52-70.

Herrington, G. & Lomax, W. (1999). *Do satisfied employees make customers satisfied?: an investigation into the relationship between service employee job satisfaction and customer perceived service quality.* Paper presented at the 28th European Marketing Academy Conference, Berlin.

Heskett, J. L., Sasser, W. E., Jr. & Schlesinger, L. A. (1997). *The service profit chain: how leading companies link profit and growth to loyalty, satisfaction and value.* New York: The Free Press.

James, L. R., Demaree, R. G. & Wolf, G. (1984). Estimating within – group interrater reliability with and without response bias. *Journal of Applied Psychology, 69,* 85-98.

Karasek, R. A. (1979). Job demands, job decision latitude, and mental strain: implications for job redesign. *Administrative Science Quarterly, 24,* 285-308.

Kets de Vries, M. F. R. & Balazs, K. (1997). The downside of downsizing. *Human Relations, 50,* 11-50.

Kozlowski, S. W. J., Chao, G. T., Smith, E. M. & Hedlund, J. (1993). Organizational downsizing: strategies, interventions and research implications. In C. L. Cooper & I. T. Robertson (Eds.), *International Review of Industrial and Organizational Psychology* (pp 263-332). New York: John Wiley & Sons.

Lazarus, R. S. & Folkman, S. (1984). *Stress, appraisal and coping.* New York, Springer.

Ryan, A. M., Schmit, M. J. & Johnson, R. (1996). Attitudes and effectiveness: examining relations at an organisational level. *Personnel Psychology, 49,* 853-881.

Parasuraman, A., Zeithaml, V. A. & Berry, L. L. (1985). A conceptual model of service quality and its implications for future research. *Journal of Marketing, 49,* 41-50.

Payne, R. L. & Morrison, D. (1999). The importance of knowing the affective meaning of job demands revisited. *Work & Stress,* 13, 208-288.

Pugh, S. D. (2001). Service with a smile: emotional contagion in the service encounter. *Academy of Management Journal, 44,* 1018-1027.

Schneider, B., Parkington, J. J. & Buxton, V. M. (1980). Employees and customer perceptions of service in banks. *Administrative Science Quarterly, 25,* 252-267.

Todd, S., Robson, A. & Lomax, W. (2000*). Evaluating the link between job satisfaction and external service quality.* Paper presented at the 29th European Marketing Academy Conference, Rotterdam.

Van der Doef, M. & Maes, S. (1999). The Job Demand-Control (-Support) Model and psychological well-being: A review of 20 years of empirical research. *Work & Stress, 13*(2), 87-114.

Wetzels M. G. M., de Ruyter J. C. & Bloemer J. M. M. (2000). Antecedents and consequences of role stress of retail sales persons. *Journal of Retailing and Consumer Services, 7,* 65-75.

Comparison of male and female manager's assessment center ratings

Tobias Eklund[1] & Per Tillman[2]*
[1] *Department of Psychology, Uppsala Universitet, Sweden*
[2] *Personnel Decisions International, Sweden*

In the current service economy, an organization's human resources are frequently touted as its most valuable asset. The competition for well-educated and competent employees is often fierce, and organizations have started using increasingly elaborate systems to recruit and develop their people. The methods are used on the assumption that ratings and evaluations of the prospective employee predict on-the-job performance (Mabon, 2002).

Many of the methods used for selection and development purposes are costly and time consuming. Moreover, differentiating a good method from a less effective one requires skilled users. Two of the most important concepts used in evaluating a method are reliability and validity. Simply put, reliability refers to the consistency of measurement, and validity refers to the extent to which the method measures what it is purported to measure, or alternatively, predicts what people claim it predicts (Clark-Carter, 1998). Perceived and de facto fairness are also important considerations when using a measurement method, and the method used should not have systematic bias in favor of one demographic group over another. Extensive research has examined differences among different groups, such as ethnic groups and gender, in relation to leadership.

Ratings of men and women

Over the past couple of decades the number of working women has increased and so has the number of women in leadership positions. Gender differences in leadership have received a lot of attention from the research community and the field can be divided into a number of sub-areas. One important question is whether or not men and women display different behaviors in leadership roles, whereas another focuses on the evaluation of women and men in leadership positions. A third such area is the examination of men's and women's effectiveness as leaders. Each of these areas can be subdivided further, and researchers have examined moderators such as profession, leadership level, and cultural influences. Alice H. Eagly is one of the more promi-

---

* *Correspondence: Per Tillman, Per.Tillman@personneldecisions.com*

nent researchers in these areas and she and her colleagues have accumulated the research on each of the aforementioned areas in three meta-analyses (Eagly & Johnson, 1990; Eagly, Makhijani & Klonsky, 1992; Eagly, Karau & Makhijani, 1995). The results of these studies are discussed below.

Gender and leadership style

There are both studies that indicate that there are differences in leadership style between men and women as well as those that suggest that such differences are absent, or not significant (e.g., Gibson, 1995; Thompson, 2000). In one meta-analysis examining 162 studies comparing male and female leaders, Eagly and Johnson (1990) found that differences in leadership style between men and women appear to be small. The authors divided the sample of the study into three categories based on methodology: laboratory studies, assessment studies, and organizational studies. Differences between men and women were bigger in laboratory and assessment studies than in organizational studies. Eagly and Johnson conclude that in the two former types of studies participants are assessed outside their normal environment, which removes the influence of previously established relationships, which they claim mutes gender effects in organizational studies. The authors claim that gender becomes a more important behavioral cue in situations where the interacting parties do not know each other, than they will in the everyday working environment. The accumulated studies in the meta-analysis focused on a variety of different leadership aspects, but it was only for those most frequently studied that differences were identified (Table 1).

Table 1: Differences in leadership style identified by Eagly and Johnson (1990)

	Women	**Men**
Laboratory studies and assessment studies	Interpersonal leadership style: Focuses on others well being, is accessible, is warm and sympathetic when interacting with co-workers.	Task-oriented leadership style: Makes a subordinate follow rules and procedures, maintain high productivity demands, clarifies differences between leaders and subordinates, acts independently.
Laboratory studies, assessment studies and organization studies	Democratic leadership style: Lets subordinates participate in decision making	Autocratic leadership style: Emphasizes attaining goals, deprives subordinates from the decision-making

The only identified gender difference in leadership style was that women tend to use a more democratic, and men a more autocratic, leadership style. Eagly and Johnson (1990) view the democratic and interpersonal, and autocratic and task-focused, leadership styles as similar. However, the democratic/autocratic leadership styles characterize a more narrow range of behaviors than the interpersonal and task focused descriptions. In their research it is clear that they do not view one particular style as more effective than another, rather, each style has its respective advantages and disadvantages, and are likely more and less effective depending on the circumstances. Furthermore, the styles should not be viewed as different ends of one continuum; for example, a high degree of task focus is not mutually exclusive with strong interpersonal skills.

Gender and ratings of leaders

Eagly, Makhijani and Klonsky (1992) conducted another meta-analysis to examine the gender differences in ratings for male and female leaders. The study includes 61 studies where all variables except gender were controlled. The results indicate a slight tendency for men to be rated more favorably than women, particularly in certain situations. In studies where there were a higher proportion of male raters, the leadership style was stereotypically male, and in professions with a high proportion of male leaders, men tended to be rated higher than women. In addition, the study indicates that women who display male leadership behaviors, and thereby contradict the stereotypically female leadership behaviors, are rated more negatively. One illustration of this phenomenon is that a leadership style that is described as 'principled' when displayed by a male is descried as 'rigid' for females. Interestingly, men who display stereotypically female leadership behaviors are not rated less favorably.

One of the fundamental issues surrounding gender difference in leadership is whether or not the differences in ratings are due to rater bias or true differences in behavior (Eagly, Karau & Makhijani, 1995). This is a particularly acute problem in organizational studies, but controlling possible extraneous variables can be difficult in assessment studies as well. Eagly, Karau and Makhijani (1995) contend that the results of the meta-analyses include many studies that keep variables that may affect the results constant, which would suggest that the influence of such factors is small.

Gender and leader effectiveness

Although Eagly and Johnsons (1990) meta-analysis indicated that men and women's leadership styles do differ in some respects, this does not necessarily mean that there are differences in how effective they are as leaders. In a meta-analysis of studies that have examined the effectiveness of male and female leaders Eagly, Karau and Makhijani (1995) included 82 studies. Their main finding was that based on these results there were no significant differences in the effectiveness of leaders based on gender. However, a more in depth analysis revealed that the effectiveness of leaders was moderated by type of leadership role. The results suggested that men were more effective in role that were described in masculine terms and that women were more effective in roles defined in feminine terms.

Furthermore, Eagly, Karau and Makhijani (1995) study showed that the organizational level also moderated the gender-effectiveness relationship. Men were found to be more effective as first line managers/leaders, whereas women were found to be more effective in middle management roles. When comparing different professions Eagly, Karau and Makhijani (1995) found one exception: military leadership. In the armed forces, men were uniformly found to be more effective. Lastly, the researchers found that men tended to be rated higher than women when there was high proportion of male raters (Eagly, Karau & Makhijani, 1995).

Cultural differences in leadership style

A majority of the aforementioned studies were conducted in the United States, and it is not certain whether or not the results can be generalized to other cultures. Gibson (1995) states that research in this area suggests that culture is an important factor that influences leadership behaviors. For instance, Swedish leaders tend to emphasize participation and power sharing to a greater extent than leaders in other countries. Gibson's study indicated that Swedish and Norwegian leaders tend to favor an interpersonal leadership style to a greater extent than American and Australian leaders. However, the gender differences identified by Eagly, Karau and Makhijani (1995) are also observed cross-culturally, lending some evidence to the argument that these differences may be internationally pervasive. In conclusion, Gibson's study shows that the differences identified by Eagly and Johnson (1990) can also be found in Sweden, but that there are also overarching differences between Swedish and American leaders where Swedish leaders of both genders tend to emphasize interpersonal leadership behaviors to a greater extent.

Selection and development methodologies

The Assessment Center methodology has its roots in German, British and American armed forces from World War II, and these methods were incorporated more broadly into organizational Human Resource practices in the 1950's (Bray & Grant, 1966; Bray & Howard, 1983). One of the pioneering organizations for the use of Assessment Centers was AT&T, and the use of Assessment Centers has gradually increased over the past five decades (Bray & Grant, 1966; Byham, 1970; Zaar & Tillman, 2003). In Sweden, Assessment

Centers have become more common since the beginning of the 1990's and is used by both domestic and international organizations. Because the method is relatively time consuming and expensive it has primarily been used for selection and development of managers and specialists (Gaugler, Rosenthal, Thornton III & Bentson, 1987), but it has also been applied in police, fire-rescue, college-student, and sales populations (Dayan, Kasten & Fox, 2002; Russell, 1985; Mabon, 2002).

The most critical quality of a selection instrument is its criterion related validity, that is, the strength of the relationship between the results of the measure and job performance (Zaar & Tillman, 2003). Schmidt and Hunter (1998) conducted a meta-analysis to compare the validities of a variety of selection methods, and found considerable variation in the validities of these methods. Some methods, such as graphology, were found to have no predictive validity, while other methods, such as cognitive tests and Assessment Centers, were found to be considerably better in predicting job performance. The accumulated research on the validity of selection methods is becoming extensive, and the results are clear with reference to which methods predict job performance well and which do not (Mabon, 2002).

Description of Assessment Center

The Assessment Center method rests on multi-trait, multi-method theory whereby the accuracy of conclusions is improved by measuring multiple traits by multiple methods, as opposed to one trait by one method. In a typical Assessment Center, a participant assumes a role in a fictitious organization and faces challenges similar to those that will be, or are, present on the job. These challenges are reflected in different job-related simulations and interviews, and psychometric tests are also included. Assessees are rated on predetermined competencies deemed critical for the target role. To ensure reliability of the ratings each competency is measured in at least two components, such as simulations, interviews and tests, but often in more than two. After completion of all assessment components, the ratings are integrated into one, overall, rating referred to as the *Overall Assessment Rating* (OAR), which is used as an indicator of the assessee's overall performance during the Assessment Center.

The types of simulations and tests included in an Assessment Center vary depending on the challenges faced and competencies needed to be successful in the target role. However, there are specific internationally established requirements that must be met in order to call a method 'Assessment Center' (International Task Force for Assessment Center guidelines, 2000). These requirements include, among others, that the assessee is rated by several raters, is rated in several assessment components, and that written and/or face-to-face simulations are included. Written simulations can be 'in-basket' exercises where the assessee is asked to respond to a number of items in writing, and face-to-face simulations can be a meeting with the assesse's boss or direct report as specified in the fictitious organization.

Assessment Center research

One of the benchmark studies on Assessment Center validity is Gaugler et al.'s (1987) meta-analysis. They summarized the results of 107 validity coefficients and state that "there is such a variety of Assessment Center procedures that a typical Assessment Center does not exist" (p. 494). They conclude that comparisons between different Assessment Centers must be made with utmost caution and consideration of their differences. Some of these differences may account for inconsistencies in validity estimates across studies. One consistent finding in Assessment Center research is the presence of high reliability and predictive validity, but low construct validity (Borman, 1982; Chan, 1996; Mabon, 2002; Schleicher, Mayes, Day & Riggio, 2002; Schneider & Schmitt, 1992). That is, Assessment Centers' OAR have been found to predict meaningful criteria, such as job performance and potential, but ratings tend to have weaker correlations for one competency across different measurement components than the correlation of different competencies within one measurement component. Some researchers have questioned these findings, and recent studies have indicated ways of improving the construct validity of Assessment Center (Jones, 1992; Arthur, Woehr & Maldegen, 2000; Woehr & Arthur, 2003).

Gender differences in Assessment Center ratings

Several studies have examined the effect of gender on Assessment Center ratings and Shore (1992) found that there were no differences in OAR, but that women tended to be rated higher on performance-style skills such as managing conflict and building relationships. In a study examining the effect of the raters, Walsh, Weinberg and Fairfield (1987) found that women received higher OAR and that there is an interaction between the gender distributions of the raters and gender such that rater groups consisting of exclusively men tend to give women higher ratings than they give men. In rater groups consisting of both women and men, there are no significant differences in the ratings of men and women. The results of a similar study by Shore, Tashchian and Adams (1997), however, indicate that there are no significant differences in ratings or interaction effect.

In sum, previous research gives a somewhat unclear picture of the influence of gender on Assessment Center ratings. Some studies (Walsh, Weinberg & Fairfield, 1987; Shore, 1992) suggest that women sometimes are rated higher than men, whereas the results of one study (Shore, Tashchian & Adams, 1997) suggests that there are no significant differences in ratings. As an additional variable, the gender distribution of the rater group may also influence the rating such that all male rater groups tend to give women higher ratings than men, which is not the case for mixed rating groups (Walsh, Weinberg & Fairfield, 1987).

Purpose and hypotheses of the present study

Purpose

The purpose of the present study is to examine whether or not there are differences in Assessment Center ratings based on the gender of the assessee, and to evaluate these differences in light of previous research and theory on gender differences in leadership.

Hypotheses

Hypothesis 1: Women will be rated higher than men on five competencies related to interpersonal leadership: manage and develop talent, foster teamwork and collaboration, build relationships, manage conflicts, and foster open communication.

Hypothesis 2: Men will be rated higher than women on the competencies: sound judgment, manage execution, and lead courageously.

No specific hypotheses for differences between men and women are presented for the remaining competencies (analyze information, strategic thinking, visionary thinking, global perspective, establish plans, influence, drive and commitment, and leadership maturity). However, we will conduct exploratory analyses to investigate differences in these competences. Similarly, although we do not hypothesize a significant difference between men and women on OAR, we will conduct exploratory analyses to examine if there are any differences in OAR in the present study.

The present study differs from previous research in some important ways. The present study is conducted within the healthcare industry and there are more female than male participants. Although no specific hypotheses are made based on these differences, the results will likely further increase our insight to the dynamics of Assessment Center ratings.

Method

The Assessment Center

The present study is based on an assessment scenario that was customized for the Swedish Health Care industry by Personnel Decisions International (PDI), a global Human Resources consulting firm. The Assessment Center consists of five to nine measurement components depending on the challenges and competencies needed for the target role. The five measurement components that were used in all cases were: behavioral interview, in-basket, Raven's Advanced Progressive Matrices (cognitive test), and Watson-Glaser Critical Thinking Appraisal (cognitive test). Some of the Assessment Centers were extended with a risk and consequence analysis, meeting with a direct report, meeting with the person's boss, the Global Personality Inventory (GPI), and/or Myers-Briggs Type Indicator (MBTI).

Assesses performance was rated on 10-17 competencies depending on the number of measurement components included. The tests were administrated the same way regardless of the number of competencies measured. Differences in performance depending on the number of competencies measured were conducted and are reported in the results section below. Ratings were made on a five-point scale, where five denotes above standard performance, three denotes meets expected standards, and one denotes below expected standards.

Participants

From the start in 1999 until May 2003 197 participants went though the Assessment Center (132 women and 65 men). Prior to the participating in the Assessment Center the participants were asked if he/she agreed to have their results being used for research. Of the 197 men and women who participated in the study, 17 people (11 women, 6 men) declined to have their results used for research purposes. The division in age and gender does not differ appreciably from the rest of the sample. Remaining in the study are 180 participants, 59 men and 121 women.

Some of the participants have gone through the Assessment Center for selection purposes, others for development purposes; however, the results are partially used to investigate future potential to advancement in the developmental Assessment Centers. That is, these evaluations also have a function as support in selection processes (Zaar & Tillman, 2003). The result in an Assessment Center could differ depending if the participant is in a selection- or development situation. It has not been possible in this study to divide the participants into the categories selection and development.

Procedure

One week before the Assessment Center the participant received preparation material sent to their homes which contains information about the Assessment Center method, they also receive a description of the fictitious organization and with a personal preparation material that is to be filled out and handed over to (PDI) before the assessment. The participant can bring the information about the fictitious organization with him/her to the Assessment Center and thereby does not have to memorize the information.

It takes about 6-10 hours to complete an Assessment Center depending on the number of measurement components. The center begins with a 30-minute introduction before initiating the various tests. The order in which the tests are carried out varies between participants for logistical reasons. Prior to the meeting simulations the participant has 30 minutes to prepare him or herself before carrying out the exercises.

After the completion of the Assessment Center all data is saved in a confidential personal file. Materials that are collected include forms with background material, the consent to participate in the center, and evaluation forms. The data is summarized in an integration and a comprehensive evaluation report of the participant's achievement. A lead coach compiles the participator result and feedback is given at the point in time that has been agreed upon. Feedback is given both to the participant and to the organization subsequent the completion of the Assessment Center.

For the present study, all participants' collected data has been used. The data is archived at PDI for at least five years after accomplished assessment. Data have been processed through integration matrices and data background forms. The more detailed data from the participant's evaluation templates has only been used when the integration matrices have been too difficult to interpret.

Sample reduction

The 17 people who dropped out have been described above. During the data processing some missing information was discovered. The explanation for this is that the lead coach in some particular factors did not think that he/she was able to give a rating on a particular competency.

Results

Effect of the number of competencies measured

Because previous research has indicated that the number of dimensions rated negatively influences the psychometric properties (Gaugler & Thornton III, 1989). The results were compared based on the number of competencies rated in the present study. No differences were found based on 10, 12, 15 or 17 dimensions rated (Table 2). Therefore, results were accumulated across number of competencies rated.

Table 2: Mean score and standard deviation on common OAR. Participants divided on number of assessed competency dimensions (10/12/15/17) and gender

Number of assessed competencies	Participants gender	N	M(SD)
10	Women	11	2.86 (.35)
	Men	3	3.30 (.70)
	Total	14	2.95 (.45)
12	Women	41	2.98 (.35)
	Men	11	2.80 (.39)
	Total	52	2.94 (.37)
15	Women	14	2.92 (.38)
	Men	6	2.97 (.21)
	Total	20	2.94 (.33)
17	Women	55	2.97 (.36)
	Men	39	2.94 (.43)
	Total	94	2.96 (.39)
Total	Women	121	2.96 (.36)
	Men	59	2.94 (.42)
	Total	180	2.95 (.38)

Comparison of Ratings of Men and Women by Competency

Hypothesis 1

Hypothesis 1 states that women were expected to be rated higher on the competencies related to interpersonal leadership: manage and develop talent, foster teamwork and collaboration, build relationships, manage conflicts, and foster open communication. The results of independent t-tests indicate that hypothesis 1 was not confirmed (Table 3). There were mean differences in the expected direction, but the differences were too small to be statistically significant. Given the power of the analyses it is unlikely that these differences are of practical significance. The largest observed difference was for foster open communication where the mean difference was .1 [t (178) = 1.43, $p >$ .05].

Table 3: Mean score and t-test results, independent groups in their respective competency dimensions in regard of Hypothesis 1

	N		M(SD)		t-test		
Competency dimension	Men	Women	Men	Women	t	df	sig. (1-tailed)
Manage and develop talent	57	121	2.88 (.52)	2.94 (.49)	.76	176	.23
Foster teamwork	57	121	2.71 (.70)	2.74 (.50)	.36	176	.36
Build relation-ships	56	109	2.88 (.50)	2.97 (.45)	1.27	163	.10
Manage dis-agreements	52	111	2.83 (.49)	2.91 (.45)	1.06	161	.15
Foster open communication	59	121	2.94 (.47)	3.04 (.43)	1.43	178	.08

Hypothesis 2

Hypothesis 2 states that men were expected to be rated higher than women on the competencies: sound judgment, manage execution, and lead courageously (Table 4). The results indicate that the hypothesis for sound judgment is confirmed [t (178) = -1.74, $p < .05$]. However, the results indicate that, contrary to hypotheses, women were rated higher, though not significantly, on manage execution and lead courageously.

Table 4: Mean score and t-test results. Independent groups in their respective competency dimensions in regard of hypothesis 2

	N		M(SD)		t-test		
Competency dimension	Men	Women	Men	Women	t	df	sig. (1-tailed)
Use sound judgment	59	121	2.89 (.53)	2.75 (.48)	-1.74	178	.04
Organize and lead business	54	121	2.68 (.63)	2.72 (.56)	.44	178	.33
Lead courageously	58	117	3.03 (.49)	3.13 (.62)	.10	173	.16

Exploratory analyses

No differences in men's and women's ratings were hypothesized OAR and the competencies: analyze information, strategic thinking, visionary thinking, global perspective, establish plans, influence, drive and commitment, and leadership maturity. However, exploratory analyses were conducted for investigate whether or not differences were present in these measures. No significant differences were found in OAR [t (178) = .08, $p > .05$] or for seven of the competencies (Table 5). However, men were rated significantly higher than women on the competencies analyze information [t (166) = -2.21, $p > .05$] and strategic thinking [t (111) = -3.38, $p > .05$].

Table 5: Test of rating differences in competencies not included in hypothesis 1 or 2

Competency dimension	N		M(SD)		t-test		
	Men	Women	Men	Women	t	df	sig. (2-tailed)
Analyze issues	58	110	2.98 (.49)	2.81 (.50)	-2.21	166	.03
Think strategically	42	71	3.24 (.56)	2.88 (.54)	-3.38	111	.001
Visionary thinking	47	81	3.00 (.68)	2.93 (.64)	-.62	126	.54
Global Awareness	43	64	2.87 (.62)	2.88 (.59)	.09	105	.93
Establish plans	54	104	2.68 (.58)	2.62 (.49)	-.69	156	.49
Champion change	46	71	2.97 (.57)	2.82 (.67)	-1.20	115	.24
Influence others	56	109	2.72 (.55)	2.74 (.47)	.19	163	.85
Drive & commitment	43	66	3.14 (.65)	3.35 (.65)	1.64	107	.10

Figure 1: Men's and women's assessment center ratings

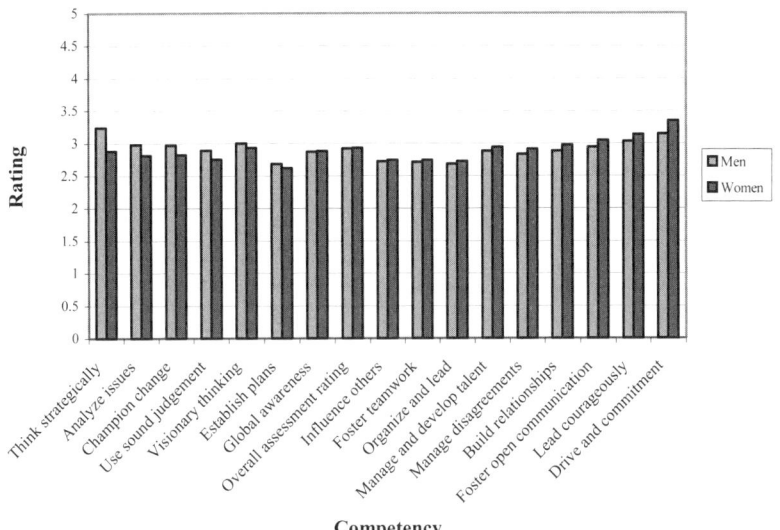

Discussion

The results suggest that there are few significant differences between men's and women's ratings examined at the competency level. Significant differences were identified in three of the 17 competencies included in the study: sound judgment, analyze information, and strategic thinking. Men were rated higher than women in all cases where significant differences were found. Only sound judgment was an a priori expected difference, whereas no significant differences were expected for analyze information and strategic thinking. Consistent with previous research and study hypothesis there were no significant differences in overall effectiveness, operationalized as OAR, between men and women. These findings indicate that although women and men do not appear to differ in terms of their overall effectiveness as leaders, men tend to receive higher ratings in the aspects of leadership related to 'thinking' skills. Upon closer examination of the data, men were found to perform significantly better than women on the two cognitive tests used in the Assessment Center [Raven: t (178) = -2.38, $p < .05$; Watson-Glaser: t (178) = -3.22, $p < .05$], suggesting that the assessees' cognitive capacity influenced their results on thinking related competencies but not others, such as interpersonal competencies.

Five of the competencies were judged to correspond closely enough to the interpersonal/democratic to warrant expectations that women would be rated higher than men based on Eagly and Johnson's (1990) findings (see hypothesis 1). This hypothesis is not supported, as there were no significant differences between men and women on the identified competencies. The results were in the expected direction, but the differences were too small to reach statistical significance. Given the size of the differences it is unlikely that these differences are of practical significance. These results are perhaps not surprising given the sample and previous findings. As mentioned previously, even when differences have been found those differences have been small (Eagly & Johnson, 1990). Furthermore, Gibson found that Scandinavians, both men and women, tend to have a more interpersonal orientation in their leadership further attenuating the any differences between genders.

Of the 17 dimensions included in the study, three were judged to correspond to Eagly's task/autocratic leadership style (see hypothesis 2), and men were hypothesized to be rated higher than women on these dimensions. Hypothesis 2 was partially supported. Men were rated higher than women on sound judgment, but not on manage execution or lead courageously where women were rated higher, though not significantly, than men. The results in the opposite direction to hypotheses are interesting given previous findings. One explanation may be that the present study used a sample from the health care industry, which was not the case in previous studies. The sample also included more women than men, which possibly may have caused differences in perspectives of women acting in male stereotyped ways.

Men were also rated higher than women on analyzing information and strategic thinking. These competencies were judged to be gender neutral, and there were no clear indicators in previous research to suggest that gender differences would emerge on these competencies. These findings could be partially be explained by the fairly large difference between men and women on the cognitive tests included in the Assessment Center; when the results from only the simulations are considered, the differences between genders on these competencies disappear. These findings are interesting within the broader context of the influence of cognitive ability on Assessment Center results. The correlation between the cognitive test scores and OAR and individual competencies are consistently low in the present study providing counter evidence to the theory that Assessment Centers are an advanced proxy for cognitive abilities tests.

Ratings on the overall measure of effectiveness, OAR, are very similar for men and women. This is interesting given that the OAR is the figure most commonly used for making recommendations for selection decisions. Furthermore, although men are rated more highly on some competencies and components in the Assessment Center, the overall effectiveness of men and women appears to be similar. Although rater biases cannot be completely ruled out, the findings suggest that the prima facia case for discrimination, difference in ratings, does not exist. However, the most central concept in assessing rater bias is that individuals with the same true score receive the same observed score. We can say little of this in the present study. It is possible, yet unlikely, that one gender's true score is higher than the other gender, but that systematic errors in ratings compensate to make the observed scores similar.

Some researchers contend that rater bias is difficult to assess accurately, but situations where rater bias is more likely have been identified. Some factors that tend to be associated with higher ratings for men include a high proportion of male raters, a high proportion of male assesses, when a male stereotypic leaderships style was the norm, and military context. In the present study, none of these conditions existed, which reduces the likelihood of systematic differences in ratings due to structural issues and that observed differences are likely a reflection of differences in true scores. However, other types of systematic rater issues cannot be ruled out.

In the present study assesses from Assessment Centers conducted for development and selection purposes were included. To the extent that the purpose of the Assessment Center influences the performance of assesses, the results of the present study may also have been influenced. Lastly, as multiple t-tests were conducted, there is a possibility that significant results were produced by chance.

The results of the present study do not describe on the job performance, but only how men and women are rated during an Assessment Center. As Eagly, Makhijani and Klonsky (1992) point out, it is possible that the assesses' behavior in the assessment situation, where they do not have already established relationships with others, may be different from their behavior on the job. Eagly, Makhijani and Klonsky (1992) argue that differences between genders are likely smaller on the job than in contained, experimental, situations because a person's gender becomes a less important behavioral cue on the job.' They argue that the leadership role becomes super ordinate the gender role in real life, and that this will serve to reduce the influence of gender on the person's behavior. This would suggest that the differences between genders are actually smaller in the assessees' everyday working situation in the Swedish health care profession.

The present study has several characteristics that need to be considered in generalizing the results. First, the study includes managers from the health care industry, and to the extent that leadership is different in other industries the generalizability may be limited. Second, the sample included more women managers than male manager. Although this is representative of the population the sample was drawn from, this is not consistent with the samples of previous research where men have tended to be in the majority (Landstingsförbundet, 2002). Eagly and Johnson (1992) found that the ratio of male to female participants may influence the results, but there have been relatively few studies conducted in settings where women are clearly in the majority to draw firm conclusions as to how this affects the results. Thirdly, the present study used chief nurses and chiefs of staff as the target roles. As the competencies required differ for different organizational levels, these results may not be generalizable to other organizational levels. Fourth, the study was based on a Swedish sample. Gibson (1995) identified some differences in leadership styles among countries, and the results of the present study may be limited to Sweden to the extent to which the dynamics causing the observed results are bound within Swedish culture.

One of the strengths of the present study is that it is based on real Assessment Center data that was used in real life. This provides a good indication of how gender differences appear in Assessment Center data. Walsh, Weinberg and Fairfield, (1987) found that Assessment Center ratings were different depending on the purpose of the Assessment Center. Thus, although many factors were not controlled in the present study, the results are likely representative of this type of Assessment Center. Future research could examine the effect of rater gender more closely, a factor that was not analyzed in the present study. Additionally, interaction effects between rater and assessee gender could help clarify the role of the rater in how Assessment Center participants are rated. Another area in need of further research is to look at differences between Assessment Centers for developmental or selection purposes, and how the purpose of the Assessment Center affects the ratings of different genders. Because Assessment Center research is scare in Sweden, addressing all areas of Assessment Centers within a Swedish context would be helpful to better understand how the application of Assessment Centers is affected by cultural differences.

References

Arthur, W. Jr., Woehr, D. J. & Maldegen, R. (2000). Convergent and discriminant validity of Assessment Center dimensions: A conceptual and empirical re-examination of the Assessment Center construct-related validity paradox. *Journal of Management, 26*, 813-835.

Borman, W. C. (1982). Validity of behavioural assessment for predicting military recruiter performance. *Journal of Applied Psychology, 67*, 3-9.

Bray, D. W. & Grant, D. L. (1966). The Assessment Center in the measurement of potential for business management. *Psychological Monographs: General and Applied, 80*, 1-27.

Bray, D. W. & Howard, A. (1983). *Personality and the Assessment Center method.* In C. D. Spielberger & J. N. Butcher (Eds.), Advances in Personality Assessment (Vol. 3), New York: Erlbaum Associates.

Byham, W. C. (1970). Assessment centers for spotting future managers. *Harvard business review, 48*, 150-167.

Chan, D. (1996). Criterion and construct validation of an assessment centre. *Journal of Organizational Psychology, 69*, 167-181.

Clark-Carter, D. (1998). *Doing quantitative research from design to report.* East Sussex: Psychology Press.

Dayan, K., Kasten, R. & Fox, S. (2002). Entry-level police candidate Assessment Center: An efficient tool or a hammer to kill a fly? *Personnel Psychology, 55*, 827-847.

Eagly, A. H. & Johnson, B. T. (1990). Gender and leadership style: A meta-analysis. *Psychological Bulletin, 108*, 233-256.

Eagly, A. H., Karau, S. J. & Makhijani, M. G. (1995). Gender and the effectiveness of leaders: A meta-analysis. *Psychological Bulletin, 117*, 125-145.

Eagly, A. H., Makhijani, M. G. & Klonsky, B. G. (1992). Gender and the evaluation of leaders: A meta-analysis. *Psychological Bulletin, 111*, 3-22.

Gaugler, B. B. & Thornton III, G. C. (1989). Number of Assessment Center dimensions as a determinant of assessor accuracy. *Journal of Applied Psychology,74*, 611-618.

Gaugler, B. B., Rosenthal, D. B., Thornton III, G. C. & Bentson, C. (1987). Meta-analysis of Assessment Center validity. *Journal of Applied Psychology Monograph, 72*, 493-511.

Gibson, C. B. (1995). An investigation of gender differences in leadership across 4 countries. *Journal of International Business Studies, 26*, 255-279.

International task force for Assessment Center guidelines (2000). *Guidelines and Ethical Considerations for Assessment Center Operations.* A report endorsed by the 28th International Congress on Assessment Center Methods, May 4, 2000, San Fransisco, California, USA, Development Dimensions International, Bridgeville, PA.

Jones, R. G. (1992). Construct validation of Assessment Center final dimension ratings: definition and measurement issues. *Human Resource Management Review, 2*, 195-220.

Landstingsförbundet (2002). Fakta om kvinnor och män i landstingen 2001. Fil nedladdad från internet: *http://www.lf.se/ag/jamstalldhet/lasvart.htm* 2003-06-19.

Mabon, H. (2002). *Arbetspsykologisk testning. Om urvalsmetoder i arbetslivet.* Stockholm: Psykologiförlaget AB.

Russell, C. J. (1985). Individual decision process in an Assessment Center. *Journal of Applied Psychology, 70*, 737-746.

Schleicher, D.J., Mayes, B. T., Day, D. V. & Riggio, R. E. (2002). A new frame for frame-of-reference training: enhancing the construct validity of Assessment Centers. *Journal of Applied Psychology, 87*, 735-746.

Schmidt, F. L. & Hunter, J. E. (1998). The validity and utility of selection methods in personnel psychology: practical and theoretical implications of 85 years of research findings. *Psychological Bulletin, 124*, 262-274.

Schneider, J. R. & Schmitt, N. (1992). An exercise design approach to understanding Assessment Center dimension and exercise constructs. *Journal of Applied Psychology, 77,* 32-41.

Shore, T. H. (1992). Subtle gender bias in the assessment of managerial potential. *Sex-Roles, 27,* 499-515.

Shore, T. H., Tashchian, A. & Adams, J. S. (1997). The role of gender in a developmental Assessment Center. *Journal of Social Behavior and Personality, 12,* 191-203.

Thompson, M. D. (2000). Gender, leadership orientation, and effectiveness: testing the theoretical models of Bolman & Deal and Quinn. *Sex Roles, 42,* 969-992.

Walsh, J., Weinberg, R. M. & Fairfield, M. L. (1987). The effects of gender on assessment centre evaluations. *Journal of Occupational Psychology, 60,* 305-309.

Woehr, D. J. & Arthur, W. Jr. (2003). The construct-related validity of Assessment Center ratings: A review and meta-analysis of the role of methodological factors. *Journal of Management, 29,* 231-258.

Zaar, C. & Tillman, P. (2003). Assessment center. För bättre ledarskap och mer framgångsrika organisatione. Stockholm: Ekerlids.

Designing a Hungarian worksite health promotion program: needs and purposes

Ágnes Juhász*

Department of Ergonomics ad Psychology, Budapest University of Technology and Economics, Hungary

The current paper presents the design, purposes and the first results of a complex, Hungarian worksite health promotion program.

"Health promotion is any event, process or activity which facilitates the protection or improvement of the health status of individuals, groups, communities or populations." (Marks, Murray, Evans & Willig, 2000, p. 325). Health promotion is the process of enabling people to increase control over and to improve their own health, in contrast to traditional medical services (The Ottawa Charter, 1986). Health promotion can be a successful method of promoting the health status and life quality of individuals, groups, communities. Health promotion makes people able to take care of their own health (Marks, Murray, Evans & Willig, 2000). To achieve its aim of preventing the occurrence of illnesses, reaching a better general life quality, health promotion can use as diverse methods as financial regulations, laws, education, promotion of communal life, organizational changes, etc. (The Ottawa Charter, 1986). Workplaces quickly became an outstanding venue for health promotion programs for several reasons (Pencak, 1991): Firstly, at the workplace the target population is easily available as we spend most of our wakeful hours at our worksite. It is especially those who work who take advantage of the traditional health services less often, while they are at the highest risk of several chronic illnesses. They thus form an important target population for preventive interventions. Last but not least, work and the workplace itself can affect the health of the employees both in positive and in negative way.

Workplace health promotion programs originated in the U.S., where company managements wanted to reduce high medical costs by offering health promotion programs to its employees since the mid-1970s. Soon workplace health promotion programs became popular in Western European countries also, as company managements recognized its efficiency in cutting costs by preventing employees from becoming ill. Besides illness prevention, workplace health promotion programs have other beneficial effects, all contributing to the increase of the company's success (improvement in the company's image,

---

* *Correspondence: Ágnes Juhász, juhasza@erg.bme.hu*

increase in productivity, decrease in the costs of employees absenteeism, improvement of workplace climate, workers attitudes toward the organization (Pencak, 1991; Sanders & Crowe, 1996). The number of such programs is continuously increasing in the U.S. and in Western Europe. In 1992 eighty-one percent of workplaces in the U.S. offered at least one health promotion program (Stokols, Pelletier & Fielding, 1995), in the United Kingdom in 1996 69% of the big companies and 40% of the small ones offered such programs (Sanders & Crowe, 1996).

Applying worksite health promotion as a practice and an approach has not become common in Hungary to date. Yet there is urgent need for this given the catastrophic public health indexes: life expectancy at birth for males in Hungary was 68.3 years in 2002, the same indicator in Sweden was almost ten years higher (77.5). Life expectancy in Europe is only lower in the post Soviet countries and in Romania (WHO, 2003). Health behaviour indicators are not better: 44% of adult men and 23% of adult women smoke in Hungary. The yearly pure alcohol consumption per capita is 9.9 liters. The number of alcoholics is around 860,000. The actual lifestyle of the Hungarians is not suitable for preserving and promoting health (Barabás, 1997). The main potential reasons for these dire indicators could reside in the recent radical political and – even more important – social changes and their consequences, such as lower standard of living, the bad conditions in health policy, the communal and moral crisis and overwork, which is very common (Makara, 1994).

Money is one of the commonly cited reasons for the absence of workplace health promotion programs in Hungary. However, correctly managed and introduced worksite health promotion programs can also be cost effective as well as through their positive effects on worker health, satisfaction, commitment, etc. A more important reason for company leaders not introducing worksite health promotion programs in Hungary could be the absence of well controlled, successful research carried out in local companies, which could serve as evidence and argument for and in support of the effectiveness of such programs. The current research would like to fill this gap by carrying out a two-year longitudinal controlled research on worksite health promotion in a Hungarian company. (This research was launched within the frameworks of an extensive Hungarian research project on the helper role models funded by the National Research and Innovation Foundation (Ministry of Education)).

The aim of this particular health promotion program is to increase the health status of the employees of a department in a telecommunication company. The longitudinal research is studying whether this purpose is effected, by comparing the physical and psychological health status, well-being, health behaviour of the employees at the starting point with those at the end of the two-year program, and also by comparing these variables with the ones measured in the control group. The research would like to compare the efficiency of the two most important approaches of worksite health promotion, namely the individual and the organizational-focused ones. The aim of the *individual focused intervention* is to help employees achieve a better health by offering skill training, health educational programs, thus improving their coping potential against workplace stress. This approach became widely used in several companies, because it is cheap and easily manageable. However its efficiency is quite low, as people do not change their lifestyle easily. The other approach, the *organization-focused intervention* lays the emphasis on the workplace, on the organization, not on the individual. The aim here is to decrease workplace demands, thus preventing the employees from becoming ill. In order to achieve this aim, this approach carries out organizational, environmental changes, which makes it more expensive, more difficult to manage and to control the results than with the individual-focused intervention. In compensation for the higher cost, the efficiency of the organization-focused programs is higher. Yet because of the above mentioned difficulties, this intervention is much less wide-spread (Mercier & Francois, 2001).

The design of the current research makes it possible to compare the efficiency of the individual-focused intervention (in the control group) with the individual + organization-focused intervention (in the experimental group).

The current paper presents in detail the results of the initial analysis carried out in the experimental group, the health problems, the needs of the employees identified by this analysis, and the purposes of the intervention tailored to the identified needs, problems.

Method

Sample

In the study we used the data of two organizational units of a telecommunication company in two different sites doing the same work. The two sites served as the experimental and the control group for the study. In the current paper we present the data of one of the sites, of 174 employees. The following *demographic variables* of the subjects were investigated: gender, age, profession, educational level, employment (manager or subordinate). 86% of the subjects were female, the mean age was 33 years (20-56 years). 87% had secondary education, 12% had higher education. Only 8% of the subjects work in managerial position. According to their marital status: 47% of the subjects live alone, 13% are divorced, 40% are married.

According to the observations (work analysis), the *main characteristics of the jobs* performed at the investigated organizational unit are: People are employees of a call centre, thus most of them are in almost continuous contact with clients. All of the subjects work with computers, facing the strains coming from computer-based work. Call centre employees have to be familiar with the continuously changing current campaigns of the telecommunication company, as providing information is one of their main tasks, which puts them under high mental load. They have to carry out their tasks under a very high time pressure because of their performance assessment, which is also based on mental tasks, politeness with the customer, achieving marketing goals. This work can be characterized in the Karasek terminology (Karasek & Theorell, 1990) as a high strain job with low control, low autonomy and high demand. Workers receive low esteem from management both in a financial and moral sense. The company, and the unit in particular, goes through frequent reorganizations, which highly influence the level of in-team social support. The employees all work in an open plan office, with all the physical and psychological demands originating from this fact. A large part of the employees work in two or three shifts.

Measures

In the study we used three different measures to investigate the health status, health behaviour, workplace stress, coping style, organizational commitment and satisfaction of the employees, namely: questionnaires, interviews and observations.

A 70-item questionnaire was created to investigate the following variables: attribution to stress and health, subjective health status, health behaviour, lifestyle, stress, work stress, well-being, job satisfaction and commitment. Items investigating stress and health attribution were formulated by using the results of a content analysis carried out on the answers given to open-ended questions in a former, preliminary research (Juhász, 2003). Health behaviours, lifestyle, subjective health status were investigated by open- and closed ended questions. Work stress was assessed by a 26-item scale enumerating the most important workplace stressors identified by job stress research. Subjects had to indicate on two 6-point scales whether the stressors were present at their workplace, and what amount of stress did they cause them (where on the scale one meant: it never occurs and it doesn't cause any stress, and six meant: it occurs almost always and causes very high level of stress). According to the analysis, the reliability of the job stress scale was satisfying (Cronbach's α was 0.86, corrected item-total correlations were between 0.3 and 0.76). Job satisfaction and commitment were investigated by closed-ended questions. Job satisfaction scale was consisted of five items. The reliability of the scale was satisfying (Cronbach's α = 0.82, corrected item-total correlations were between 0.49 and 0.73). Organizational commitment was measured by an 8-item scale, with a good reliability (Cronbach's $\alpha = 0.73$).

In order to obtain more in depth, more qualitative data besides the quantitative data from the questionnaire, we asked volunteers to take part in 30 minute interviews about job stress and coping. Forty-three employees took part in the interviews. The results of the interviews are not presented in this paper.

Besides the above mentioned two measures, four hour structured observations were also carried out on twenty volunteers in order to have more detailed and objective information on the job tasks, stressors, individual and collective coping style of the employees. The results of the observations are not presented in this paper.

Procedure

An oral briefing was held in small groups about the study, the aims and the methods before the investigation has started. Questionnaires were completed electronically (Intranet) during working hours. Observations and interviews were also carried out during working hours at the workplace.

The current paper presents the results of the primary (before intervention) survey on the subjective health status, lifestyle, health behaviour, work stressors, organizational commitment and satisfaction of the employees in the experimental group. The aim of this survey and analysis is to identify the most important health, lifestyle problems, the most important demands, organizational problems of the subjects, on which future health promotion interventions (individual and organization-focused) should concentrate. In the following part of the paper we will present only the results that are the most interesting and important for the future intervention program, and in the last chapter we will discuss the potential intervention methods aimed at the identified problems.

As the purpose of this analysis is to present the descriptive data of the investigated sample, no specific hypotheses were formed. The presented results are mainly based on investigation of frequencies, central tendencies, dispersion of the answers.

The statistical analysis was made by the program SPSS 11.0.

Results

Subjective health status of the sample

As the main aim of health promotion programs is to promote the health of the employees, an experimental study has to evaluate the subjects' health status before and after intervention. We used subjects' self-reports in order to have data more on subjective than on objective health status.

According to the answers given to the questionnaire 25% of the subjects have an illness currently under medical treatment. 14% have been inpatients during the last year. The majority of the subjects (55%) visited their doctor once or twice last year. The most common reasons for seeing the doctors were: because of a specific symptom or complaint (47%), and for medical check-up (29%).

The questionnaire also listed the 18 most common symptoms related to psychological stress, and subjects had to mark those they regularly have. The sample reported to have 3.5 symptoms in average (SD: 2.3). The most frequently mentioned symptoms were: fatigue, frequent headache and depression. Fatigue could be connected to shift work.

Table 1 presents the frequencies of the *symptoms* in the sample in percentages of the subjects reporting a particular symptom. (As one subject could report several symptoms, the sum of the percentages exceeds 100).

Table 1: Symptoms of the subjects

Symptom	Frequency
Frequent cold	18.7%
Frequent headache	35.1%
Allergy	25.2%
Fatigue	58.9%
Stomach problems	20.7%
Constipation	13.8%
Joint pain	20.7%
Limb pain	14.9%
Dizziness	14.4%
Depression	25.9%
Anxiety	14.9%

Subjects evaluated their general and current health status by giving answers to questions like: "How often do you consider yourself to be in good health?", and "How would you describe your present health status?". 9% of the subjects always, 64% mostly, 24% often and three percent rarely consider themselves healthy. 6% of the subjects described their present health status to be bad, 40% described it to be medium, 47% good and 6% excellent. These results show that most of the subjects are in medium or good health.

Well-being of the subjects was measured by a four-item questionnaire, with a 4-point minimum and 16-point maximum total. Mean point at the scale was 10.31 (standard deviation: 1.76). According to this, the sample's average well-being is closest to the medium anchor of the scale.

Health behaviour

As individual-focused health promotion programs concentrate mainly on lifestyle changes, it was necessary to investigate the sample's health behaviours at the starting point of the research. All data on health behaviour is based on self-reports.

As many of the subjects work in shifts, not getting enough *sleep* can be an important health risk. As it appears in the data: the average in sleeping hours on working days is slightly less than the ideal (6.97 hours), on days off it is 8.63 hours.

Forty-four percent of the sample *smoke*, which is much worse than the incidence in the population, especially because in this sample the majority of the subjects were female. (The incidence of smoking in the Hungarian female population is 23%, WHO, 2004).

Alcohol consumption does not seem to be an important problem for the sample: most of the subjects (59.9%) consume alcoholic drinks only a few times a year, 14.8% drink monthly, also 14.8% weekly. Compared with the data for the general Hungarian female population, we can establish that in the investigated sample the ratio of teetotallers (10.7%) and heavy drinkers (0.7%) is also lower.

Sedentary lifestyle is a common problem in white-collar jobs. In the current sample only 24.3% of the subjects engage regularly in physical exercise (several times a week or daily). One fourth never exercise, and 50.7% only do exercise occasionally. These ratios are similar to the general ones for Hungary (Kopp & Skrabski, 1995).

Attributions for health quality

Investigating common sense views about health, and the attributions given for good health quality can be important in planning health promotion interventions, health education campaigns, as it is practical to know the participants' preliminary theories, notions, beliefs, in order to be able to connect or contrast them to the new information given by the program.

Table 2 presents the attributions subjects had for health quality: subjects had to divide 100 points between the answer categories given to the question *„What can be good health status attributed to in your opinion?"*

Table 2: Attribution of health

Attribution	Average answers
Lifestyle	36.58
Relationships	24.84
Harmony	19.58
External factors	9.85
Work	20.84
Money	10.72

According to the results, work itself can have a significant role in health promotion. A Further task of the research should be to investigate which particular characteristics of work are health promoting, and which are health damaging.

Work stress

Stress is one of the major health risks in our modern society. It also constitutes the focus point of many of the workplace health promotion programs, especially the organization-focused ones, so it is important to investigate the quantity of the stress subjects are currently experiencing, and the main work-related stressors.

The frequency of answers the subjects gave to question: *"How stressful is your work?"* is as follows: 5% of the subjects found their work to be not at all, 20% somewhat, 45% moderately, 18% very much and 2% extremely stressful.

Occupational stress was also investigated by a 26-item questionnaire. Average experienced work stress on the job stress questionnaire was 62.49 (standard deviation: 24.47), where the possible minimum points would be 26, the possible maximum 156.

The *most common stress factors* for the sample were: low salary, little remuneration, unfavourable physical conditions at the workplace, no opportunity for promotion.

The *most important stressors* for the sample were: low salary, little remuneration, too much work, not enough time for completing the tasks, and unfavourable physical conditions at the workplace.

More than *forty-four percent* of the sample thinks that many or most of the potential stress factors listed in the questionnaire affect their health in a negative way often, or most of the time.

Non-work factors also have an important role in increasing the general stress level experienced by the subjects. Highest stress apart from work is caused by financial problems (average: 3.72 on a 6-point scale).

Subjects had to evaluate their general stress level on a 5-point scale. The frequency of answers is as follows: 4% found their general stress level to be very low, 15% low, 53% medium, 25% high and 2% extremely high.

Work seems to have a more important role in experienced stress than family. Dividing 100% between the stress inducing potential of work and that of the family, subjects gave 60% to work and 41% to the family in average.

Organizational satisfaction and commitment

As workplace health promotion programs can have beneficial side effects like increase in job satisfaction and organizational commitment, it is important to investigate these variables at the starting point as well.

Job satisfaction was measured on a 5-point scale by a 5-item questionnaire. The maximum total point is: 25. The average of the sample on this scale was: 16.3 (standard deviation: 3.19). It seems that the sample is only a little bit more satisfied than the medium anchor of the scale.

Organizational commitment was measured by an 8-item questionnaire on a 5-point scale. The maximum total points was 40. The average total point in the sample was 26.65 (standard deviation 5.83). The average commitment is slightly higher than medium anchor of the scale.

Determinants of health status

Correlation statistical analysis has been carried out to investigate what are the possible determinants of health status, by identifying the correlates of subjective health in order to have deeper insight in the phenomena, and to prepare future interventions.

Stress seems to be an important variable in this sense as there was significant negative correlation between the general health state and *the experienced stress-level* ($r = -0.34**$), and between the actual health state and the experienced stress level ($r = -0.39**$)

Number of symptoms and work stress ($r = 0.26**$), and the number of symptoms and the experienced stress level ($r = 0.38**$) were also correlated with each other.

Health attribution was also connected to the subjective health status: there was significant difference in attributing health to work between those having a treated illness, and those not having such. Those who do not have an illness attribute heath more to work, than those who have illnesses ($t = -2.69$, $p<0.05$).

However because of the nature of correlation, no conclusion on causal relationships can be made.

Discussion

According to this investigation the *subjective health status* of the majority of the sample is acceptable, although 9% were currently in bad health, and 25% had an illness currently under medical treatment. They could form the principal target group for health promotion interventions. Analysis of the symptoms revealed that symptoms related to depression, depressive mood are the most common in the sample. This result can help shape the course of future health promotion interventions.

The *lifestyle* of the sample is worse with regard to its effects on health by several points than the national Hungarian average (which is already poor, see above). The ratio of smokers is especially high.

Twenty percent of the investigated employees are experiencing very high or extremely high *work stress,* underlining the importance of workplace health promotion interventions. Investigating the most important job stressors can help in the design of the organizational-focused interventions. The importance of stress as a target of future interventions can also be highlighted by the correlations between stress and subjective health status.

The practical importance of this study lies in focusing our attention on the principal problems in the workplace environment, work organization and the employees' lifestyle, which may be connected to current or future physical and mental health problems of the workforce. This therefore enables the formulation of a preventive intervention program fitted to the target population's needs. The secondary – but just as important – practical returns of the study were bringing the issue of health, workplace stress, healthy lifestyle, and healthy work environment to the consciousness of both the management and the workforce. Positive effects of this awareness have already been noticed in some of the latest measures of the management (e.g., competing for a prize for purchasing sports implements).

However we must take into account some possible limitations of the study resulting from the research methodology. One possible limitation could be the problem of plain responding to the questionnaire. Given the frequent reorganisations and cutting down at the investigated organisation, employees might have been afraid of sincerely reporting their workplace stressors and complaints, notwithstanding that they filled out the questionnaires anonymously with self-chosen identification numbers. The interviews contradicted this supposition: employees were happy to talk about their problems, and saw this research as a sign of the organisation's improving employee care. Yet a limitation of the study can be that the health status and the lifestyle of the sample were only investigated by self-report, thus giving way to possible subjective distortions.

Next study steps - future intervention

Next study steps will be the analysis of the data of the control group, and after the final data analysis to create and to introduce preventive health promotion programs – treating health and lifestyle problems identified by the primary investigation – to the two groups: individual-focused programs to the control group and individual and organisational focused programs to the experimental group. Short-term effects of the program will be evaluated by comparing the results of the primary investigation with the final investigation, and by comparing the data of the experimental group with the control group.

Individual focused intervention

The aim of this intervention is to promote healthy lifestyle among the employees. The actual programs will be developed after the final evaluation of the primary investigation. Health and lifestyle problems discovered so far are smoking, sedentary lifestyle, not enough rest (fatigability) and depression.

Programs addressing these and other, to be identified problems will be established (e.g., relaxation training, exercise at the workplace, health education on smoking, psychological counselling).

Organizational focused intervention

The aim of organizational focused intervention is to decrease or eliminate the potentially harmful workplace demands thus preventing health problems. Work and workplace problems identified so far are: time pressure, low esteem of the employees' work, unfavourable physical conditions at the workplace, no adequate performance appraisal, no support for social relationships at the workplace and low autonomy at work.

Further work problems affecting health, and their appropriate interventions will be identified by health-promotion focus groups formed by employees.

Conclusion

The paper presented the concept and the first data of a two-year workplace health promotion program. The published data gave an insight into the current health status, actual lifestyle and workplace circumstances of the experimental group. The identified (and to be completed) problems will serve as the basis for designing a complex workplace health promotion program. Analysis of the internal correlations between the indicators can help in understanding the causes of the actual problems and symptoms, thus enabling future interventions to be more appropriate and effective.

References

Barabás, K. (1997) A nemzet egészsége a nemzet legfőbb kincse. [Health of the nation is the most important treasure of the nation]. In Z. Benkő (Ed.), *„Mert életem millió gyökerű"*. *Egészségfejlesztés-Mentálhigiéne. ["Because my life has million roots". Health promotion – Mental health promotion]*. Szeged: JGYTF Kiadó.

Juhász Á. (2003). *Common sense views about stress and health – indications for health promotion.* Poster presented at the XIth European Congress on Work and Organizational Psychology, 14-17 May, Lisbon, Portugal.

Karasek, R. & Theorell, T. (1990). *Healthy Work. Stress, Productivity, and the Reconstruction of Working Life.* Basic Books, HarperCollinsPublishers.

Kopp, M. & Skrabski, Á. (1995). *Magyar lelkiállapot. [Hungarian mood]. Budapest:* Végeken Kiadó.

Makara, P. (1994) Egészségvédelem Magyarországon: A kihívás természete. [Health protection in Hungary: the nature of the challenge]. In Z. Benkő (Ed.), *Az egészségneveléstől az egészségfejlesztésig. [From health education to health promotion]*. Szeged: JGYTF Kiadó.

Marks, D.F., Murray, M., Evans, B. & Willig, C. (2000). Health psychology. *Health promotion, 15,* 325-346

Mercier, M. & Francois, M. (2001). *Approche psychoergonomique du stress au travail. 3. Prévention/gestion du stress: analyse bibliographique.* Les notes scientifiques et techniques de l'INRS. Publication réalisée dans le cadre du projet INRS 'Stress au travail'. Institut National de Recherche et de Securite. Janvier, 2001.

The Ottawa Charter (1986). In L. Barić (Ed.), *Health promotion and health education in practice (module 2). The organisational model.* Forwarded by I. Kickbusch, WHO EURO Barns Publications, 1994.

Pencak, M. (1991). Workplace health promotion programs. An overview. *Nursing Clinics of North America, 26*(1), 233-240.

Sanders, D. & Crowe, S. (1996). Overview of health promotion in the workplace. In A. Scriven & J. Orme (Eds.), *Health Promotion. Professional Perspectives* (pp. 199-211). London: Macmillan Press Ltd.

Stokols, D., Pelletier, K. R. & Fielding, J. E. (1995). Integration of Medical Care and Worksite Health Promotion. *JAMA, 273*(14), 1136-1142.

WHO (2004). European Health for All Database. http://hfadb.who.dk/hfa

Managers' subjective role projects during the initial phase of an organizational change process

Monica Nyström[*]
Medical Management Centre, Karolinska Institute, Sweden
Work and Organisational Psychology Unit, Umeå University, Sweden

Health care organisations exist in dynamic and complex economic, technological, and political contexts and are under pressure to continuously adapt to new needs and demands. The managerial role is especially important as an 'organisational tool' to ensure successful organisational adaptation to changes and smooth implementation of change interventions. Lower-level managers serve as integrating organisational mechanisms, but they can also behave in ways that are damaging to the organisational system. Thus, it is important to be able to understand and predict the behaviour of individual managers during change periods.

Managers often experience organisational change as difficult and stressful as it puts pressure on their roles. Organisational role theory (Kahn, Wolfe, Quinn, Snoek & Rosenthal, 1964; Katz & Kahn, 1978) describes an interpersonal role process where role behaviour is seen as an effect of external (organisational) and interpersonal pressures. The role process is influenced by the personal attributes of the actors involved and the nature of their relations. The manager is both a role sender and a receiver and the way individual managers perceive and make sense of other actor's expectations on the role is assumed to influence their role behaviour. Discrepancies in expectations of the role can be sources of role stress. Role conflict, role ambiguity, and role overload are concepts that are of particular interest during dynamic periods when the role is put under pressure.

Role conflict exists when one role expectation makes the fulfilment of another role expectation difficult or impossible, including the focal person's own expectations. Role ambiguity is defined as the "absence of adequate information required for satisfactory accomplishment of one's role" (Kahn et. al., 1964, p. 103). Two major types of role ambiguity have been defined. 'Task ambiguity', caused by lack of information concerning the proper definition of the job, its goals, and permissible means for implementing them has been further divided into ambiguity regarding the scope of responsibilities, the role behaviours necessary to fulfil one's responsibilities, and whose ex-

[*] *Correspondence: Monica Nyström, monica.nystrom@lime.ki.se*

pectations for role behaviour that must be met. The second type of role ambiguity is related to the socio-emotional aspect of the role, that is, ambiguity regarding the consequences of role behaviour. Present and future ambiguity represents a time dimension, where future ambiguity has been connected to most negative effects for role incumbents (French & Caplan, 1973; Kahn, 1980; Kahn & Byosiere, 1992). Role overload occurs when the total demands and expectations on the focal person overpower the capacity of the individual (Kahn, 1980). This overload can be qualitative, when the person does not have the qualities or competence that is required, or quantitative, when time stress and high workload coincide. Thus, an organisational change period might involve higher role ambiguity, new role conflicts, and temporary or long-term role overload for managers. It could also involve more or less role negotiation (Graen & Scandura, 1987) and social re-construction of the role.

Role theory has been criticized for not distinguishing clearly between objective and subjective variables (French & Caplan, 1973), and role conflict, role ambiguity and role overload are concepts that have subjective components. Subjective data can provide more specific information on the managers' cognitive models of role content and role context in relation to these concepts. Even though there is an assumed connection between cognition and action, the manager's process of cognitive sense-making of the role context and of changes in role expectations during dynamic periods has not been studied extensively.

Hosking and Morley (1991) use the term 'project' in their model of 'skilful organizing processes'. This term can be used for the description of managers' subjective roles. When managers describe their role important, work-related projects should emerge. A 'project' is defined as "more or less social, cognitive, and political processes in which actors attempt to construct changes in ways that will 'add value' to their lives" (Hosking & Morley, 1991, p 227). Thus, a role project is formed partly by the individuals, by the context and by the specific situation, and the processes that evolve among these elements. To capture some of the dynamic features of this process a time perspective is important. When managers describe their role situation they are assumed to refer to the past, present and future, a kind of emergent role history that affects their present and future sense-making and role construction. In role terms this will also contain their reflections on their own behaviour in relation to role content and context.

The purpose of the present study was to describe managers' subjective role projects and strategies during initial organisational change phases, leading to a more detailed description and understanding of the subjective side of the managerial role. Managers from five day-care units undergoing organizational changes participated in the study. Changes can provide both opportunities and threats and affect or initiate a project. Past and present projects are assumed to form a manager's subjective role through processes of reflection and construction. Thus, a subjective role is formed and re-constructed retrospectively by present and past projects, which in turn serve to form a dynamic opinion about oneself and the kind of role projects one gets involved in.

Four basic categories, also consistent with organisational role theory, were chosen to describe managers' subjective role projects: *'purposes/goals'*, *'action/action strategies'*, *'situations/events'* and *'actors'*. Goals are seen as emergent and retrospective constructions where the managers are assumed to reflect and construct models that can explain their own and other people's behaviour. Constructed goals can be used as a framework for future reflections. Purposes/goals are also related to role behaviour as the intentions of a role sender to send certain expectations and of a role incumbent to behave in certain ways. Situations/events represent contextual information. Actions and action strategies are related to intended or described role behaviour. Role senders and receivers represent the actors in different situations. These categories formed the basis for a description of subjective role projects, together with cognitive processes of reflection and construction (Figure 1).

Figure 1: Hypothetical model of basic categories in a subjective role project

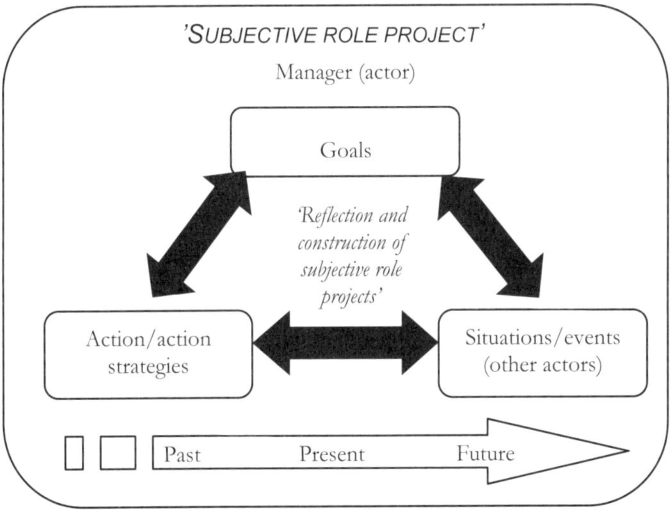

The research questions concerned finding potential indications of role projects, possibly according to the hypothetical project structure, and finding out if the variation between managers could be described. In order to capture the qualitative aspects of the role projects a special judgement technique was used for the analyses. Three judges familiar with bottom-up analyses made qualified judgements of the material, allowing for several interpretative perspectives.

Method

Participants

Five managers of day-care centres, two male (B, D) and three females (A, C, E), working in a middle size Swedish municipality participated in the study. The managers were responsible for units ranging from five to six wards, each with a staff of 3-4 persons and 15-18 children. The total number of subordinates varied from 22 to 32. All managers had 15-20 years experience working in childcare, and 7-17 years of experience working in a supervisory role. During the 1990's the government which finances childcare required cutbacks and restructuring because of an economic downturn. This resulted in organisational changes that increased the managerial responsibility to several geographically separated units, reduced the staff, and increased the number of younger children at the units. Thus, at the time of the study the managers' scope of responsibility increased to incorporate more units, staff, and children.

Empirical material

The empirical material consisted of transcribed, open interviews of 1-1½ hours with five childcare managers concerning their work situation, 4-6 weeks before the organisational changes were implemented. The managers were instructed to describe their work role and situation in general, and then specifically asked to describe the aspects of their work situation that presently were most important to them. The interviewer had work experience from the managerial role in childcare, so that the language and terms of the profession were easily understood. Follow-up questions were aimed at encouraging the participants to talk about their role and provide more information. No specific questions about role components were posed, but some questions were used to help the managers to focus on the subject of the study. Questions included for example "What recent important situations/events in your work have you encountered? How have you interpreted and dealt with these situations? How do you plan to handle them?"

The judges

Three judges from different departments at a university (social welfare, anthropology, education) more or less familiar with hermeneutics, phenomenology, ethnographic, and/or narrative methods, interpreted the transcribed interviews to ensure reliability, but also to allow openness for different interpretative perspectives on the complex verbal material.

Procedure

First, the structure and information of the organisational changes were presented to the judges. Then they were asked to go through the five transcribed interviews one by one. Their instructions were to search for potential projects based on the hypothetical model of the subjective role (Figure 1) and summarize their analyses for each manager, one at a time.

Content analyses

The recorded narrative summaries made by the judges were transcribed and analysed. Two independent classifiers partitioned summaries into propositions (i.e., a distinguishable part of the text that is a bearer of meaning and forms natural semantic units) and classified them according to a two-dimensional classification scheme with three levels in each dimension. The first dimension had three system levels – organisational, social, and individual – while the second was a time dimension of past, present and future.

Three levels of analyses were then used: subjective role projects, detailed role element and analyses relating data to a project-construction process. In the first analysis classification was done according to system levels and then guided by the tense of the action or event and placed within the time dimensions. Propositions containing the judges' comments unrelated to the interview text were not further used. Propositions placed in the same category by both classifiers (i.e., not all propositions were used) were sorted into classes of similar content, and potential subjective role projects and labels for proposition classes were suggested.

In order to investigate and describe differences between individual managers based on the qualitative database, it was necessary to construct categorization schemes and models. In a second step, all judges' propositions were further analysed using a detailed categorization scheme, resulting in detailed representations of the managers' role situations. This scheme involved a time dimension, role project categories (Figure 1), further divided into subcategories (Table 1). Propositions were classified into one of the basic role categories, then into past, present or future and subcategories proposed. Data that at least two judges agreed on were used to capture more details on the role content in order to analyze variation between managers.

Finally, data from both levels of analyses were categorised into model terms to test if the model could be used to capture some of the dynamics in a project-construction process.

Results

Subjective role projects

In the narrative summaries the judges confirmed their support for the existence of role projects in the managers' interview data. Role project analyses were then based on data found in all three judges' summaries, to ensure reliability. Results supported the existence of role component categories (Figure 1) and showed that all managers pursued two role projects, except for manager C who had only one. The identified role projects were connected to the ongoing organisational changes, with one major project concerning how to handle the new situation, while the second project concerned the ongoing changes and/or their potential effects. The projects concerned:

Handling the organisational changes (Manager A, B, C, D, E)

Searching for social support in the new role situation (Manager A)

Handling their own and others employment situations (Manager B, E)

Keeping the control of the social climate (Manager D)

Manager A emphasized the importance of interaction and communication with her staff. To enhance this interaction she planned to structure her own situation, delegate tasks, direct more and 'become more autocratic'. Her second project concerned the social support that she tried to find in order to cope with difficulties in the new situation. Her general strategy can be described as a 'rational structuring and finding social support strategy'.

Manager B used a 'rational structuring and influencing people strategy' as he tried to structure his own work and his interaction and communication with staff. He had been occupied with relocation of staff, using a strategy where he made promises and directed the changes in detail. His own employment had been at stake and he tried to influence decision makers by clearly expressing his wishes.

Manager C did not act much, but reflected and waited for the new change situation to unfold. This was complemented by a check of the current status of her staff's expectations of her role, basically a 'check current status and wait and see strategy'. Her extensive 'non-actions' were complemented with reflections on her own goals for the role.

Manager D used many strategies to try to increase the future efficiency in his units. He communicated frequently with his staff and tried to coordinate, structure, and delegate tasks to them. He used his authority to be directive. He focused on keeping control over the situation, especially the 'work climate' and emerging staff conflicts. His general strategy can be described as a 'rational structuring, planning and controlling strategy'.

Manager E had a 'delegating and an intensive personal interaction strategy' and focused on keeping rather extensive, personal contact with her staff. She planned to get to know each new staff member and to delegate tasks. She was occupied with staff relocations, but her main focus was to give support and show empathy and consideration for the affected individuals.

Thus, the main projects all managers pursued concerned how to handle the upcoming organisational changes. The managers' detailed actions and action strategies were further classified into eight general project strategies: 1) Rational structuring (A, B, D), 2) Finding social support (A), 3) Influencing people (B), 4) Checking current status (C), 5) Waiting (C), 6) Planning and controlling (D), 7) Delegating (E), 8) Keeping an extensive personal interaction (D).

The managers' ways of dealing with insecurity in the new situation were then related to a role project process, with three phases: initial, middle, and end phase. When a new situation with extensive changes arises, insecurity is or rapidly becomes quite high. This process can be expressed in a series of questions that need to be answered during the initial change period:

1) First, are the changes large enough to be perceived or recognized as requiring substantial action on the part of managers? Do the changes represent threats or opportunities or both?

2) Once changes are recognized other questions arise. What does the change issue concern and what are the possible demands and dilemmas it creates? Is there a need for social networking, mobilizing influence, or negotiation in order to understand the changes, relate them to one's own situation, and/or engage people for future actions?

3) When things become clearer a project containing strategic actions arises, focusing on new questions. What is the change issue related to? What are one's interests and aims concerning this change issue? What actors and what time frames are relevant? What action strategies should be used and specific actions taken in order to protect one's interests and reach one's aims?

Can this way of representing the process of constructing role projects explain the managers' various ways of thinking? If so, where in this process did the five managers find themselves during the initial change period? The time aspect in all propositions that related situations, action strategies, and goals was analyzed, indicating the complexity of relations and the dynamics of the projects. Depending on these results and the clarity in their projects and strategies, the managers were placed in different phases of a project-construction process (Figure 2).

Manager C was placed in phase 1, not knowing for sure if this new situation was a threat or an opportunity, exploring the present situation, while waiting for more information that could give guidance. Managers A and B were in the beginning of phase 2, conducting analyses and working with issue structuring, while they looked for support or mobilized influence. Managers D and E seemed less vague about their interests, demands, dilemmas, and action strategies. Manager D had rather clear projects, an extended time frame, and actions already underway.

Some of these results can be explained by external factors or experiences, since manager D had more time at his disposal, and manager E already had relevant experience working with several units and closing them down. Another hypothesis is that progress in the project-forming process is connected to the use of more proactive strategies for managers in Phase 3 and a more reactive strategy in phase 1. Exhibiting a proactive conflict management style in relation to workplace uncertainty has been found to decrease the negative impact of role conflicts, while exhibiting a reactive style has the opposite effect (Tidd, 2002). Thus, the process model highlighted the kind of issue-structuring or sense-making the managers focused on during the initial change period.

Figure 2: The five managers' locations in the role project-construction process

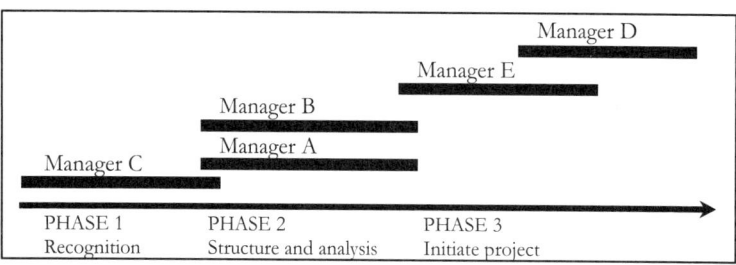

When answers to the project-related questions become clearer, the role project will probably take a more consistent form and become less vague. Finally, project owners can clearly state what they want to achieve, their overall action strategies, specific actions planned, when they will act, and where hindrances and problems are likely to occur. This process of forming subjective role projects can probably occur at a faster or slower pace depending on the situation and the individual manager's knowledge and capacities. Even though the sequence can be rapid, even almost simultaneous, it was possible to describe the managers within a three step process with a recognition phase, a structure and analysis phase and a project initiating phase (Figure 2).

Detailed role elements

The categorization scheme was further developed in order to assess role variation in greater detail. Concepts from Hosking and Morley's (1991) model were used (threats, opportunities, project goals) and subcategories of the basic role components in Figure 1 were proposed and tested. This resulted in a categorization scheme of role elements used to identify similarities and dissimilarities among the managers (Table 1). A mix between qualitative and quantitative categorization was used.

These role descriptions were based on each judge's entire description and contained more details, more or less related to present and past role projects. There were also comments made by the judges that were not directly related to the interview text, but that indicated variation among the mental models the judges used in their interpretations.

The results clarified relations between specific situations, action strategies, goals, and time dimensions within each project. Ten situation-threats (S), three situation-opportunities (O), ten actors (R), one personal aspect (P), nine action strategies (A), and nine purposes/goals (G) represented subcategories of role project components used to describe variation between managers. Table 1 presents part of the results (for more extensive results, see Nyström 2004) supported by at least two judges. Categories identified by only one judge were not included (S1, O1, O2, G3, G4). The analysis was a qualitative test of the role project, and is open to new or additional interpretations based on richer data.

Table 1: Variation in role element categories among the five managers (at least two judges agreed on the existence of a category in the manager's verbal protocols)

Subjective role categories	Manager:	A	B	C	D	E	∑
SIT./	S1 Fragmentation						0
EVENTS	S2 Problems/conflicts among people staff/parents/ manager	1	1	1			3
Threats							
	S3 Subordinates absence from work/relocation of staff		1			1	2
	S4 Contact with field activities/staff	1				1	2
	S5 Administrative demands/fulfilling						0
	S6 Organizational decisions/dealing with changes	1	1	1	1	1	5
	S7 The manager's own expectations on higher levels	1	1			1	3
	S8 Changes in managerial role/re-employment/new demands		1			1	2
	S9 The manager's own support	1					1
	S10 Difficulties with role aspects				1		1
SIT. /	O1 Opportunities – org.						0
EVENTS	O2 Opportunities – social						0
Opportunities	O3 Opportunities – personal			1	1	1	3
ACTORS	R1 Manager	1	1	1	1	1	5

							Σ
	R2 Staff	1	1	1	1	1	5
	R3 Parents	1	1		1		3
	R4 Children			1	1		2
	R5 Supervisors	1				1	2
	R6 District staff		1			1	2
	R7 Colleagues			1	1	1	3
	R8 Family – on			1		1	2
	R9 Friend			1			1
	R10 Other *						0
PERSONAL	P1 Personal aspects	1	1	1	1	1	5
ACTION-	A1 Direct and influence				1		1
STRATEGIES	A2 Delegate and let staff influence	1			1		2
	A3 Give support and help			1		1	2
	A4 Emphasize performance standard and goals				1		1
	A5 Structure and increase efficiency	1			1	1	3
	A6 Communication/interaction with staff	1	1	1	1	1	5
	A7 Get support – networking	1	1	1	1	1	5
	A8 Managerial role aspects – general	1	1				2
	A9 Non-actions	1	1	1		1	4
GOALS	G1 Personal goals – managerial role	1	1	1	1	1	5
	G2 Goals concerning staff	1				1	2
	G3 Goals concerning childcare						0
	G4 Administrative goals						0
	G5 Official goals	1	1				2
	G6 Project goals		1			1	2
	G7 Future states/neutral						0
	G8 Future states/opportunities						0
	G9 Future states/threats			1	1		2
Σ		19	19	14	16	22	90

* politicians

The results were in line with the project model and its components. They also gave additional information on previous situations and projects and descriptions of the manager's personal aspects, like traits, emotions, values and preferences. Data provided very specific individual details but also similarities among managers.

The managers mainly perceived the organisational changes as threats. They all reported an increased feeling of insecurity, as their role was about to change, and would involve new demands, problems and dilemmas, but differed in their interpretation of the changes. All managers involved themselves and their staff in their projects and discussed their own personal goals in relation to the managerial role. They all had action strategies involving communication and interaction with staff and attempts to get support through networking activities, but differed in their approaches. Further studies on how previous projects are connected to the present ones can be of interest for an understanding the subjective role, but was beyond the scope of the present study.

The role project-construction process

Differences among managers' role projects and strategies during a change period can have an effect on the social and organisational role context. Hosking and Morley stressed that it is important for managers to possess skilful organizing processes and even defined leadership as "a more or less skilful process of organizing, achieved through negotiation, to achieve acceptable influence over the description and handling of issues within and between groups" (1991, p. 250). Thereby they highlight the importance of being skilful when forming role projects and choosing action strategies for implementation. If one combines Hosking and Morley's ideas with the present role project approach one can draw the conclusion that a manager skilful in organizing processes should:

be involved in networking, mobilizing and building relationships *i.e., be able to get support and use influence when needed*

know what they themselves are trying to protect and promote *i.e., have clear role projects*

know when, how, and why to negotiate *i.e., have clear action strategies*

have issue-specific and process-knowledge (for example: knowing who to go to in order to build understandings, through whom to mobilize influence, and why negotiation is important in the process) *i.e., have personal aspects and action strategies that express this kind of knowledge.*

have capacities that are tied to the demands of their tasks, i.e., have personal aspects and action strategies that contain these capacities.

Thus, the final analyses combined data from the two earlier analyses and classified them according to the components of Hosking and Morley's model, expressed in the skilful organizing processes above.

Results showed that Managers D and E had the clearest projects and actions strategies followed by A and B, while Manager C expressed more uncertainty. Being able to get support from a network of people using political and social processes was an option all managers discussed. For example, manager A lacked support but planned to get support from colleagues and supervisors and to investigate staffs' thoughts, wishes and demands, while manager E had searched and gotten support from the personnel assistant, colleagues, staff and family. She planned regular communication with her staff and to have an introduction-day where she would bring in a consultant to help facilitate the change process.

It is interesting that no one said that they had clear support from their supervisors and only Manager A talked about seeking her supervisors' support, while Manager B tried to influence them. Reasons for these results are indicated by the critique and the unfulfilled expectations concerning district-level staff and supervisors, expressed by Manager A, B and E. Within an organisational system it ought to be important to receive support from supervisors with more power and influence, but colleagues seemed to be the support option for these managers.

Other important aspects of social and political processes involved in handling organisational change on a unit level were networking with and getting support from staff. Managers D and E had an advantage, since they had discussed and already received support from their staff. Manager B had talked to some staff concerning relocation, while manager A planned to investigate their views. Manager C did not mention this in relation to her actions, but expressed the goal of having a dialogue with her staff.

Issue-specific knowledge and process-knowledge concerned projects, threats and opportunities. Managers were probably helped in pursuing their role projects by knowing the background of and reasons for the organisational change, and by having previous experiences of organisational change, working with many units, of handling social aspects, and by having some knowledge of one's own role during a change period. Some of this knowledge is indicated in the results since all managers had more or less elaborated ideas on action strategies. For example, manager A had many ideas about how to deal with the change situation, but was unclear about the limits of her role and had difficulty dealing with conflict. Manager B knew how organisational decisions were made and had experience working with larger units, but found relocation of staff and knowing how to answer their questions about relocation difficult. Manager C was aware of role demands from politicians and parents, and was used to dealing with changes, but did not really grasp what her managerial tasks would be after the re-organisation. Manager D knew reorganisation decisions came from politicians and higher officials in order to increase efficiency and had a lot of ideas. He looked into the sensitive interpersonal issues, listened and organized, but was afraid of losing control. Manager E knew the changes concerned money, had considerable experience and enjoyed having responsibility, but she did not like administrative tasks and had difficulties to keep a distance to her job.

According to the results managers D and E seemed to show the highest skilfulness in organizing processes during the initial change period, 4-6 weeks before implementation. They had more clearly formed their up-coming role projects and were more pro-active in their choice of action strategies for implementation. However, this could easily change with time, as the new role projects become clearer to managers A, B, and C.

The use of a model aided a qualitative description of variation among managers and the detailed role element categories were be placed within the role project-construction process discussed earlier. Thus, a dynamic process model of subjective role projects was proposed (Figure 3).

Figure 3: A model of the role project-construction process with the specific role elements for manager E

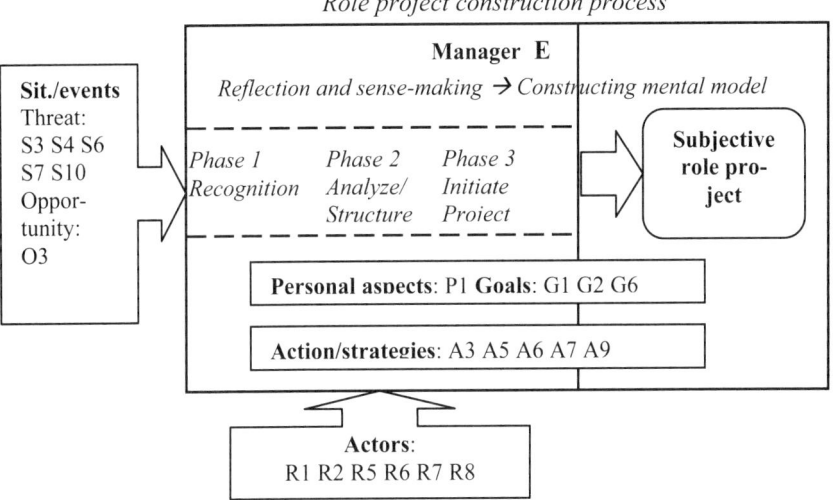

The model is based on an input-output model with the dynamic perspective of the project-construction process, combined with the role element categorization scheme from table 1. In the model, the reflection, sense-making, and construction processes used during the three phases were complemented with detailed role element categories for each manager. An example is given for manager E (Figure 3). Specific action strategies, actors, and goals will eventually form the managers' subjective role project, triggered by situations, mainly those perceived as threats.

Discussion

The purpose of the study was to describe managers' potential subjective role projects and strategies during initial phases of an organisational change process, leading to a more detailed description and understanding of the subjective side of the managerial role. Results showed that the model of subjective role projects (Figure 1) can be used to describe important aspects of the subjective role in great detail. The approach can also be used to describe similarities and dissimilarities in role content and in perceptions of the role context among the managers, as well as indicate differences in the development of role projects.

Variation was described on three levels. Subjective role projects were based on the corresponding data from all judges, leaving out much information. The detailed role elements were based on the three judges' entire summary data increasing the scope of information used. Finally, data from both the above levels were categorized into a model of the project-construction process to capture some of the dynamics of role projects.

Using qualitative, verbal data always introduces the issue of reliability, especially for describing variation among managers. The managers' verbal statements can be interpreted differently, as was the case when the three judges analysed the interview transcripts. This suggests why it is important to gather several perspectives on the interpretation of the complex qualitative data base. It also reduces the risk of missing important information in the analyses. Several independent classifiers were also used in the analyses of the judges' narrative summaries to insure higher reliability.

The results can be connected to role theory concepts. During the first phases of the change process the knowledge of the organisational changes and their effects was vague. Role ambiguity was high among managers and probably remained high until they had tested their interpretation of and planned strategies for the new situation. Role ambiguity concerned insecurity about what the managerial role would involve in the future and what role expectations the new organisational situation would bring.

All forms of task ambiguity were found in the managers' role descriptions. Socio-emotional role ambiguity regarding consequences of role behaviour can be tied to the managers' concerns about their own ability to meet staff demands. Future ambiguity is probably higher in organisational change periods, especially before the actual impact is clear. This was exemplified by the future-oriented focus of the role projects and the managers' concern about their ability to handle the new situation and live up to situational demands. A concern for the future, whether it concerned their own role, the staff's situation or childcare in general, was also found. The managers tried to meet the new ambiguous situation by seeking social support and building supportive networks. Manager D fought to remain in control. Research on the impact of large-scale organisational changes has indicated that individuals with high levels of perceived control experienced less stress, despite high levels of role ambiguity (Hansen, 2001). If role ambiguities persist or if too many changes succeed each other for these managers it can result in negative outcomes found in other studies: low job satisfaction, lowered self-confidence, stress, feelings of futility and alienation and lowered efficiency at work (French & Caplan, 1973; Kahn et al., 1964).

To some extent the managers found themselves in a role negotiation period due to the insecurity of their own employment and placements, and some managers tried to influence supervisors and others in their role set. Networking activities were a priority, especially as support from supervisors was perceived as missing. The managers therefore searched for social support elsewhere, such as from colleagues, friends, family and staff. Connections between role ambiguity and stress highlights the importance of finding a strategy, individual as well as organisational, for handling insecurity during change processes. Research has found that constant organisational change leading to prolonged conflicts at work places can be a primary cause to burnout (Eriksson, Starrin & Janson, 2003) and anxiety for reorganisations at the workplace was a primary organisational factor that explained high rates of sick leave for municipal employees in Sweden (Szücs, Hemström & Marklund, 2003). Organisational and social support might reduce potential negative effects, especially in the first phases of the change process.

The new organisational situation, perceived mainly as a threat, resulted in role stress and strain and was especially evident in relation to ongoing structural effects, such as re-employment of managers and the relocation or firing of employees. A potentially stressful situation or episode does not actually create distress unless it is appraised as threatening (Folkman, Lazarus, Dunkel-Schetter, DeLongis & Gruen, 2000) and threat appraisal is an important subjective aspect in the assessment of role stress (Siegall, 2000). The strong impact of the organisational changes on the subjective role projects is in line with organisational role theory, but how the actual situation was interpreted was very personal, stressing the benefits of using subjective data.

The conclusion is that the concept of 'subjective role projects' can contribute to role theory by describing the detailed subjective role content in relation to a specific role context. A role project is a dynamic mental scheme that combines different aspects of role content. It acts as a mediator between the situations in the role context and the effects in the form of role problems, such as role conflict and role ambiguity. The role project approach can then be used to describe and understand how managers approach and make sense of a new situation, and thereby create an organisational awareness of potential role problems during change periods.

References

Eriksson, U. B., Starrin, B. & Janson, S. (2003). *Utbränd och emotionellt utmärglad.* Lund: Studentlitteratur.

Folkman, S., Lazarus, R. S., Dunkel-Schetter, C., DeLongis, A. & Gruen, R. (2000). The dynamics of a stressful encounter. In T. E. Higgins (Ed.), *Motivational science: Social and personality perspectives. Key reading in social psychology* (pp. 111-127). Philadelphia, PA, US: Psychology Press.

French, J. R. P. & Caplan, R. D. (1973). Organizational stress and individual strain. In A. J. Marrow (Ed.), *The failure of success*. New York: American Management Association.

Graen, G. B. & Scandura, T. A. (1987). Toward a psychology of dyadic organizing. *Research in Organizational Behavior, 9*, 175-208.

Hansen, M. J. (2001). *Individual reactions to a large-scale organizational change in a healthcare organization.* Dissertation, Loyola University of Chicago, US.

Hosking, D. & Morley, I. E. (1991). *A social psychology of organizing. People, processes and contexts.* New York: Harvester Wheatsheaf.

Kahn, R. L. (1980). Conflict, ambiguity, and overload: Three elements in job stress. In D. Katz, R. L. Kahn & J. S. Adams (Eds.), *The study of organizations.* San Francisco: Jossey-Bass Inc.

Kahn, R. L. & Byosiere, P. (1992). Stress in organizations. In M. D. Dunnette and L. M. Hough (Eds.), *Handbook of industrial and organizational psychology* (2nd ed., vol. 1, pp. 75-170). Palo Alto, CA: Consulting Psychologists Press.

Kahn, R. L., Wolfe, D. M., Quinn, R. P., Snoek, J. D. & Rosenthal, R. A. (1964). *Organizational stress: Studies in role conflict and ambiguity.* New York: Wiley.

Katz, D. & Kahn, R. L. (1978). *The social psychology of organizations* (3rd ed.). New York: Wiley.

Nystrom, M. (2004). *Contrasting perspectives on the subjective managerial role.* Unpublished manuscript.

Siegall, M. (2000). Putting the stress back into role stress: Improving the measurement of role conflict and role ambiguity. *Journal of Managerial Psychology, 15*(5-6), 427-435.

Szücs S., Hemström Ö., & Marklund S. (2003). Organisatoriska faktorers betydelse för långa sjukskrivningar i kommuner. *Arbete och Hälsa, No 2003-6,* 1-40. Arbetslivsinstitutet, Stockholm, Sweden.

Tidd, S. T. (2002). *Conflict style and coping with role conflict: An extension of the uncertainty model of work stress.* Dissertation, Vanderbilt University, US.

Demands and organizational stress reactions in hospitals

Holger Pfaff[1], *Jürgen Lütticke*[2], *Nicole Ernstmann*[3], *Frank Pühlhofer*[1] & *Peter Richter*[4]

[1] *Division of Medical Sociology, University of Cologne, Germany*
[2] *Federal Association of the AOK, Germany*
[3] *Center for Health Services Research, University of Cologne, Germany*
[4] *Institute of Work-, Organizational-, and Social Psychology, Technical University of Dresden, Germany*

The aim of this study is to evaluate the organizational coping concept on hospital conditions. Within this concept it is assumed that environmental stressors and demands cause organizational stress reactions on different levels of a hospital and that the impact of these stressors and demands is moderated by organizational resources and coping capacities. The study was conducted in February 2002 among medical staff of $n = 35$ wards in three German hospitals. Stress and demands are operationalised by an objective measure (patient days per full-time-equivalent employee), stress reactions are operationalised by work flow problems and decreasing affective commitment, and both culture of trust and perceived supervisor support serve as indicators for moderating organizational resources. By analyzing the relationship between demands and stress reactions in a first step and comparing the interrelationship of demands and stress reactions in terms of different moderating influences in a second step, central assumptions of the underlying concept could be confirmed by exploration. Future multilevel analysis will have to clarify whether the interactions between demands, stress reactions and organizational resources are influenced by individual or organizational characteristics.

Introduction

As a consequence of socio-economic changes in the majority of European countries, most countries have adopted a series of strategies to increase cost-effectiveness in health service provision. Health system reforms are increasingly focusing on the role of hospitals. Restructuring hospital services in-

---

* *Correspondence: Holger Pfaff, holger.pfaff@medizin.uni-koeln.de*

This study is supported by a grant of the German Federal Ministry of Education and Research, grant no 01 HW 0112

cludes a number of institutional and functional changes aimed at increasing the quality and responsiveness of service provision. New concepts draw specific emphasis on reducing inefficiencies by designing a system that is both patient focused and efficient in the delivery of health care. Trends in hospital capacity and utilization show changes with fewer beds being used more intensively (World Health Organization, 2002).

The ongoing changes in health care organizations lead to increasing job demands. The individual consequences on employees' health and well being due to increasing job demands and the impact of individual buffering factors are subject to many studies. There is much evidence for the interactive effect of perceived control on the relationship between job demands and individual health due to the interest in Karaseks (Karasek, 1979) demand-control model (e.g., see Terry & Jimmieson, 1999; Van der Doef & Maes, 1999 for reviews). There is additional empirical support that job demands and job control should be conceptualized as having both individual- and group-level-foundations (Van Yperen & Snijders, 2000). Concerning the association between job demand and individual health the effect of effort-reward-imbalance (Siegrist, 1996) has been examined and empirically supported lately (e.g., Siegrist 1996; Larisch, Joksimovic, von dem Knesebeck, Starke & Siegrist, 2003). Another distinction can be made by separating job demands and job resources in terms of their specific outcomes. Job demands are then related to exhaustion and lack of job resources is related to disengagement (Demerouti, Bakker, Nachreiner & Schaufeli, 2001). Further moderating factors on the interaction between job demands and their adverse consequences are e.g., perceived organizational support (Rhoades & Eisenberger, 2002), and perceived supervisor support (Eisenberger, Stinglhamber, Vandenberghe, Sucharski & Rhoades, 2002). When taking into account the specific characteristics of human service organizations like hospitals (Hasenfeld & English, 1974; Ulich 2002), it can be argued that in application on human service organizations the basic concepts of the demand-control model must be adapted (Söderfeldt, Söderfeldt, Muntaner, O'Campo, Warg & Ohlson, 1996).

This paper proposes an alternative concept for the interrelationships between different hospital dimensions: the organizational coping concept. In contrast to the models mentioned above which examine individual consequences of job demands it focuses on demands and stress reactions on the organizational level and on organizational resources that moderate the interrelationship of demands and stress reactions. Our central aim is to evaluate this concept by exploring the moderating influence of organizational resources on the relationship between demands and organizational stress reactions.

Organizational coping

According to the organizational coping concept (Pfaff, 2003) all organizations have to face environmental stressors and demands. It is assumed that these stressors lead to unfavorable stress reactions within the organization (e.g., financial crisis, work flow problems) on condition of deficient organizational coping skills. The coping capacity of a hospital determines the negative effects of environmental demands on this hospital (Figure 1).

Figure 1: The organizational coping concept

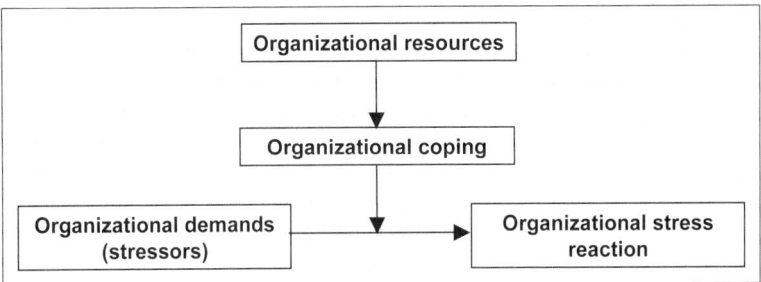

According to this concept the success of an organization depends on the way an organization copes with demanding situations and how it is able to gain and organize resources in order to cope effectively and efficiently with stressful situations. Thus, organizational stress is a result of the interaction between demands and coping resources.

Organizational resources are human resources, social capital (trust, supportive relationship), cultural resources (knowledge base), technical resources (IT), and the organizational network (Badura & Hehlmann, 2003). There is no organizational stress given, if the coping resources exceed the demands. If the coping resources are – quantitatively and qualitatively – insufficient to cope adequately with the demanding situation the organization is 'stressed'. Organizational stress reactions are then likely on all levels of the enterprise: finance (financial crisis, low ROI), customer (patient dissatisfaction, low image), employee (turnover, absenteeism, low commitment), organization (work flow problems, lack of planning) and learning (low level of organizational learning).

Staff work load is an objective indicator for organizational demand. The measurement of job stressors and strains varies from self-report instruments, observational approaches to physiological indicators. However, the importance of the identification and more frequent use of objective measures has been underlined (Hurrell, Nelson & Simmons, 1998). Admissions per full-time-equivalent employee and patient days per full-time-equivalent employee are two alternative indicators to measure staff work load. In order to take into account the fact that the admissions per full-time-equivalent employee do not include the average length of stay, we conducted the analyses with patient days per full-time-equivalent employee as indicator for the organizational demand.

We expect that increasing staff work load stresses the ward system. Assuming that coping capacities are on a low level the demands might lead to increasing problems of work flow management. Under the pressure of high organizational demand there is less time for 'quality'. In other words: Stress 'soaks up' communication. In times of stress there is less time to communicate and less time to plan and coordinate. Work flow problems are the consequences. In the current economic situation only a certain amount of hospitals are supposed to be able to cope effectively with the occurring problems. Therefore we assume a positive relationship between staff work load and work flow problems. Beside the work flow level we expect the increasing demands to have a negative impact on the employees' commitment. Given the hypothesized interactions we assume a moderating role of the organizational resources supportive leadership and culture of trust.

Methods: Study design

The study presented is part of the multi-centre study 'Hospital management with biopsychosocial scores', which was granted by the German Federal Ministry of Education and Research (grant no 01 HW 0112). The aim of the project was to develop, measure, and evaluate psychosocial, survey based performance measures for the strategic stakeholder management in hospitals. The reported study was conducted in three German hospitals, two of them in Western Germany and one in Eastern Germany. To test the hypothesis that staff work load is a determinant of both work flow problems and employees' commitment the individual data has been aggregated on the ward level. 35 wards of different types of hospital sizes and units have been included in the study (Table 1 and table 2).

Table 1: Hospital types and number of included wards

	Number of wards	%
General hospital	18	51.4
Specialized hospital	17	48.6

Table 2: Units and number of included wards

	Number of wards	%
Gynecology	6	17.1
Psychiatry	5	14.3
Cardiology	4	11.4
Surgery (visceral and vessels)	4	11.4
Internal medicine (general)	9	25.7
Surgery (general)	7	20.0
Total	35	100.0

Two data bases have been matched together: the data base of the hospital management (patient days per full-time-equivalent employee in 2001) and the results of an employee survey conducted in February 2002. Employees filled out a paper-and-pencil questionnaire on employee stress and resources. Data collection started in February 2002 and was performed according to Dillman's Total Design Method. The survey was conducted over seven weeks and included three reminders. The response rate was 62%. Data from $n = 375$ nurses has been included in the analysis. Data from further medical staff (e.g., physicians, physical therapists) could not be matched to single wards. Thus it had to be excluded from the analysis.

Methods: Measurement

The indicator 'patient days per full-time-equivalent employee' has been calculated by multiplying length of stay in 2001 with the number of cases in 2001 and dividing the product by the number of full-time-equivalent employees (FTE) in 2001. The variable 'work flow problems' represents the mean of the individually perceived work flow problems of the ward employees participating in the study. The scale measuring the individually perceived work flow problems includes three aspects of work flow: at first a global impression of the quality of work organization (e.g., "The right hand doesn't 't know what the left hand is doing"), secondly two indicators for failures in effective work flow-management (perceived patient waiting times and perceived changes in patient scheduling), and thirdly the evaluation of the cooperation process between wards and within the ward (Cronbach's $\alpha = .83$). The scale 'affective commitment' (Allen & Meyer, 1990) measures the emotional attachment and identification with the hospital with seven items. The moderating factor organizational culture was measured by a self developed four item scale organizational 'culture of trust' (Cronbach's α = .89) which assesses the level of trust and reciprocal agreement in the hospital staff (e.g., "In our hospital we trust each other"). The scale 'perceived supervisor support' stems from the University of Michigan and was used in Germany by Udris & Rimann (1999). The three item scale (Cronbach's α = .91) measures the potential emotional support a supervisor is able to give. Statistical analysis included descriptive measures (mean, standard deviation, minimum, maximum) and the calculation of Spearman correlations to test both the interaction of demands and work flow problems and the interaction of demands and employees' affective commitment. In a second step the variables culture of trust and perceived supervisor support were subdivided by their means into two groups of wards with high and low level resources. Bivariate regressions were calculated separately for the groups to explore the moderating role of culture of trust and perceived supervisor support. The effects are demonstrated graphically by the interaction of the regression lines. The explorative approach helps to clarify if there is some, at least weak, evidence to believe that the relationship between staff work load and organizational stress reactions could be moderated by organizational resources like culture of trust or social support.

Results

Table 3 shows the descriptive statistics for both main and moderating variables. Table 4 shows the correlation coefficients between the main variables. There is a significant positive correlation between patient days per full-time-equivalent employee and work flow problems (r = .53). This indicates that increasing numbers of patient days per full-time-equivalent employee are associated with increasing work flow problems. There is a non-significant negative correlation between patient days per full-time-equivalent employee and affective commitment (r = -.21) indicating that growing numbers of patient days per full-time-equivalent employee are only moderately associated with decreasing affective commitment.

Table 3: Descriptive statistics

	M	**SD**	**Min**	**Max**	**N**
Patient days per full-time equivalent employee	526.10	196.46	140.60	1240.20	32**
Work flow problems*	2.73	0.37	2.19	3.47	35
Affective commitment*	2.51	0.24	2.04	2.90	35
Culture of trust*	2.20	0.21	1.77	2.73	35
Perceived supervisor support*	2.94	0.34	2.19	3.50	35

* Items rated on continuous scales from 1 = strongly disagree to 4 = strongly agree
** N results from missing data of three wards
N = number of wards

Table 4: Correlation coefficients

	Work flow problems	**N**	**Affective commitment**	**N**
Patient days per full-time equivalent employee	.534**	32	-.21	32

** marked Spearman correlation coefficient is significant on the level of $p < 0.01$

N = number of wards

Figure 2 shows the interrelationship between patient days per full-time equivalent employee and work flow problems separately for high and low level of culture of trust. Figure 3 illustrates the same interrelationship separately for high and low level of perceived supervisor support. When comparing the predicted slopes for high and low level of resources it is obvious that the regression lines show less slope in both cases of high level of resources. This indicates that on condition of a high level of culture of trust or perceived supervisor support, the negative impact of increasing demands could be reduced.

Figure 2: Bivariate regression between patient days per full-time equivalent employee and work flow problems for high and low level of culture of trust (* p <.05)

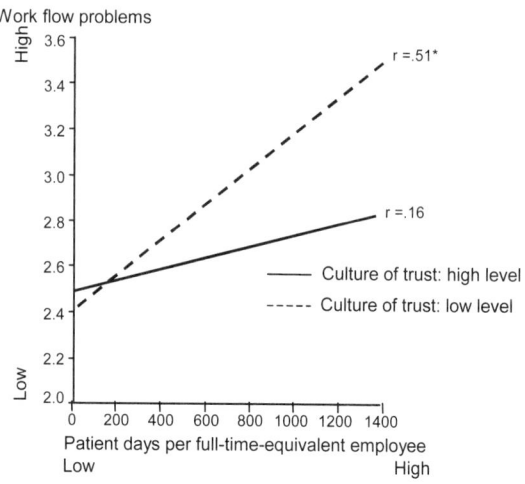

Figure 3: Bivariate regression between patient days per full-time equivalent employee and work flow problems for high and low level of perceived super-visor support

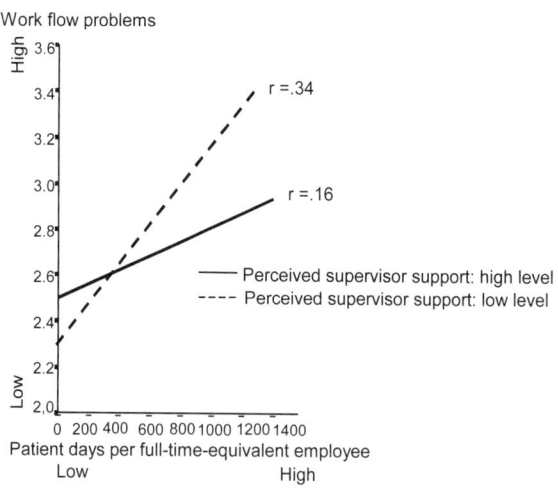

Figure 4 demonstrates the interrelationship between patient days per full-time equivalent employee and affective commitment in terms of high and low level of culture of trust in an explorative way. Figure 5 shows the same interrelationship separately for high and low level of perceived supervisor support. It can be seen in figure 5 that high levels of culture of trust are potentially able to minimize the negative effects of increasing demands on employees' affective commitment. Concerning the perceived supervisor support as organizational resource (figure 5), the impact of high levels of the resource is rather negligible.

Figure 4: Bivariate regression between patient days per full-time equivalent employee and affective commitment for high and low level of culture of trust

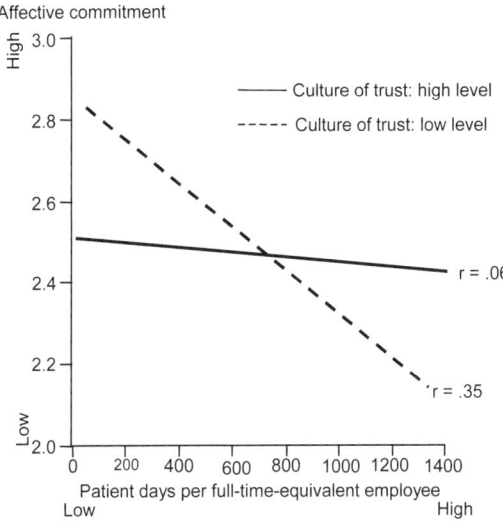

Figure 5: Bivariate regression between patient days per full-time equivalent employee and affective commitment for high and low level of perceived supervisor support

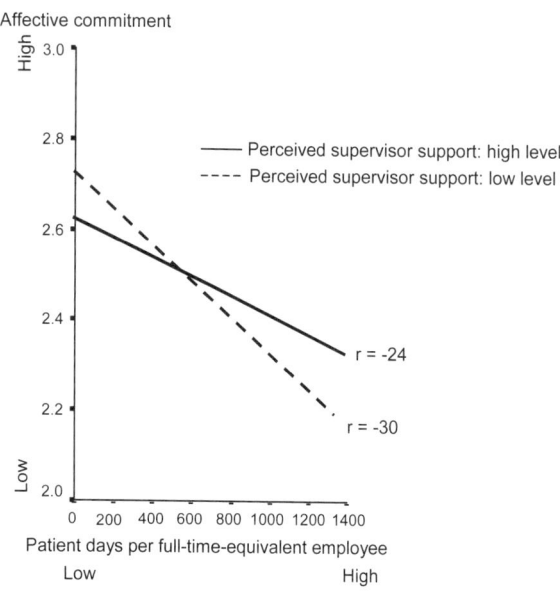

Discussion

There is an interrelationship between staff work load and work flow problems indicated by the positive correlation coefficient. The impact of organizational resources on this interrelationship is demonstrated by the disordinal interaction of their graphs. Both culture of trust and perceived supervisor support decrease the negative consequences of increasing staff demands on work flow problems. The correlation between staff work load and affective commitment appears to be in conflict with the predictions of the organizational coping concept. The strength of the association is unconvincing. But the division of the wards into those with more and those with less organizational resources shows the impact of those resources. Given the situation of low levels of resources, the impact of demands on the employees' affective commitment is visible. Increasing job demands are therefore probably associated with decreasing affective commitment on condition of organizational resources not being sufficient to cope adequately with the situation.

There are certain methodological difficulties to be considered for the interpretation of the results. The full-time equivalent employee-ratio should be risk-adjusted for the case mix of relevant patient characteristics in future analyses of the data. Age, comorbidity, need for care and further inpatient characteristics are supposed to have a significant effect on internal processes like work flow problems of the medical staff. There are some further pitfalls in using aggregated data. A relationship on the level of the aggregates could not necessarily be translated onto the level of individual behavior (ecological fallacy). There is a risk of information loss in our analysis which could eventually lead to false interpretation of the results if one wants to draw conclusions from the relationship on the aggregated data level to relationships on the individual level. Determinants of staff work load are admission rate (external cause), average length of stay, and personnel policy (internal cause). Staff work load is therefore an objective independent variable. Staff work load leads to an overload within the wards and – as a consequence – to organizational problems. Considering the methodological weakness of the explorative analysis, the tentative conclusion is that high staff work load could lead to a situation in which stress 'soaks up' communication, in which there is no time for quality, and hence in which suboptimal work flow conditions and information gaps are more likely.

Conclusion

Increasing organizational demands lead to organizational stress reactions like serious work flow problems and decreasing affective commitment. These hypotheses were tested in an ecological study with 35 research units (wards). The result was that there is a positive, significant correlation between staff work load and work flow problems and a non-significant positive relationship between staff work load and affective commitment. The interrelationships could both be possibly influenced by the resources culture of trust and perceived supervisor support. As the main theoretical conclusion the result of our analysis – the methodological difficulties of this explorative study in mind – underlines the assumptions of the organizational coping concept.

The methodological conclusion implies the necessity of bigger sample sizes of wards and employees within each ward in future studies. Our aim is to combine the chosen correlational approach with the recommended multilevel analysis approach in future studies (e.g., Snijders & Bosker, 1999) to additionally explore the postulated cause-effect-relationships on different levels of the organization.

As a practical conclusion hospitals should appreciate 'time for quality' as a mean to reach learning capacities which enable the ward and the whole system to cope effectively and efficiently with the pressure of a competitive environment. If there is not enough time to think about the appropriateness and usefulness of how work is organized in and between the wards the result might be a pathogenic coping strategy which is ineffective in the short run and dangerously inefficient and burnout producing in the long run. Hospital management should therefore institutionalize a jour fixe 'quality time' to escape the vicious circle of overload and inefficient coping actions.

References

Allen, N. J. & Meyer, J. P. (1990). The measurement and antecedents of affective, continuance and normative commitment to the organization. *Journal of Occupational Psychology, 63*, 1-18.

Badura, B. & Hehlmann, T. (2003). *Betriebliche Gesundheitspolitik*. Berlin: Springer.

Demerouti, E., Bakker, A. B., Nachreiner, F. & Schaufeli, W. B. (2001). The job demands-resources model of burnout. *Journal of Applied Psychology, 86*(3), 499-512.

Eisenberger, R., Stinglhamber, F., Vandenberghe, C., Sucharski, I. L. & Rhoades, L. (2002). Perceived supervisor support: Contributions to perceived organizational support and employee retention. *Journal of Applied Psychology, 87*(3), 565-573.

Hasenfeld, Y. & English, R. A. (1974). *Human Service Organization*. Ann Arbor: University of Michigan Press.

Hurrell, J. J., Jr., Nelson, D. L. & Simmons, B. L. (1998). Measuring job stressors and strains: Where we have been, where we are, and where we need to go. *Journal of Occupational Health Psychology, 3*(4), 368-389.

Karasek, R. A. (1979). Job demands, job decision latitude, and mental strain: Implications for job redesign. *Administrative Science Quarterly, 24*, 285-306.

Larisch, M., Joksimovic, L., von dem Knesebeck, O., Starke, D. & Siegrist, J. (2003). Berufliche Gratifikationskrisen und depressive Symptome. Eine Querschnittsstudie bei Erwerbstaetigen im mittleren Erwachsenenalter. *Psychotherapie, Psychosomatik, Medizinische Psychologie, 53*(5), 223-228.

Pfaff, H. (2003). Organisationsentwicklung – ein Thema für das deutsche Gesundheitswesen. In Kassenärztliche Bundesvereinigung (Ed.), *Neue Vertrags- und Versorgungsformen – Impulse setzen durch Qualitätsmanagement* (pp. 13-32). Köln: Kassenärztliche Bundesvereinigung.

Rhoades, L. & Eisenberger, R. (2002). Perceived organizational support: A review of the literature. *Journal of Applied Psychology, 87*(4), 698-714.

Siegrist, J. (1996). Adverse health effects of high-effort/low-reward conditions. *Journal of Occupational Health Psychology, 1*(1), 27-41.

Snijders, T. A. B. & Bosker, R. J. (1999). *Multilevel Analysis: An introduction to basic and advanced Multilevel Modelling*. London: Sage.

Söderfeldt, B., Söderfeldt, M., Muntaner, C., O'Campo, P., Warg, L.-E. & Ohlson, C.-G. (1996). Psychosocial work environment in human service organizations: a conceptual analysis and development of the demand-control model. *Social Science Medicine, 42*(9), 1217-1226.

Terry, D. J. & Jimmieson, N. L. (1999). Work control and employee well-being: A decade review. In C.L. Cooper & I.T. Robertson (Eds.), *International Review of Work and Organizational Psychology* (pp. 95-148). Chichester: Wiley.

Udris, I. & Rimann, M. (1999). SAA und SALSA: Zwei Fragebögen zur subjektiven Arbeitsanalyse. In H. Dunckel (Ed.), *Handbuch psychologischer Arbeitsanalyseverfahren* (pp. 397-420). Zürich: vdf.

Ulich, E. (2002) (Ed.). *Arbeitspsychologie in Krankenhaus und Arztpraxis*. Bern: Huber.

Van der Doef, M. & Maes, S. (1999). The job demands-control (-support) model and psychological well-being: A review of 20 years of empirical research. *Work and Stress, 13*, 87-114.

Van Yperen, N. W. & Snijders, T. A. B. (2000). A multilevel analysis of the demands-control-model: Is stress at work determined by factors at the group level or the individual level? *Journal of Occupational Health Psychology, 5*(1), 182-190.

World Health Organization (2002). *The European Health Report. WHO regional publications*. European series, 97 (p. 117). Copenhagen: WHO Library Cataloguing in Publication Data.

Hospital restructuring and downsizing and psychological burnout among nursing staff: A longitudinal study

Ronald J. Burke[*]
Schulich School of Business, York University, Canada

The health care system in most developed countries has undergone significant restructuring during the past decade (Aiken, Sochalski & Anderson, 1996; Aiken & Fagin, 1997). These changes have been undertaken without a clear sense of how best to bring them about or the impact they would have on hospital functioning and effectiveness (Sochalski, Aiken & Fagin, 1997; White, 1997). Organizational restructuring and downsizing is a complex and difficult task (Kets de Vries & Balazs, 1997). A small but growing literature suggests that such changes fail to reach their objectives (usually financial) about half the time (Burke & Nelson, 1998; Cascio, 1993, 1998; Cameron, Whetten & Kim, 1987). Negative employee reactions, termed survivor sickness (Noer, 1993), are observed in an even greater number of cases (Burke & Leiter, 2000; Burke & Nelson, 1998). Survivor sickness is a constellation of attitudes and behaviours including low morale, diminished commitment, heightened cynicism and mistrust and increased anger.

An increasing number of studies have examined hospital downsizing and restructuring in North America. These studies, without exception, highlight the presence of survivor sickness among nursing staff and raise questions about hospital functioning (Armstrong-Stassen, Cameron & Horsburgh, 1996; Burke & Greenglass, 2000; Baumann, O'Brien-Pallas, Deber, Donner, Semogas & Silverman, 1995; Davidson, 1997; Havlovic, Bouthillette & van der Wal, 1998; Richard Ivey School of Business, 1997; Woodward, Shannon, Cunningham, McIntosh, Lendrum, Rosenblum & Brown, 1999).

[*] *Correspondence: Ronald Burke, rburke@schulich.yorku.ca*

This research was supported in part by the Social Sciences and Humanities Research Council of Canada, the School of Business, York University and the Department of Psychology, York University. The study would not have been possible without the cooperation of the Ontario Nurses' Association. Esther Greenglass contributed to the design of the study, Graeme Macdermid participated in data collection and Lisa Fiksenbaum assisted with data analysis.

Many nurses believe that deterioration in working conditions has jeopardized patients' well-being. A survey (Dialogue on Health Reform, 1996) reports that 85% of 20,000 registered staff nurses, members of the Ontario Nurses' Association, believe that understaffing due to budget cuts and downsizing has reached the point that unsafe conditions exist for patients. Ninety-four percent believed that the health-care system needed reform. The impact on nurses of these changes has been considerable. With fewer qualified staff to care for patients, the workload for nurses has significantly increased (Baumann et al., 1995). Nurses are reporting higher stress levels, high job insecurity levels and poor morale (Baumann et. al., 1995). Work overload has been a significant predictor of job dissatisfaction and poor mental health outcomes in nurses (Armstrong-Stassen, Cameron & Horsburgh, 1996; Burke & Greenglass, 2000). RNs are increasingly being replaced by less well-trained practical nurses and nursing assistants. The increasing use of unregulated generic workers is an additional stressor for nurses (Richard Ivey School of Business, 1997).

Nurses' psychological well-being is deteriorating as a result of these wide-spread changes in the workplace. Nurses speak of the effects of layoffs on the surviving nurses in the system (Havlovic, Bouthillette & van der Wal, 1998). Working longer hours, doing more, missing breaks, dealing with concerned patients' families, nurses are worn down (Baumann et. al., 1995). Given the climate of widespread restructuring, downsizing and job cutbacks, job insecurity can be expected to be a major factor affecting nurses' psychological well-being.

This research has also identified particular restructuring and downsizing-related stressors which can influence nursing staff satisfaction and well-being as well as interfere with hospital effectiveness. For example, workload has emerged on an important stressor during these transitions (Armstrong-Stassen, Cameron & Horsburgh, 1996; Greenglass, Burke & Fiksenbaum, 2001). In addition, levels of hospital support provided to staff during these trying times has been found to have positive relationships with self-reported satisfaction and well-being among nursing staff (Burke & Greenglass, 2001).

Figure 1 presents the research framework used in this study. Five blocks of predictor variables were included and examined in a particular order. The first block of predictors ($n = 1$) was the 1996 measure of one of the three psychological burnout components (e. g., emotional exhaustion). The second block of predictors were individual demographic characteristics ($n = 6$) and included age, marital status and level of education. The third block consisted of work situation characteristics ($n = 5$) such as hospital size, years working in present unit and work-status (full-time and part-time). These three blocks were considered as control variables in the analyses of the data. The fourth block of predictors consisted of restructuring and downsizing stressors ($n = 3$)

and included workload as well as the effects of both nursing staff bumping procedures and the use of less qualified, lower paid nursing staff to perform more routine patient care duties. The final block of predictors included the measures of hospital and union support ($n = 2$).

Figure 1: Research framework

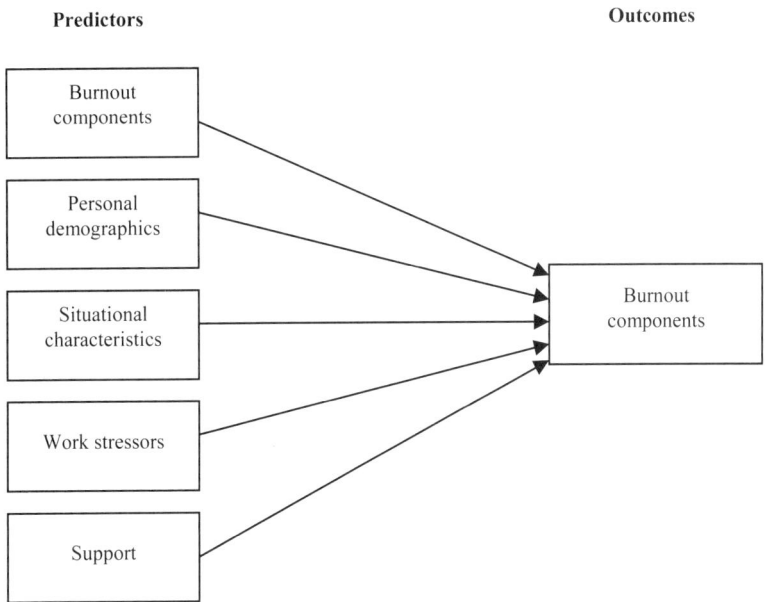

Predictors

Outcomes

- Burnout components
- Personal demographics
- Situational characteristics
- Work stressors
- Support

Burnout components

Method

Procedure

The sample is part of a longitudinal study of the effects of hospital restructuring and downsizing in Ontario on hospital-based nursing staff and their perceptions of hospital functioning. The first wave questionnaire was mailed in November 1996 to 3,892 randomly selected members of the Ontario Nurses' Association (total membership about 40,000) at their home addresses. The study was introduced as an independent research effort not as a union-sponsored initiative. This resulted in 1,363 completed and returned questionnaires, a response rate of 35% when questionnaires returned because the respondent had moved were eliminated. Three years later (November, 1999), a second survey was sent to the same 3,892 individuals at their 1996 addresses. A total of 925 questionnaires were returned, a 27% response rate, when questionnaires returned because the respondent had moved were eliminated. The relatively low response rate likely resulted from asking women responsible for household tasks to complete a lengthy questionnaire. Three sub-groups of respondents were present: individuals who were no longer employed any where in 1999 ($n = 107$), individuals who were employed in 1999 but no longer as hospital-based nursing staff ($n = 74$) and individuals still employed as hospital-based nursing staff in 1999 ($n = 744$). Three hundred and ninety-three staff nurses (53%) had completed questionnaires in 1996 and again in 1999 and form the basis of this study.

Respondents

Table 1 shows the demographics of the sample. There was considerable diversity on most items. Respondents were mainly women (97%), about one half of the sample worked full time, about half of the sample had some type of supervisory duties, over 80% had an RN degree-either college or hospital based, about 80% were married or living with a partner and about 84% had children. On average, respondents had been employed in their current units about 9 years and in their current hospital about 15 years. The average age of respondents was 45. Respondents lived and worked in communities and hospitals of various sizes. Finally, respondents worked in a variety of nursing units, with about two-thirds in medical/surgical, intensive care/coronary, emergency and obstetrics. The 1996 and 1999 samples were representative of the overall union membership in terms of age, gender and full-time versus part-time work status.

Table 1: 1996 Demographic characteristics

	N	%		N	%
Nursing unit			**Marital status**		
Medical/surgical	99	25. 4	Married, living together	313	79. 8
Intensive care/coronary	68	17. 4	Single, widowed, divorced, separated	79	20. 2
Emergency	46	11. 8	**Education**		
Obstetrics	40	10. 3	RNA diploma	7	1. 8
Continuing care/Geriatrics	26	6. 7	RN – college	193	49. 2
Operating room	25	6. 4	RN – hospital	131	33. 4
Pediatrics	23	6. 2	BA	59	15. 0
Psychology	22	5. 9	MA	2	. 5
Oncology	19	4. 9	**Years in unit**		
Recovery room	16	4. 1	1-5	103	26. 3
Medical/Surgical short stay	12	3. 1	6-10	133	34. 1
Other	79	20. 2	11-15	78	19. 9
Children			16-20	38	9. 7
Yes	328	83. 5	Over 20	39	10. 0
No	65	16. 5	**Age**		
Community size			Under 25	5	1. 2
1,000,000+	48	12. 6	26-35	101	26. 6
500,000-1,000,000	41	10. 8	36-45	142	37. 4
250,000-500,000	86	22. 6	46-55	108	28. 5
100,000-250,000	65	17. 1	56 and over	24	6. 3
50,000-100,000	68	17. 8	**Years in hospital**		
Less than 50,000	73	19. 2	1-5	27	6. 9
Sex			6-10	117	29. 8
Women	379	97. 4	11-15	85	21. 7
Men	10	2. 6	16-20	70	17. 9
Work status			over 20	93	23. 7
Full time	193	49. 7	**Years in nursing**		
Part time	195	50. 3	1-5	16	4. 1
Supervision duties			6-10	54	13. 8
Yes	184	47. 3	11-15	85	21. 6
No	205	52. 7	16-20	73	16. 7
Hospital size – beds			Over 20	164	41. 8
400+	93	23. 8	**Changed units**		
251-400	116	29. 7	Yes	56	14. 4
151-250	81	20. 8	No	332	85. 6
125-150	27	6. 9			
Less than 125	73	18. 7			

Measures

Psychological burnout components

Emotional exhaustion was measured by five items (α = .90), part of the General Burnout Questionnaire, developed by Schaufeli, Leiter, Maslach and Jackson (1996). Respondents indicated how often they experienced particular feelings on a seven point scale (0 = never, 6 = every day). A sample item was "I felt emotionally drained from my work".

Professional efficacy was measured by a six-item scale (α = .73), from the General Burnout Questionnaire. One item was "At my work, I felt confident that I am effective at getting things done".

Cynicism was measured by a five-item scale (α = .82) from the General Burnout Questionnaire. "I have become more cynical about whether my work contributes anything".

Personal and Situational Demographics were measured by a variety of single item measures. These included: years employed on current nursing unit, years employed in present hospital, years employed as a staff nurse in a hospital setting, whether job included supervisory duties, current nursing unit, whether respondent had changed units during the past year, size of hospital (i.e., number of beds), size of community where hospital was located, hours worked per week, highest level of education qualification, marital status, parental status and gender.

Restructuring and Downsizing Stressors

Workload was measured by four items (α = .69). "The changes on my unit have made my job more demanding". "My workload has increased as a result of the lack of resources".

Staff Bumping, the replacement of shorter-tenured nursing staff or the longer-tenured nursing staff, was measured by three items (α = .57). Respondents indicated their agreement with each statement (1 = strongly agree, 3 = neither agree nor disagree, 5 = strongly disagree). One item was "Changes in nursing staff as a result of bumping have had a negative effect on patient care". Nurses with more hospital tenure were given priority over nurses with less hospital tenure in the event of job loss.

Impact of Generic Workers was measured by two items (α = .69). Respondents indicated their agreement with each on a five point scale. A sample item was "The use of generic workers to perform nursing duties has resulted in a deterioration of patient care".

Support

Hospital support was measured by an eight item scale ($\alpha = .91$) taken from Eisenberger, Huntington, Hutchinson and Sowa (1986). Respondents indicated their agreement with each item on a seven point scale (1 = strongly disagree, 7 = strongly agree). Items included: "This hospital really cares about my well-being". "This hospital values my contribution to its well-being".

Union support was measured by four items ($\alpha = .77$). Respondents indicated their agreement with each item on a 5 point scale. One item was "My union in this hospital improves working conditions for nurses".

Results

Testing the Research Framework

The research framework (see Figure 1) was tested using hierarchical multiple regression analysis. The first variable entered was the 1996 measure of a particular psychological burnout component (e. g., emotional exhaustion). The second block of variables entered were personal demographics ($n = 6$). The third block of predictors entered were the work situation characteristics ($n = 5$). These three blocks of predictors served as control variables, before considering the relationships of work stressors and measures of support on the 1999 measures of psychological burnout. The fourth block of predictors were the work stressors likely to be influenced by the restructuring and downsizing ($n = 3$). The final block of predictors were the measures of hospital and union support ($n = 2$).

When a block of predictors accounted for a significant amount or increment in explained variance ($p < .05$), specific measures within such blocks having independent and significant relationships with a criterion measure ($p < .05$) were reported along with their respective βs.

Regression Analyses

Table 2 shows the results of hierarchical regression analyses in which the three psychological burnout components were separately regressed on the five blocks of predictors (see Figure 1).

Table 2: Predictors of 1999 Psychological burnout

Burnout components	R	R^2	ΔR^2	p
Emotional exhaustion (*n* = 343)				
Emotional exhaustion (. 40)	. 52	. 27	. 27	. 001
Personal demographics	. 53	. 28	. 01	NS
Situational characteristics	. 53	. 28	. 00	NS
Work stressors	. 62	. 38	. 00	. 001
Workload (. 29)				
Support	. 63	. 40	. 02	. 05
Hospital (-. 12)				
Professional efficacy (*n* = 343)				
Professional efficacy (. 38)	. 41	. 17	. 17	. 001
Personal demographics	. 44	. 17	. 02	NS
Situational characteristics	. 45	. 20	. 01	NS
Work stressors	. 45	. 20	. 00	NS
Support	. 48	. 23	. 03	. 01
Hospital (. 18)				
Cynicism (*n* = 343)				
Cynicism (. 44)	. 53	. 28	. 28	. 001
Personal demographics	. 53	. 28	. 00	NS
Situational characteristics	. 54	. 29	. 01	NS
Work stressors	. 57	. 33	. 04	. 001
Workload (. 17)				
Support	. 60	. 36	. 03	. 001
Hospital (-. 18)				

The following comments are offered in summary. First, each 1996 measure of a particular burnout component had significant and positive relationships within their 1999 measure. Second, personal demographic factors and work situation characteristics failed to account for significant increments in explained variance on any of the burnout components. Third, work stressors associated with hospital restructuring accounted for significant increments in explained variance on two of the burnout components (emotional exhaustion, cynicism). Workload had significant and independent relationships with both of these burnout components (β = .29 and .17 respectively). Finally the support variables accounted for a significant increment in explained variance under three burnout components. Hospital support had independent and significant relationship with all three burnout components (β = .12, emotional exhaustion; β = .18, professional efficacy; β = -.18, cynicism).

Two other observations are worth noting. First, the 1996 measure of a given burnout component was the strongest predictor of this measure three years later. This pattern suggests a good deal of stability in these measures over the three year time period. Second, workload and hospital support had generally consistent relationships with the 1999 burnout components, but in opposite directions as hypothesized.

Discussion

The research framework underlying the study received considerable support and findings consistent with those of other researchers. First, psychological burnout levels were fairly consistent over time and nursing staff indicating higher burnout in 1996 were also more likely to report greater burnout in 1999. Others have observed stability in burnout components over time, typically over a shorter time period (see Schaufeli & Enzmann, 1998). An organization that makes no effort to address the causes of burnout is likely to face consistent levels of self-reported burnout overtime.

In addition, consistent with other research results (e. g., Armstrong-Stassen, Cameron & Horsburgh, 1996; Greenglass, Burke & Fiksenbaum, 2001), workload issues, along with levels of organizational support during the transition process, influenced levels of burnout (also see Burke & Leiter, 2000). Thus, particular experiences of nursing staff during hospital restructuring and downsizing are likely to have important effects on nursing staff reactions to these transitions and their well-being.

Specific findings were consistent with previous conclusions (Schaufeli & Enzmann, 1998). Thus, exhaustion was related to workload (a job demand) and efficacy was related to hospital support (a resource) while cynicism was related to both.

Hospital support as predicted was found to reduce the effects of job demands on burnout components. Union support produced no such effects. The healthcare restructuring was implemented in a top-down unilateral manger. The role of the nurses union was to ensure that changes in job assignments and job losses were consistent with the terms of the collective agreement. In essence the nurses union had little power and influence in the restructuring and downsizing exercise.

What needs to be done now?

First, the health care system needs to understand the events of the past five years and how these have impacted on hospitals and their staffs. Second, a commitment needs to be made by the health care system and hospital leadership to rebuild staff morale that has been damaged in this process (Nelson & Burke, 1998). Third, efforts and resources must be devoted to revitalizing hospitals, units and staff (Aiken, Smith & Lake, 1994). This is a long term process (Burke & Nelson, 1997; Noer, 1993).

Hospitals are then faced with the huge challenge of turning around nursing staff reactions to previous restructuring and downsizing initiatives that were managed in a top-down, unilateral way, lacking a clear vision of what the hospital was doing, why and where it was heading, with minimal effort to rebuild badly damaged staff morale, tattered levels of trust and reconfigured nursing units (Marmor, 1998; Reinhardt, 1996).

Some practical suggestions can be developed. Senior hospital leadership must embrace and champion efforts to revitalize their organizations (Sochalski & Aiken, 1999). Such efforts will necessarily involve time, money and other resources. The involvement of staff associations or unions in such initiatives has considerable merit. The acknowledgement of the present circumstances and the articulation of what the hospital would like to achieve must be clear and reinforced. Various forums to convey these messages must be created.

Hospital support has emerged as perhaps the most significant single factor in helping nursing staff handle these difficult transitions. Nursing staff, more than any other group within the hospital, have been disproportionately affected by these changes (Saltman & Figueras, 1998). Critical elements include a respect for staff, being responsive to staff needs and suggestions and investing in them (Baer, Fagin & Gordon, 1996). There is likely to be a need for management and supervisory development in support of this priority.

References

Aiken, L. H. & Fagin, C. M. (1997). Evaluating the consequences of hospital restructuring. *Medical Care, 35*, 1-4.

Aiken, L. H., Sochalski, J. & Anderson, G. F. (1996). Downsizing the hospital nursing workforce. *Health Affairs, 15*, 88-92.

Aiken, L. H., Smith, H. L. & Lake, E. T. (1994). Lower medicare mortality among a set of hospitals known for good nursing care. *Medical Care, 32*, 721-787.

Armstrong-Stassen, M., Cameron, S. J. & Horsburgh, M. E. (1996). The impact of organizational downsizing on the job satisfaction of nurses. *Canadian Journal of Nursing Administration, 9*, 8-32.

Baer, E. D., Fagin, C. M. & Gordon, S. (1996). *Abandonment of the patient: The impact of profit-driven health care on the public.* New York: Springer.

Baumann, A., O'Brien-Pallas, L., Deber, R., Donner, R., Semogas, D. & Silverman, B. (1995). The process of downsizing in selected Ontario acute care hospitals: Budget reduction strategies and planning process. *Quality of Worklife Research Unit. University of Toronto, Working Paper series*, 95-4.

Burke, R. J. & Greenglass, E. R. (2000). Organizational restructuring: Identifying effective hospital downsizing processes. In R. J. Burke & C. L. Cooper (Eds.), *The organization in crisis* (pp. 284-303). London: Blackwell Publishers.

Burke, R. J. & Greenglass, E. R. (2001). Hospital restructuring and nursing staff well-being: The role of perceived hospital and union support. *Anxiety, Stress and Coping, 14*, 93-115.

Burke, R. J. & Leiter, M. P. (2000). Contemporary organizational realities and professional efficacy: Downsizing, reorganization and transition. In P. Dewe, M. P. Leiter & T. Cox (Eds), *Coping and health in organizations* (pp. 232-258). London: Taylor & Francis.

Burke, R. J. & Nelson, D. L. (1997). Downsizing and restructuring: Lessons from the firing line for revitalizing organizations. *Leadership and Organization Development Journal, 18*, 325-334.

Burke, R. J. & Nelson, D. L. (1998). Downsizing, restructuring and privatization: A North American perspective. In M. K. Gowing, J. D. Kraft & J. C. Quick (Eds), *The new organizational reality: Downsizing, restructuring and revitalization* (pp.21-54). Washington, D. C.: American Psychological Association.

Cameron, K. S., Whetten D. A. & Kim, M. U (1987). Organizational effects of decline and turbulence. *Administrative Science Quarterly, 32*, 222-240.

Cascio, W. F. (1993). Downsizing: What do we know? What have we learned? *Academy of Management Executive, 7*, 95-104.

Cascio, W. F. (1998). Learning from outcomes: Financial experiences of 311 firms that have downsized. In M. K. Gowing, J. D. Kraft & J. C. Quick (Eds.), *The new organizational realty: Downsizing, restructuring and revitalization* (pp. 55-70). Washington, D. C.: American Psychological Association.

Davidson, H. (1997). The effects of health care reform on job satisfaction and voluntary turnover among hospital-based nurses. *Medical Care, 35*, 634-645.

Dialogue on Health Reform (1996). Toronto: Ontario Nurses'Association.

Eisenberger, R., Huntington, R., Hutchison, S. H. & Sowa, D. (1986). Perceived organizational support. *Journal of Applied Psychology, 71*, 500-507.

Greenglass, E. R., Burke, R. J. & Fiksenbaum, L. (2001). Workload and burnout in nurses. *Journal of Applied and Community Psychology, 11*, 211-215.

Havlovic, S. J. Bouthillette, F. & van der Wal, R. (1998). Coping with downsizing and job loss: Lessons from the Shaugnessy Hospital closure. *Canadian Journal of Administrative Studies, 15*, 325-332.

Kets de Vries, M. F. R. & Balazs, K. (1997). The downside of downsizing. *Human Relations, 50*, 11-50.

Marmor, T. R. (1998). Hope and hyperbole: The rhetoric and reality of managerial reform in health care. *Journal of Health Services Research and Policy, 3*, 62-64.

Nelson, D. L. & Burke, R. J. (1998). Lessons learned. *Canadian Journal of Administrative Sciences, 15*, 372-381.

Noer, D. (1993). *Healing the wounds: Overcoming the trauma of layoffs and revitalizing downsized organizations.* San Francisco: Jossey-Bass.

Reinhardt, V. E. (1996). Spending more through 'cost control': Our obsessive quest to gut the hospital. *Health Affairs, 15*, 145-154.

Richard Ivey School of Business (1997). *Leading the management of change: A study of 12 Ontario hospitals.* London, Ont: Richard Ivey School of Business.

Saltman, R. B. & Figueras, J. (1998). Analyzing the evidence on European health care reforms. *Health Affairs, 17*, 85-108.

Sochalski, J. & Aiken, L. H. (1999). Accounting for variation in hospital outcomes: A cross-national study. *Health Affairs, 18*, 68-82.

Sochalski, J., Aiken, L. H. & Fagin, C. M. (1997). Hospital restructuring in the United States, Canada, and Western Europe: An outcomes research agenda. *Medical Care, 35*, 13-25.

Schaufeli, W. S. & Enzmann, D. (1998). *The Burnout companion to study and practice: A critical analysis.* London: Taylor & Francis.

Schaufeli, W. S., Leiter, M. P., Maslach, C. & Jackson, S. E. (1996). *MBI – General Survey.* Palo Alto, CA.: Consulting Psychologist Press, Inc.

White, K. (1997). Hospital restructuring in North America and Europe. *Medical Care, 35*, 7-12.

Woodward, C. A., Shannon, H. S., Cunningham, C., McIntosh, J., Lendrum, B., Rosenblum D. & Brown, J. (1999). The impact of re-engineering and other cost reductions strategies on the staff of a large teaching hospital. *Medical Care, 37*, 556-569.

Withdrawal and burnout in health care: On the mediating role of lack of reciprocity

Wilmar Schaufeli[*1], *Vicente González-Romá*[2], *José-Maria Peiró*[2], *Sabine Geurts*[3] *& Inés Tomás*[2]

[1] *Department of Social and Organizational Psychology, Utrecht University, The Netherlands*
[2] *Research Unit on Work and Organizational Psychology, University of Valencia, Spain*
[3] *Department of Work and Organizational Psychology, University of Nijmegen, The Netherlands*

The main purpose of this article is to illustrate the role that a lack of reciprocity between employee's investments and outcomes plays in the development of burnout and withdrawal. Buunk and Schaufeli (1999) have pointed out that reciprocity plays a key role in social and organizational life, and that establishing reciprocal relationships is essential for the individual's health and well-being. They argue that the strong and universal preference for reciprocal relationships is a deeply rooted psychological mechanism that may have fostered survival and reproductive success in our evolutionary past. The notion of reciprocity is also crucial in equity theory (Adams, 1965) that postulates that employees pursue equity in their exchange with the organization. That is, employees agree to make specific contributions to an organization (e.g., skills, experience, time, and effort) for which they expect the organization to provide benefits (e.g., payment, fringe benefits, promotion prospects, and a supportive climate) that are proportional to their contributions. Classic equity theory (Adams, 1965) assumes that people's evaluation of the balance between investments and benefits is primarily based on *social* comparisons, that is, comparisons with real or hypothetical others. Pritchard (1969), however, argued that inequity could easily well arise from the lack of correspondence between investments and benefits relative to one's own *internal* standards, or between demands and resources, for that matter. Following Pritchard's line of reasoning, we define reciprocity as the equality of perceived investments and benefits *relative to one's internal standards* (*cf.* Schaufeli, Van Dierendonck & Van Gorp, 1996). A lack of reciprocity is experienced when the costs of the exchange with the organization outweigh

---

[*] *Correspondence: Wilmar Schaufeli, w.schaufeli@fss.uu.nl*

The writing of this paper was supported by a grant from the Spanish Ministry of Education and Culture (#SAB1998-0206).

the benefits received back in return: in that case the expectation of reciprocity remains unfulfilled.

Mental bookkeeping

Theories on job stress often assume that a discrepancy or mismatch between some kinds of investments and benefits, or demands and resources *directly* leads to poor employee health and well-being, without assuming intermediate cognitive processes. For instance, the Effort-Reward Imbalance (ERI) model (Siegrist, 1998, p.192) claims that "...lack of reciprocity between costs and gains (i.e., high cost/low gain conditions) defines a state of emotional distress (...) and associated strain reactions", but lack of reciprocity is not included in the model as a mediator. Instead it is assumed that an imbalance between efforts (i.e., high job demands) and rewards (i.e., salary, esteem, job stability, promotion prospects) directly leads to autonomic arousal and associated physical strain reactions such as cardiovascular disease, as well as to burnout (Bakker, Killmer, Siegrist & Schaufeli, 2000). In a similar vein, the Job De- mand-Control-Support (JDCS) model (Karasek & Theorell, 1990) assumes that the interplay between high job demands and poor job control directly leads to psychological strain, such as burnout (De Rijk, Le Blanc, Schaufeli & De Jonge, 1998). Again, without including an intermediate cognitive process variable such as lack of reciprocity into the model. In sum: both models as- sume that the discrepancy between efforts and rewards (ERI) or between demands and resources (JDCS) is responsible for poor employee health and well-being (e.g., burnout) but they do *not* assume a cognitive evaluative proc- ess that assesses the relative impact of the positive (i.e., rewards, resources) and the negative (i.e., efforts, demands) characteristics of the job.

We believe that including reciprocity as a process variable into job stress models may help to illuminate the psychological mechanisms involved. Basi- cally, we assume that an employee's global sense of reciprocity results from his or her 'mental bookkeeping' of costs and gains that go into and result from the relationship with the organization. Job demands are considered 'investments' in the sense that they require the expenditure of effort, time, energy, and skill, whereas, for instance, supportive leadership behavior is viewed as a 'benefit' that results from the exchange relationship with the organization. These two variables are selected in the present study because job demands and social support play a crucial role in most job stress models, including the ERI-model and the JDCS-model.

In case the result of the 'mental bookkeeping' is negative, that is, when a lack of reciprocity is experienced (whether or not after various failed attempts to restore the balance), employees may nevertheless not wish to leave the or- ganization. The choice for this coping strategy – leaving the field – will namely depend, among other things, on the perceived availability of alternative employment opportunities (Rusbult & Farrell, 1983). When employees perceive barriers to leave the work situation, for instance because of high unemployment rates, they are 'forced' to stay in their jobs. At the time the current study was carried out unemployment rates in Spain were quite high. According to the Statistical National Institute, in the year that the current study was conducted 32% of the working population in the service sector was unemployed. So that it is likely that many employees in our study were 'locked in' their jobs. In addition, other pull factors may play a similar role, such as a high need for secure jobs. Typically, Spanish employees strongly favor stable, tenured jobs in the civil service. For instance, 62% of a representative sample of Spanish workers indicated that job security was "(very) important" to them so that job security ranked second on a list containing fifteen job characteristics, just after a good income (Orizo, 1991). In addition, 65% of a representative sample aged between 16 and 30 years from the Valencian region, where the current study was carried out preferred a job as a civil servant to a permanent contract in a private enterprise (Garcia-Montalvo, Pieró & Soro, 2003).

Consequences of perceived lacking reciprocity

When employees experience a lack of reciprocity at work, they not only will feel bad but they will also be motivated to restore the balance (Adams, 1965). More specifically, cognitive withdrawal (i.e., turnover intention and reduced commitment) as well as behavioral withdrawal (i.e., absenteeism) are means available to restore reciprocity. For instance, in their social-psychological theory of absenteeism Chadwick-Jones, Nicholson and Brown (1982) argued that absenteeism should be considered as negative exchange behavior: employees are withholding their presence from work to make up for workload pressures, stress, or other negative aspects of their jobs. Indeed, several studies have shown that employees report sick more often the greater the lack of reciprocity they perceive in their exchange with the organization (e.g., Geurts, Buunk & Schaufeli, 1994a; 1994b).

In addition to behavioral withdrawal, lacking reciprocity is also expected to lead to cognitive withdrawal; i.e., propensity to leave the job and reduced organizational commitment. From a social exchange perspective it can be assumed that the more employees feel that their investments into the organization outweigh the benefits they received back in return, the less attached they will feel to the organization and thus the more they will reduce their levels of commitment and the more they will be willing to leave the organization. This was supported by Syroit, Lodewijkx, Franssen and Gertsel (1993), who found that employees reduced their levels of organizational commitment in response to unfulfilled expectations of reciprocity in the employment relationship. Furthermore, Geurts, Schaufeli and Rutte (1999) observed a direct relationship between lack of reciprocity and registered absenteeism, whereas an indirect effect was observed (via feelings of resentment) on poor organizational commitment and turnover intention. In a somewhat similar vein, studies on organizational fairness have provided empirical support for poor organizational commitment as reaction to perceived unfairness in organizations (e.g., Rutte & Messick, 1995). Finally, it has been shown that lack of reciprocity is positively related to intention to leave the organization (e.g., Rosin & Korabik, 1995).

As noted before, a lack of reciprocity is also associated with psychological strain. More specifically, we expect that a lack of reciprocity is positively related to burnout. In accordance with the literature, we conceive burnout as a multidimensional construct that consists of emotional exhaustion, depersonalization, and reduced personal accomplishment (Maslach, Schaufeli & Leiter, 2001). Emotional exhaustion refers to the depletion of emotional resources in response to high job demands; depersonalization refers to an impersonal and cynical attitude towards recipients of one's care; and reduced personal accomplishment refers to the tendency to evaluate oneself negatively with regards to one's accomplishments at work. Buunk and Schaufeli (1993, 1999) have argued that lacking reciprocity in interpersonal caregiver-recipient relationships as well as in employee-organization relationships is related to burnout. They point out that investing in a social exchange relationship without receiving appropriate outcomes is frustrating and highly energy consuming. The resulting emotional exhaustion is dealt with by reducing investments, that is, by developing a detached, cynical, and impersonal ('depersonalized') attitude in an attempt to restore reciprocity. An attitude like this is dysfunctional because it increases failures, deteriorates work performance and thus fosters a sense of diminished personal accomplishment. A series of studies among nurses, mental health care professionals, teachers, police officers, prison guards, and mental retardation staff have confirmed the positive relationship between lacking reciprocity with the organization and burnout (for an overview see Buunk & Schaufeli, 1999).

The research model

In figure 1 our research model is displayed. The signs indicate the expected direction of the relationships.

As can be seen from figure 1, not only indirect paths via lack of reciprocity are assumed, but also *direct* paths linking demands and burnout, and linking supportive leadership and cognitive withdrawal, respectively. In other words the model assumes that lack of reciprocity '*partially*_mediates' the relationship between job demands and supportive leadership on the one hand, and cognitive and behavioral (i.e., absenteeism) withdrawal and burnout on the other hand.

Figure 1: The research model

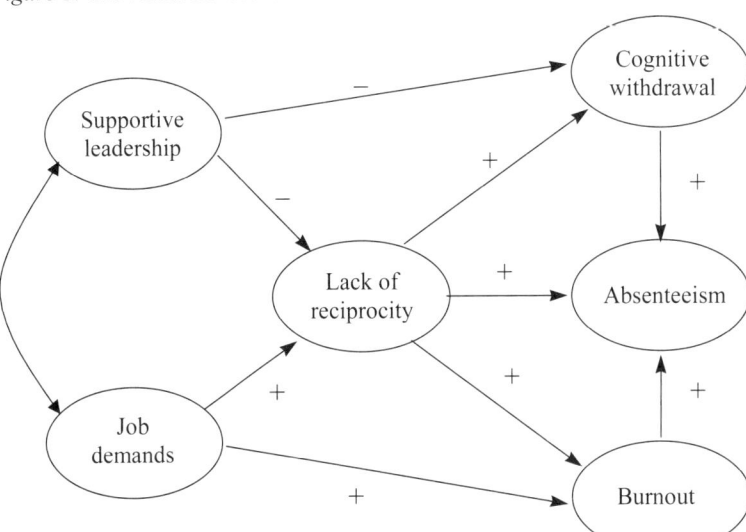

Job demands such as work-overload and role problems have been identified as major determinants of various stress reactions or strains, including burnout (for overviews see; Lee & Ashforth, 1996; Schaufeli & Enzmann, 1998, pp. 82-83). In addition, because of the particular relevance for the medical setting, the present study includes environmental demands such as poor physical climate and the exposure to toxic substances, radiation, and biological agents (Tan, 1991). Thus, we expect a positive relationship between job demands and burnout (see figure 1).

Research findings also suggest that supportive leadership behaviors are associated with stronger organizational commitment (e.g., Glisson & Durick, 1988), and a lower propensity to leave the organization (Rosin & Korabik, 1995). Thus, we expect that supportive leadership is negatively related to cognitive withdrawal from the organization (see figure 1).

Our research model not only assumes that lack of reciprocity is related to absenteeism, but also that cognitive withdrawal is affecting levels of absenteeism. Based on the so-called withdrawal model of absenteeism (Johns, 1997) it is expected that the loosening of the attachment to the organization precedes actual absenteeism. Indeed, several meta-analyses report sample-sized-weighted correlations between organizational commitment and absenteeism that range from -0.10 to -0.12 (e.g., Mathieu & Zajac, 1990). Hence, a weak positive relationship is expected between cognitive withdrawal and absenteeism.

Finally, our research model assumes that burned-out employees are more likely to be absent because their symptoms – particularly emotional exhaustion – interfere with attendance at the job. It has been found across ten studies (Schaufeli & Enzmann, 1998, p. 91) that the relationship between absenteeism and emotional exhaustion is most consistent (r's about .15), followed by depersonalization (r's about .10). Reduced personal accomplishment was related to absenteeism only in three studies with an average explained variance less than 1%. Accordingly, we expect small, positive effects of burnout on absenteeism.

Gender differences

Our study includes male as well as female health-care workers. It seems that structural differences exist in the absence behaviors of men and women. For instance, VandenHeuvel and Wooden (1995) report that absence behavior of women is more sensitive to external pressure to the workplace, whilst absence behavior of males is more sensitive to factors internal to the workplace. Results from a large-scale epidemiological study seem to concur with these findings since it was observed that low levels of job control, job demands, and social support were associated with higher rates of sickness absenteeism among males, but not among females (North, Syme, Feeney, Shipley & Marmot, 1996). Although it seems that absenteeism is related to different factors in male and female employees, study results are not entirely conclusive. Therefore, we will investigate our research model also separately for each sex.

Method

Participants and procedure

A sample of 1,000 subjects was drawn from a population of 35,805 employees who were employed by the Regional Public Health Service (RPHS) in the Valencian region in Spain by means of a two-stage randomized procedure. In the first stage, 250 work teams were randomly selected. Next, in the second stage, four members of each work team were sampled; one of them being the team supervisor, the remaining three were randomly selected from the team. A professional interviewing agency approached about 1,000 employees on their jobs and asked them to fill out the questionnaire. The total number of usable questionnaires returned was 932.

Team supervisors responded to a slightly different questionnaire in which items on supervisor's supportive behaviors were worded as self-perceptions (i.e., "I coach my employees adequately so that they can do a proper job") rather than as employees' perceptions (i.e., "Your supervisor coaches you so that you can do your job properly"). Because our research model includes supportive leadership behaviors as perceived by subordinates, team supervisors are excluded, leaving a total sample of 721 non-supervisor employees. Female respondents who were on maternity leave were excluded (see below), so that a final sample of $n = 715$ remained. With regard to gender, 63.1% of these employees were women. The study sample average age was 41.1 years ($SD = 9.6$), and the average organizational tenure was 14.3 years ($SD = 8.3$). Twenty-three percent were physicians, 33% were nurses, 15% were nursing auxiliaries, 14% were maintenance personnel, and the remaining 15% worked in administrative or technical jobs.

Measures

Supportive leadership behaviors (SLB). Following Yukl (1990), three supportive leadership behaviors were measured: acknowledgment, consideration and communication. Each type of behavior was measured by three items: the *acknowledgment* scale refers to the extent to which the supervisor acknowledges the employees' efforts, work outcomes, and initiatives (e.g., "My supervisor acknowledges my initiatives for improving work"). The *consideration* scale refers to the extent to which the supervisor shows interest in subordinates and trusts them (e.g., "My supervisor shows interest in us as persons"). The *communication* scale indicates the extent to which the supervisor informs subordinates about the organization, the job, and other relevant issues (e.g., "My supervisor informs us about the issues that may affect us"). Each employee was asked to rate his/her supervisor using a 5-point Likert scale ranging from 1 (*'strongly disagree'*) to 5 (*'strongly agree'*). Cronbach's α of the three SLB scales were as follows: acknowledgment: 0.94, consideration: 0.89, and communication: 0.89.

Job demands. Two scales were used to measure different job demands. The first 3-item scale (Camman, Fichman, Jenkins & Klesh, 1979) assessed perceived *work overload* (e.g., "The amount of work I have to do is excessive"). Items were scored on a 5-point Likert scale ranging from 1(*'strongly disagree'*) to 5 (*'strongly agree'*). Cronbach's α for this scale was 0.83. The second scale assessed perceived job stress and consisted of 11 items that were selected from the Occupational Stress Indicator (OSI; Cooper, Sloan & Williams 1988). Subjects were asked to indicate how demanding different aspects of their jobs are, such as the physical work environment (e.g., noise, heat), shift work, poor work team climate, and the risk of being exposed to radiation, toxic substances, or biological agents. Items were scored on a 5-point Likert scale ranging from 1 (*'not at all'*) to 5 (*'very much'*). In order to investigate the dimensionality of the job stress scale, a principal component analysis with subsequent varimax rotation was carried out that included all 11 items of the scale. Two components emerged with Eigenvalues greater than 1 explaining 48% of the variance in total. Six items that referred to role stress (i.e., role conflict and role ambiguity) and to the social-communicative aspects of the job (i.e., the organization's political gossip, discrimination, and favoritism) loaded high (i.e., equal or greater than 0.50) on the first component that was labeled *organizational demands*. The remaining five items that referred to various working conditions (physical dangers, poor environmental conditions shift work, and physical and mental effort) loaded high on the second component that was labeled *demanding_working conditions*. The α coefficient for the first component was 0.83, whereas it was slightly lower for the second component (0.66).

Perceived lack of reciprocity was measured by a 3-item scale that was used previously in studies on absenteeism (e.g., Geurts, Schaufeli & Buunk, 1993) and burnout (e.g., Van Dierendonck, Schaufeli & Buunk, 1996): (1) "I invest more in my work than what I get out of it"; "Considering what I'm paid for my work, I put too much effort into it"; "What I do in my work is in balance with what I'm paid for" (reversed). Subjects responded using a 5-point Likert scale ranging from 1 (*'strongly disagree'*) to 5 (*'strongly agree'*). The α coefficient was 0.76.

Burnout. For reasons of economy, all three burnout dimensions (i.e., *emotional exhaustion, depersonalization and lack of personal accomplishment*) were measured by three items each. Items were selected from the Maslach Burnout Inventory (Maslach & Jackson, 1986) on their face-validity (Peiró, González-Romá, Tordera & Mañas, 2001). The response scale ranged from 1 (*'never'*) to 5 (*'always'*). Cronbach's α for the three scales were 0.79 (emotional exhaustion), 0.71 (depersonalization) and 0.76 (lack of personal accomplishment).

Cognitive withdrawal was assessed by three indicators: propensity to leave the organization, propensity to leave the unit, and poor organizational commitment. *Propensity to leave the organization* was measured by a 3-item self-constructed scale (e.g., "If a private health care organization would offer me a job with the same pay and status that I have now, I would quit my present job") with a 5-point Likert answering format ranging from 1 (*'strongly disagree'*) to 5 (*'strongly agree'*). Coefficient α was 0.69. *Propensity to leave the unit* was measured by a single item ("When I'm offered the same job conditions, I'd rather work in a different RPHS unit"), using a similar response scale. *Organizational commitment* was measured by three items (e.g., "I share the goals of my organization") that were selected from the scale developed by O'Reilly and Chatman (1986). The response scale was identical to the one used in both propensity to leave scales. Coefficient α was 0.82.

Absence frequency (i.e., the number of absence episodes during the previous 18 months preceding the interview as registered in the organization's files) was chosen as an indicator of behavioral withdrawal. Absence frequency measures are more stable than time lost measures and it is believed that the former best reflects voluntary absence; that is, absences in which employees have some freedom of choice in deciding whether or not to stay away from work (Hammer & Landau, 1981). For administrative reasons only absences longer than two days were registered into the RPHS personnel files because under the current law, all absences longer than two days have to be certified by the employee's family physician. Spanish employees are fully financially compensated for their absence at work. As noted before, female respondents who were on maternity leave were excluded from further analysis.

Because the distribution of absenteeism measures was truncated, the absence frequency measure showed high levels of kurtosis (5.84) and skewness (2.13). Therefore, the following transformation was applied: ln (absence frequency + 1) (Aiken & West, 1991). After this transformation levels of kurtosis (0.13) and skewness (.98) were acceptable for using the estimation method described below.

Analysis

Structural equation modeling (SEM) methods as implemented by LISREL 8 (Jöreskog & Sörbom, 1993) were used to test the hypothesized model. Maximum likelihood (ML) estimation methods were used and the input for each analysis was the variables covariance matrix. As the ML method assumes multivariate normal observed variables, this distributional assumption of the data was tested. The tests of univariate and multivariate normality yielded by PRELIS 2.30 indicated that the observed variables could not be considered as strictly normal. However, simulation studies that have analyzed the robustness of ML estimators to violations of distributional assumptions when the observed variables are discrete (e.g., Muthén & Kaplan, 1985) reported that when the sample sizes are reasonable, the non-normality of the data is not expected to produce incorrect parameter estimates. Moreover, not much distortion of the ML χ^2 goodness-of-fit statistic is to be expected with non-normal ordered categorical variables, if they show a moderate departure from normality, that is, most variables having univariate skewness and kurtosis in the range -1.0 to +1.0 (Muthén & Kaplan, 1985). All the variables in our study but one showed a moderate departure from normality; only propensity to leave the unit showed a kurtosis statistic (-1.15) outside the aforementioned range.

The goodness-of-fit of the models was evaluated using absolute and relative indices. The absolute goodness-of-fit indices calculated were the χ^2 goodness-of-fit statistic, the Adjusted Goodenss-of-Fit Index (AGFI, Jöreskog & Sörbom, 1989), and the Root Mean Square Error of Approximation (RMSEA, Browne & Cudeck, 1993). For AGFI no critical values exist, whereas values for RMSEA smaller than 0.08 are indicative of an acceptable fit, and values greater than 0.1 should lead to model rejection (Browne & Cudeck, 1993). The relative goodness-of-fit indices computed were the Non-Normed Fit Index (NNFI) and the Comparative Fit Index (CFI), the two incremental fit indices recommended by Marsh, Balla and Hau (1996). For both indices, values greater than 0.90 are considered as indicating a good fit (Hoyle, 1995).

Before testing the hypothesized structural model (see figure 1), we tested the implied measurement model to ascertain whether the observed variables measured by means of questionnaires were adequate indicators of their corre-sponding latent variables, and whether these latent variables could be consid-ered distinct constructs (Anderson & Gerbing, 1988). The measurement model showed an adequate fit to data ($\chi^2 = 331.5$, $df = 80$, $p < 0.01$; AGFI = 0.91; RMSEA = 0.069; CFI = 0.93; NNFI = 0.91). The parameter estimates obtained revealed that the model latent variables were discriminable con-structs, and that all factor loadings were statistically significant ($p < 0.01$), except the loading of lack of personal accomplishment ($\lambda = 0.01$[1]). Therefore, this observed variable was removed from the measurement (and further) model(s). When the measurement model was re-estimated, a slightly im-proved goodness-of-fit indices was obtained ($\chi^2 = 216.9$, $df = 67$, $p < 0.01$; AGFI = 0.93; RMSEA = 0.057; CFI = 0.96; NNFI = 0.94).

Results

Descriptive statistics and correlations among the study variables are displayed in table 1. As expected, the correlation coefficients obtained showed that lack of reciprocity was negatively associated with the three supportive leadership behaviors (SLB), and positively related to the three job demands variables.

---

[1] *All parameter estimates throughout the paper are standardized.*

Table 1: Means, standard deviations and correlations among the study variables

Variables	M	SD	1	2	3	4	5	6	7	8	9	10	11	12	13	14
1. Acknowledgement	3.2	1.3	--													
2. Consideration	3.6	1.2	.82**	--												
3. Communication	3.2	1.2	.76**	.76**	--											
4. Role overload	3.0	1.1	-.08*	-.07	-.07	--										
5. Organizational demands	3.0	1.0	-.33**	-.31**	-.32**	.24**	--									
6. Demanding working conditions	2.9	0.9	-.18*	-.17**	-.15*	.28**	.51**	--								
7. Lack of reciprocity	3.7	1.0	-.14**	-.14**	-.14**	.31**	.26**	.30**	--							
8. Depersonalization	1.8	0.8	-.14**	-.11**	-.07	.12**	.22**	.21**	.07*	--						
9. Emotional exhaustion	3.0	0.9	-.09*	-.09*	-.07*	.42**	.37**	.46**	.38**	.25**	--					
10. Personal accomplishment	2.0	0.8	-.14**	-.14**	-.10**	-.06	.10**	-.03	-.08*	.27**	-.03	--				
11. Propensity to leave the organization	2.0	0.9	-.27**	-.24**	-.26**	.13**	.29**	.16**	.14**	.20**	.16**	.10**	--			
12. Propensity to leave the unit	2.5	1.5	-.24**	-.22**	-.21**	.13**	.23**	.16**	.10**	.22**	.17**	.14**	.28**	--		
13. Organizational commitment	3.6	1.0	.31**	.28**	.31**	-.12**	-.36**	-.23**	-.22**	-.13**	-.22**	-.18**	-.35**	-.20**	--	
14. Absenteeism	0.4	0.5	-.03	-.03	-.06	.04	.04	.01	.02	.00	.09*	-.05	.02	.06	-.02	--

$*p < .05; **p < .01$

215

Furthermore, and again as expected, lack of reciprocity was negatively related to organizational commitment, and positively related to propensity to leave the organization and the unit. Also in accordance with our expectations, the correlation coefficient between lack of reciprocity, and depersonalization and emotional exhaustion were positive. Finally, lack of reciprocity was not correlated with absenteeism. Only emotional exhaustion showed a statistically significant correlation with absenteeism.

The hypothesized model showed a satisfactory fit to data ($\chi^2 = 299.8$, $df = 81$, $p < 0.01$; AGFI = 0.92; RMSEA = 0.06; CFI = 0.94; NNFI = 0.92). The parameter estimates obtained (see figure 2) showed that SLB was negatively related to cognitive withdrawal (-0.51, $p <. 01$), but contrary to our expectations it was not related to lack of reciprocity (-0.02, *n.s.*). Job demands were positively related to lack of reciprocity (0.48, $p < .01$) and burnout (.73, $p < 0.1$). As expected, lack of reciprocity was positively related to cognitive withdrawal (0.27, $p <. 01$) and burnout (0.18, $p < .01$), but it was not related to absenteeism. Besides, neither cognitive withdrawal nor burnout were significantly related to absenteeism (0.03 and 0.08, respectively).

Figure 2: Standardized parameter estimates for the structural parameters of the hypothesized model

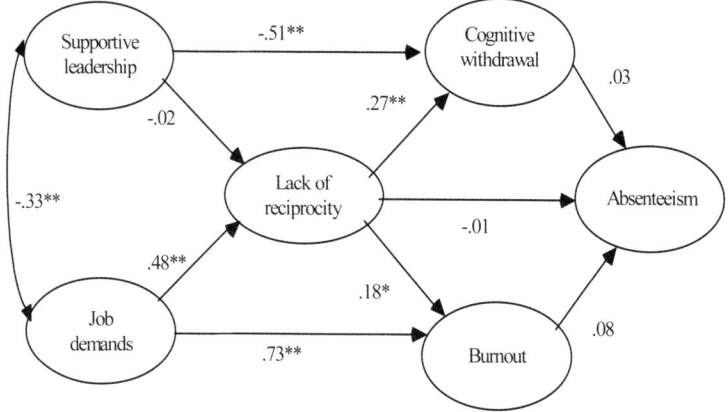

Note: ** p<0.01; * p<0.05.

As to the hypotheses referring to the mediating role of lack of reciprocity, these results pointed out that lack of reciprocity did *not* mediate the impact of SLB on cognitive and behavioral withdrawal and burnout, because SLB and lack of reciprocity were not related. Lack of reciprocity *partially* mediated the relationship between job demands and burnout, because job demands and lack of reciprocity were significantly related, and the relationship between lack of reciprocity and burnout was still significant when the impact of job demands on burnout was simultaneously estimated. However, lack of reciprocity did not mediate the relationship between job demands and absenteeism, because the relationship between lack of reciprocity and absenteeism was not significant. To ascertain whether lack of reciprocity mediated the impact of job demands on cognitive withdrawal, the hypothesized model was re-estimated including the coefficient estimating the impact of job demands on cognitive withdrawal. This model showed a good fit to data ($\chi^2 = 245.8$, $df = 80$, $p <. 01$; AGFI = 0.93; RMSEA = 0.055; CFI = 0.95; NNFI = 0.94). The new coefficient estimating the impact of job demands on cognitive withdrawal was statistically significant (0.50, $p < .01$), and the coefficient estimating the impact of lack of reciprocity on cognitive withdrawal lost its statistical significance (0.02, $p > .05$). The difference in fit between both nested models was statistically significant ($\Delta\chi^2 = 54$, $\Delta df = 1$, $p < 0.01$). Hence, these results revealed that lack of reciprocity did *not* mediate the relationship between job demands and cognitive withdrawal.

As argued in the introduction, absence behaviors of males and females should be studied separately as well. Therefore we performed a multi-group analyses including the male ($n = 264$) and female ($n = 451$) subsamples. The research model showed an acceptable fit to the data of ($\chi^2 = 393.2$, $df = 162$, $p < 0.01$; AGFI = 0.95; RMSEA = 0.045; CFI = 0.94; NNFI = 0.92) with largely comparable path coefficients for both subsamples. Only in three cases these path coefficients differed significantly: (1) supportive leadership → lack of reciprocity was – as expected – significantly negative for males but insignificant for females; (2) job demands → lack of reciprocity was significantly stronger positive for females; (3) burnout → absenteeism was significant and positive for males and insignificant for females. When the model was re-estimated with all structural parameters – except these three – constrained to be equal, and the non-significant relationships of cognitive withdrawal → absenteeism and lack of reciprocity → absenteeism fixed to zero, its fit was satisfactory ($\chi^2 = 394.6$, $df = 171$, $p < 0.01$; AGFI = 0.96; RMSEA = 0.04; CFI = 0.94; NNFI = 0.93). The difference in fit between both multi-group models was not statistically significant ($\Delta\chi^2 = 1.4$, $df = 9$, $p > 0.05$). This points to the fact that the parameter restrictions as imposed in the final model could be maintained. In this final model, the path coefficient linking burnout to absenteeism was 0.17 ($p < 0.05$) in the male subsample and 0.01 ($n.s.$) in the female subsample. In other words, the expected positive relationship between burnout and absenteeism was observed among male employees only.

Discussion

Although the hypothesized model (see figure 1) fitted well to the data, the current study did not confirm the central mediating role of lack of reciprocity. In fact, lack of reciprocity only (partially) mediated the relationship between job demands and burnout. That is, high job demands are associated with lack of reciprocity (an unfavorable perceived imbalance between investments in and outcomes from the organization), which, in its turn is associated with burnout (emotional exhaustion and depersonalization). Another possible mediating effect of lack of reciprocity disappeared when an alternative model was fitted to the data that included a direct path between both variables involved (job demands and cognitive withdrawal). Unfortunately, lack of reciprocity did neither play a mediating role with respect to both remaining outcome variables in the model (i.e., cognitive withdrawal and absenteeism) nor with respect to supportive leadership. Below we will discuss these somewhat disappointing results. On the other hand, strong direct relationships were found between job demands and burnout, and between non-supportive leadership and cognitive withdrawal (i.e., organizational commitment and propensity to leave). In other words, employees who experience high job demands report high levels of burnout, whereas those who have poor support from their supervisors show an increased tendency to withdraw from the organization.

Lacking relations with absenteeism

We can only speculate why absenteeism is not related to any of the structural variables in the model, except weakly to burnout in the male subsample. For instance, employees in health care might feel highly responsible for their patients so that they will not easily desert them and stay absent from work. An additional reason for not reporting sick might be that health care workers feel quite committed to their colleagues; staying home means an increased workload for those who remain on the job. Statistically speaking, this could mean that the variability in absence is too low to allow for significant relationships with other variables in the model (restriction of range).

It is quite remarkable that emotional exhaustion is significantly and positively related to absenteeism, whereas the remaining cognitive variables (depersonalisation, organizational commitment and propensity to leave) are not. So perhaps health care workers overcome cognitive barriers relatively easy and do not report sick because of loyalty to their patients and to their colleagues. In contrast, high levels of emotional exhaustion make it much more difficult for them to go to work, despite their loyalties. However, also the correlation of emotional exhaustion with absenteeism is weaker in this study ($r = 0.09$) than typically found (about $r = 0.15$) (Schaufeli & Enzmann, 1998, p. 91). The loyalty and high commitment of health care employees to other people is illustrated by a study of Garden (1991) who showed that in the human services 'feeling types' who are characterized by concern for other people outnumber 'thinking types' who tend to neglect other people by a ratio of four to one. Interestingly, in business environments this ratio is exactly opposite and 'thinking types' are four times more common.

Gender differences

Our multi-group analysis in which males and females were distinguished pointed to the fact that structural differences exist in the absence behavior of men and women[2]. This agrees with VandenHeuvel and Wooden (1995), who showed that absenteeism in women is more strongly related to external pressures such as life events, whereas in males absenteeism is more strongly influenced by work related factors, such as job satisfaction. Instead of job satisfaction as in the study of VandenHeuvel and Wooden (1995), we included burnout but the results are similar: burnout is associated with absenteeism in males but *not* in females. This also agrees with the results of a recent Dutch national population study that showed that – despite higher prevalence rates – mental health in working women was *not* predictive for future absenteeism, whereas in males it was (Laitinen-Krispijn & Bijl, 2000). Of course, the results of our analyses need replication, but at least for the time being they suggest that in future research on absenteeism men and woman should be studied separately.

Direct effects of job demands and supportive leadership

It appeared that job demands and unsupportive leadership have relatively strong direct relationships with burnout and cognitive withdrawal, respectively. This is in line with the recently developed Job-Demands Resources (JD-R) model (Demerouti, Bakker, Nachreiner & Schaufeli, 2001). This model distinguishes between two sets of variables, job demands and job resources, which have different effects on particular outcome measures. Job demands are those aspects of the job (physical, psychological, social, or organizational) that require sustained effort and are therefore associated with certain physiological and psychological costs. Job resources refer to those aspects of the job that either/or (1) reduce job demands; (2) are functional in achieving work goals; (3) stimulate personal growth, learning and development. More specifically, the JD-R model assumes that demanding aspects of work, such as work overload may lead to chronic overtaxing and the draining of energy and eventually exhaustion – the core symptom of burnout. On the other hand, lacking resources (i.e., not being acknowledged or treated with consideration by one's supervisor, or being poorly informed) precludes actual goal accomplishment and thus may cause failure and frustration and may eventually result in disengagement and withdrawal from work. Hence, two processes seem to be at work: the former being energetically in nature, the latter motivational (*cf.* Bakker, Demerouti & Schaufeli, 2003). As in the study of Demerouti et al. (2001), we observed relatively strong direct relationships between job demands and burnout (exhaustion) and between job resources and cogni-

---

[2] *Women (M = 0.4; SD = 0.5) show higher absenteeism rates then men (M = 0.3; SD = 0.4); $t (647) = 2.95$, $p < .01$. Also the variance in absence rates is significantly higher for woman: $F (450, 263) = 1.56 (p < .001)$.*

tive withdrawal (disengagement). A likewise negative relationship between demands and resources was observed in our study as in the study of Demerouti et al. (2001): the higher the job demands, the less supportive the leadership is perceived (and vice versa). This negative correlation might be interpreted in two ways: either job demands are so high because leadership is inadequate, or because of high job demands leadership is bound to be inadequate.

In addition, a relatively strong and positive relationship was observed in our alternative model between job demands and cognitive withdrawal. That is, when health care employees experience high demands, they are less committed to the organization and they think more about quitting their jobs. Probably, this direct effect reflects a protective reaction akin to burnout (Maslach, Schaufeli & Leiter, 2001). In a way, both burnout (especially the depersonalization component) and cognitive withdrawal are ways of mentally distancing oneself from the job in order to cope with the high demands. Reducing one's identification with the job counteracts the potential negative effects of high job demands. Indeed, small but significant positive correlations have been found between work overload and organizational commitment, for instance (e.g., Mathieu & Zajac, 1990).

Study limitations

One obvious limitation of the current research is that the research design is cross-sectional. Hence, the postulated relationships – as hypothesized in figure 1 – cannot be interpreted causally. Secondly, internal consistency of the demanding working conditions scale was slightly lower (0.66) than the criterion for Cronbach's α of 0.70 that is generally considered to be sufficient (Nunnaly, 1978). However, it is unlikely that this might have had a negative impact on the fit of the model to the data since two other indicators of the latent job demands variable (i.e., work overload and organizational demands) were included that showed sufficient internal consistencies. Thirdly, it appeared that the fit of the model increased significantly when personal accomplishment was removed as an indicator of burnout. This is not very surprising since both remaining burnout dimensions – emotional exhaustion and depersonalization – are stronger interrelated than each of them with personal accomplishment. For instance, a meta analysis based on 47 studies showed that emotional exhaustion and depersonalization were correlated 0.64, whereas correlations with personal accomplishment were only -0.33 and -0.36, respectively (Lee & Ashforth, 1996). Furthermore, there is accumulating evidence that depersonalization develops in response to emotional exhaustion and that personal accomplishment largely develops in parallel with these two burnout dimensions (Maslach, Schaufeli & Leiter, 2001; Schaufeli & Enzmann, 1998, p. 117-119). Fourthly, because the number of employees per team that was included in the current study was relatively small (i.e., about 3) we could not use multi-level analysis. However, in future research this powerful tool should be used to test similar models, provided that the number of participants suffices. In doing so, "shared job strain" (Semmer, Zapf & Greif, 1996) – the proportion of strain that different members of a team have in common – and "affective tone" (George, 1996) – the collective work team affective climate (see also González-Romá, Peiró, Subirats & Mañas, 2000) – can be studied. This approach increases the validity of strain measures because it eliminates idiosyncratic perceptions of individual employees.

Practical implications

As far as prevention of job related strain is concerned results of the current study points to the crucial importance of reducing job demands instead of increasing supportive leadership. By reducing job demands burnout might be prevented, both directly because less energy has to be spent on the job, as well as indirectly because perceptions of lack of reciprocity are counteracted. In addition, reducing job demands might increase the identification with the organization, thus increasing organizational commitment and decreasing the propensity to leave. Ultimately, as multi-group analyses suggest, the reduction of burnout might decrease absenteeism – at least in men. Various ways of organization-based strategies to modify job demands have been described such as job redesign, participative management, flexible work schedules, and the design of physical settings (e.g., Quick, Quick, Nelson & Hurrell, 1997, pp. 163-185). On the other hand, increasing supportive leadership – for instance through Management Development programs – cannot assumed to be likewise successful. According to our findings, increasing supportive leadership would only decrease cognitive withdrawal; an effect that is also obtained when job demands are decreased. Thus increasing supportive leadership does not have a unique effect.

But instead of directly tackling high job demands or unsupportive leadership it is also possible to change equity perceptions of employees. For instance, Van Dierendonck, Schaufeli and Buunk (1998) showed that employees who participated in small-scale stress management groups that concentrated on changing the employee's 'balance of give and take' had lower exhaustion scores and were less absent at the one year follow-up compared to those in the control group who did not participate.

Final note

The current study suggests that perceptions of lack of reciprocity do only matter to a limited degree. Such perceptions seem to be directly related only to burnout symptoms. In addition, lack of reciprocity is – albeit only in males – indirectly related to registered absenteeism through burnout. Obviously, the employee's 'mental bookkeeping' of job demands and job resources may have a limited negative psychological impact. The current study sheds some light on the intervening cognitive process that is involved in the stress process and that has been largely neglected by today's leading approaches in the field such as the Effort-Reward Imbalance model (Siegrist, 1998) and the Job Demands-Control Support model (Karasek & Theorell, 1990).

References

Adams, J. S. (1965). Inequity in social exchange. *Advances in Experimental Social Psychology, 2*, 267-299.

Aiken, L. S. & West, S. G. (1991). *Multiple regression: Testing and interpreting interactions*. Newbury Park, CA: Sage.

Anderson, J. C. & Gerbing, D. W. (1988). Structural equation modeling in practice - a review and recommended 2-step approach. *Psychological Bulletin, 103*, 411-423.

Bakker, A. B., Demerouti, E. & Schaufeli, W. B. (2003). Dual processes at work in a call centre: An Application of the Job Demands – Resources Model. *European Journal of Work and Organizational Psychology, 12*, 393-417.

Bakker, A. B., Killmer, C. H., Siegrist, J. & Schaufeli, W. B. (2000). Effort-reward imbalance and burnout among nurses. *Journal of Advanced Nursing, 31*, 884-891.

Browne, M. W. & Cudeck, R. (1993). Alternative ways of assessing model fit. In K. A. Bollen & J. Scott Long (Eds.), *Testing structural equation models* (pp. 136-162). Newbury Park, CA: Sage.

Buunk, B. P. & Schaufeli, W. B. (1993). Burnout: A perspective from social comparison theory. In W. B. Schaufeli, C. Maslach & T. Marek (Eds.), *Professional burnout: Recent development in theory and research* (pp. 53-69). Washington, DC: Taylor & Francis.

Buunk, B. P. & Schaufeli, W. B. (1999). Reciprocity in interpersonal relationships: An evolutionary perspective on its importance for health and well-being. *European Review of Social Psychology, 10*, 260-291.

Camman, C., Fichman, M., Jenkins, D. & Klesh, J. (1979). *The Michigan Organizational Assessment Questionnaire*. Unpublished Manuscript. University of Michigan, Ann Arbor, Michigan.

Chadwick-Jones, J. K., Nicholson, N. & Brown, C. (1982). *Social psychology of absenteeism*. New York, NY: Praeger.

Cooper, C. L., Sloan, S. J. & Williams, S. C. (1988). *Occupational Stress Indicator. Management guide*. Oxford: ASE, NFER-NELSON.

Demerouti, E., Bakker, A. B., Nachreiner, F. & Schaufeli, W. B. (2001). The Job Demands – Resources model of burnout. *Journal of Applied Psychology, 86*, 499-512.

De Rijk, A., Le Blanc, P. M., Schaufeli, W. B. & De Jonge, J. (1998). Active coping and need for control as moderators of the job demand-control model: Effects on burnout. *Journal of Occupational and Organizational Psychology, 71*, 1-18.

Garcia-Montalvo, J., Pieró, J. M. & Soro, A. (2003). *El observatorio sobre la transición de los jóvenes en la Comunidad Valenciana* [A lookout on the transition of the youth in the Valencian community]. Valencia: Fundación Banciaixa, IVE.

Garden, A. M. (1991). The purpose of burnout: A Jungian interpretation. *Journal of Social Behavior and Personality, 6*, 73-93.

George, J. M. (1996). Group affective tone. In M. A. West (Ed.), *Handbook of work group psychology* (pp.77-94). Chichester: John Wiley and Sons.

Geurts, S. A., Buunk, A. P. & Schaufeli, W. B. (1994a). Health complaints, social comparisons and absenteeism. *Work and Stress, 8*, 220-234.

Geurts, S. A., Buunk, A. P. & Schaufeli, W. B. (1994b). Social comparisons: a structural modeling approach. *Journal of Applied Social Psychology, 24,* 1871-1890.

Geurts, S. A., Schaufeli, W. B. & Buunk, B. P. (1993). Social comparison, inequity, and absenteeism among bus drivers. *European Work and Organizational Psychologist, 3,* 191-203.

Geurts, S. A. E., Schaufeli, W. B. & De Jonge, J. (1988). Burnout and intention to leave among health-care professionals: A social psychological approach. *Journal of Social and Clinical Psychology, 17,* 341-362.

Geurts, S. A. E., Schaufeli, W. B. & Rutte, C. (1999). Absenteeism, turnover intention and inequity in the employment relationship. *Work & Stress, 13,* 253-267.

Glisson, C. & Durick, M.(1988). Predictors of job satisfaction and organizational commitment in human service organizations. *Administrative Science Quarterly, 33,* 61-81.

González-Romá, V., Peiró, J. M., Subirats, M. & Mañas, M. A. (2000). The validity of affective workteam climates. In M. Vartiainen, F. Avallone & N. Anderson (Eds.), *Innovative Theories, Tools and Practices in Work and Organizational Psychology,* (pp. 97-109). Göttingen, Germany: Hogrefe & Huber Publishers.

Hammer, T. H. & Landau, J. (1981). Methodological issues in the use of absence data. *Journal of Applied Psychology, 66,* 574-581.

Hoyle, R. H. (1995) The structural equation modeling approach: Basic concepts and fundamental issues. In R. H. Hoyle (Ed.), *Structural equation modeling, concepts, issues, and applications* (pp. 1-15). Thousand Oaks, CA: Sage.

Johns, G. (1997). Contemporary research on absence from work: Correlates, causes and consequences. *International Review of Industrial and Organizational Psychology, 12* 115-174.

Jöreskog, K. G. & Sörbom, D. (1989). *LISREL VII: Analysis of linear structural relationships by maximum likelihood, instrumental variables, and least squares methods.* Mooresville, IN: Scientific Software.

Jöreskog, K. G. & Sörbom, D. (1993). *LISREL 8: User's Reference Guide.* Chicago, Ill: Scientific Software International.

Karasek, R. & Theorell, T. (1990). *Healthy work: Stress productivity, and the reconstruction of working life.* New York, NY: Basic Books.

Laitinen-Krispijn, S. & Bijl, R. V. (2000). Mental disorders and employee sickness absence: the NEMESIS study. *Social Psychiatry & Psychiatric Epidemiology, 35,* 71-77.

Lee, R. T. & Ashforth, B. E. (1996). A meta-analytic examination of the correlates of the three dimensions of job burnout. *Journal of Applied Psychology, 81,* 123-133.

Marsh, H. W., Balla, J. R. & Hau, K. T. (1996) An evaluation of incremental fit indices: A clarification of mathematical and empirical properties. In G. A. Marcoulides & R.E. Schumacker (Eds.), *Advanced structural equation modeling, issues and techniques,* (pp. 315-353). Mahwah, NJ: Lawrence Erlbaum.

Maslach, C. & Jackson, S. E. (1986). *Maslach Burnout Inventory: Second edition.* Palo Alto, CA: Consulting Psychologists Press.

Maslach, C., Schaufeli, W. B. & Leiter, M. P. (2001). Job burnout. *Annual Review of Psychology, 52,* 397-422

Mathieu, J. E. & Zajac, D. M. (1990). A review and meta-analysis of the antecedents, correlates, and consequences of organizational commitment. *Psychological Bulletin, 108,* 171-194.

Muthén, B. & Kaplan, D. (1985). A comparison of some methodologies for the factor analysis of non-normal Likert variables. *British Journal of Mathematical and Statistical Psychology, 38,* 171-189.

North, F. Syme, S. L., Feeney, A., Shipley, M. J. & Marmot, M. G. (1996). Psychosocial work environment and sickness absenteeism among British civil servants: The Whitehall II study. *American Journal of Public Health, 86,* 332-340.

Nunnaly, J. C. (1978). *Pychometric theory.* New York: Academic Press.

O'Reilly, C. & Chatman, J. (1986). Organizational commitment and psychological attachment. The effects of compliance, identification and internalization on prosocial behavior. *Journal of Applied Psychology, 71,* 492-499.

Orizo, F. A. (1991). *Los nuevos valores de los españelos* [The new values of the Spaniards] Madrid: Fundación Santa Marie.

Peiró, J. M., González-Romá, V., Tordera, N. & Mañas, M. A. (2001). Does role stress predict burnout over time among health care professionals? *Psychology & Health, 16,* 511-525.

Pritchard, R. D. (1969). Equity theory: A review and critique. *Organizational Behavior and Human performance, 4,* 176-211.

Quick, J. C., Quick, J. D., Nelson, D. L. & Hurrell, J. J. (1997). *Preventive stress- management in organizations.* American Psychological Association: Washington, DC.

Rosin, H. & Korabik, K. (1995). Organizational experiences and propensity to leave: A multivariate investigation of men and women managers. *Journal of Vocational Behavior, 46,* 1-16.

Rusbult, C. E. & Farrell, D. (1983). A longitudinal test of the investment model: The impact on job satisfaction, job commitment, and turnover of variations in rewards, costs, alternatives, and investments. *Journal of Applied Psychology,* 68, 429-438.

Rutte, C. G. & Messick, D. M. (1995). An integrated model of perceived unfairness in organizations. *Social Justice Research, 8,* 239-261.

Semmer, N., Zapf, D. & Greif, S. (1996). 'Shared job strain': A new approach for assessing the validity of job stress measurements. *Journal of Occupational and Organizational Psychology, 69,* 293-310.

Schaufeli, W. B. & Enzmann, D. (1998). *The burnout companion for study and practice: A critical analysis.* London: Taylor & Francis.

Schaufeli, W. B., Van Dierendonck, D. & Van Gorp, K. (1996). Burnout and reciprocity: towards a dual-level social exchange model. *Work & Stress, 10,* 225-237.

Siegrist J. (1998). Adverse health effects of effort-reward imbalance at work. In C. L. Cooper (Ed.), *Theories of organizational stress* (pp. 190-204). Oxford University Press.

Syroit, J., Lodewijkx, H., Franssen, E. & Gerstel, I. (1993). Organizational commitment and satisfaction with work among transferred employees: An application of referent cognitions theory. *Social Justice Research, 6,* 219-234.

Tan, C. C. (1991). Occupational health problems among nurses. *Scandinavian Journal of Work Environment and Health, 17,* 221-23

VandenHeuvel, A. & Wooden, M. (1995). Do explanations of absenteeism differ for men and woman? *Human Relations, 48,* 1309-1329.

Van Dierendonck, D., Schaufeli, W. B. & Buunk, B. P. (1996). Equity among human services professionals: Measurement and relation to burnout. *Basic and Applied Psychology, 18,* 429- 451.

Van Dierendonck, D., Schaufeli, W. B. & Buunk, B. P. (1998) The evaluation of an individual burnout intervention program. *Journal of Applied Psychology, 83,* 392-407.

Yukl, G. A. (1990). *COMPASS: The Managerial Practices Survey.* New York: Author/Manus Associates.

Job burnout among Austrian psychotherapists

Julia Hickel[*], Christian Korunka
Faculty of Psychology, University of Vienna, Austria

Maslach and Jackson (1986) defined burnout as "…a syndrome of emotional exhaustion, depersonalization, and reduced personal accomplishment that can occur among individuals who do 'people work' of some kind" (p.1). A very intense type of 'people work' and at the same has only rarely been investigated in the context of burnout is psychotherapy. The aim of this study was to analyze job burnout among Austrian psychotherapists. Resources and work demands of psychotherapists were analyzed in relation to burnout. The study is based on the well-known demand-control-support model of Karasek (1979).

Psychotherapy is an intense form of relationship work dealing very often with clients with severe psychological and psychiatric disorders. It is offered mainly as individual psychotherapy in an – isolated – independent private practice, resulting therefore in a very specific form of a work setting in human service work. Intense personal interaction work is the key context and content of this work (Büssing & Glaser, 2000).

With regard to job resources, psychotherapy typically allows for good control of most of the working environment. (e.g., the number of clients in private practice). On the other hand, private support has to be the main source of social support in this work (especially in isolated private practice settings).

Few studies deal with burnout and distress among psychotherapists. Some were based on small and unrepresentative samples. In one of the earlier studies in this field, Guy, Poelstra and Stark (1989) found a noticeable rate of personal distress in a representative sample of American psychotherapists, and a significant negative relation between personal distress and the quality of patient care. Ackerley, Burnell, Holder and Kurdek (1988) observed high burnout rates in about one third of their representative sample of psychotherapists. In their study the highest burnout rates were found in psychotherapists with little individual training therapy, lack of control in their work settings, and an overcommitment to their clients.

---

[*] Correspondence: Christian Korunka, christian.korunka@univie.ac.at

Both Raquepaw and Miller (1989) and Dupree and Day (1995) found higher burnout rates in psychotherapists working for agencies or institutions, as compared to psychotherapists working in private practice. A similar result was observed by Vredenburgh, Carlozzi and Stein (1999) for counseling psychologists. In most of the studies cited so far, younger, less experienced psychotherapists showed higher burnout rates as compared to older, more experienced therapists. Those psychotherapists working mainly with severe disorders, i.e., disorders with a generally limited therapeutic success rate (e.g., patients with heavy substance abuse, psychoses), have a potential for higher burnout rates (Elman & Dowd, 1997). Client demands in general (high expectations, reduced motivation, resistance) are sources of stress in this work (Brentup, 2002).

Depressed emotional states of the therapists could be on one hand an outcome of intense work with severely disturbed clients, but offer on the other hand a potential for enhanced empathy (Gilroy, Carroll & Murra, 2002). Compassion fatigue could also be a sign of chronic lack of self care (Figley, 2002). Personal distress of the psychotherapists may decrease the quality of care offered to their clients (Guy et al., 1989).

The job profile of psychotherapy reflects specific qualities and resources. It may be seen as a specific form of meaningful relationship work, offering a good chance to find existential significance (Malach Pines, 2002). 'Passionate commitment' may be related to high job satisfaction, low burnout and high personal accomplishment (Dlugos & Friedlander, 2001). Clinical case consultation/supervision, support from peers, spouses and friends and careful planning of the caseload are empirically confirmed adequate coping strategies (Coster & Schwebel, 1997; Kramen-Kahn & Downing Hansen, 1998).

The moderation of control and social support in the relation between job demands and emotional job outcomes (i.e., burnout) is the focus of the well-known and heavily investigated demand-control-support model (Karasek, 1979; Karasek & Theorell, 1990; van Vegchel, de Jonge, Söderfeldt, Dormann & Schaufeli, 2004). The demand-control-support model postulates the most adverse health effects for a combination of high psychological demands, low control, and low social support. Although the model may be used as a general framework for the investigation of burnout, it has to be taken into consideration that every occupation has a specific risk profile for burnout (Bakker, Demerouti, Taris, Schaufeli & Schreurs, 2003). For instance, patient demands are the most important determinants of burnout in general practitioners (Bakker, Schaufeli, Sixma, Bosveld & van Dierendonck, 2000).

Therefore, the demand-control-support dimensions need to be adapted for the specific working conditions of psychotherapists for this study on burnout.

As already stated, most psychotherapists work in independent private practice settings. In these settings, job demands objectively result both from the number of therapy hours per week, and from the structure of client disorders. Based on our own knowledge of the job characteristics in this field, and also from discussions with experts (trainers) and practitioners, we expect high emotional demands for psychotherapists providing more than 20-25 therapy hours each week. Similarly, high emotional demands are to be expected when working with a high number of clients with severe disorders, i.e., disorders where a comparatively low success rate has to be expected.

Job control in psychotherapeutic work may result from potential control over the client selection, the number of clients per week, the time schedule for each psychotherapeutic process, and the general planning of working hours and therapy processes.

In private (single) practices, social support is available mainly from friends and family members, and only partly from colleagues. In general, clinical case supervision is a well-proven and widely accepted institutionalized form of support of psychotherapeutic work. As a result of the high quality standards in Austrian psychotherapy (as a result from a 'psychotherapeutic law' and high educational standards) it can be assumed that most of the psychotherapists are making use of regular supervision processes of their own work.

The objectives of this study are:

to determine the general burnout degree of Austrian psychotherapists.

to analyze empirically confirmed 'risk factors' for burnout in a representative sample of Austrian psychotherapists (considering gender, age, various psychotherapeutic-methodical orientations, and work practice settings such as private practice and institutions).

to adapt and test Karaseks´ demand-control-support model as a predictor for job burnout in psychotherapists.

Study design and methods

Psychotherapy in Austria

Since 1991 Austria has a psychotherapy law defining high quality standards of psychotherapeutic training and practice. From an educational perspective, psychotherapy is a secondary profession, in addition to a primary profession in the field of human service work (e.g., psychology, medicine, social work). In practice, after finishing the intense training process (typically 5-6 years) psychotherapists switch very often from their primary profession to psychotherapy and start to work as independent psychotherapists. The Austrian

Ministry of Health maintains a list of licensed psychotherapists. Most of the occupational more active licensees are also members of the Austrian Professional Association for Psychotherapy (ÖBVP) (a noticeable part of the licensed psychotherapists do not practice psychotherapy.) Therefore, to reach a representative sample of occupationally active psychotherapists, a contact via the professional association is necessary.

Most of the therapists are working in independent private practice, or in a mixed form of private and institutional psychotherapy. Austrian psychotherapists represent a wide range of different methodical orientations. Clients of licensed psychotherapists may claim a partial refund of their therapy costs from their medical insurance.

Participants

A questionnaire and a stamped return envelope were included in a regular association newsletter sent out to the 2,410 psychotherapists who are also members of the Austrian Professional Association for Psychotherapy (ÖBVP). A reminder email was sent four weeks later to those association members with internet access. Study participation was anonymous. 458 questionnaires were usable for statistical analysis. The return rate was 19%, a just acceptable value for this type of study.

The sample consists of 330 (72%) women and 128 (28%) men. 16% of the psychotherapists were under 40 years old, 53% between 40 and 50 years, and 31% older than 50 years. The average amount of job experience is 11 years. As expected, the psychotherapists have a wide range of theoretical orientations, with 21% systemic orientated psychotherapy, 21% person/client centered psychotherapy, 14% gestalt therapy, 14% psychoanalysis, and 5% behavioral therapy as the most common subsamples. Nearly 40% of the psychotherapists live in Vienna.

For the above mentioned sample characteristics, which also included also the home province of the psychotherapists, data from the Ministry of Health and the professional association were available for comparison. χ^2-distribution tests were calculated for comparing the analysis sample with the total samples of association members and licensed psychotherapists. No significant differences were found in these indicators. Thus, it can be stated that the analysis sample is representative for Austrian psychotherapists with regard to the distribution of sex, age, theoretical orientation, and home province.

Instruments

Burnout was measured with the German language version of Maslach Burnout Inventory (MBI-D, Büssing & Perrar, 1992). In line with Büssings' conceptualization of MBI-D emotional exhaustion and depersonalization were considered as the two dimensions for analysis of burnout in the present study. Emotional exhaustion and depersonalization are generally considered to be the core dimensions of burnout (Demerouti, Bakker, Nachreiner & Schaufeli, 2001).

Data on job perceptions and sociodemographic data were collected by a specially developed questionnaire based on scales used by Orlinsky, Ambühl and Andreoli (1989). Job demands were measured both by the total number of psychotherapy hours per week, and by a client symptom severity index. Job control was measured by a scale consisting of five items: control of client selection, number of clients, time schedules, duration of psychotherapies and general working conditions. Social support was measured by a scale consisting of five support resources relevant for psychotherapeutic work: support by colleagues, friends, partner, family and general support. Additionally, the psychotherapists were asked if they made use of regular clinical supervision.

All the scales used in this study indicated acceptable internal consistencies (burnout frequency of symptoms: EE: $\alpha = 0.86$, DP: $\alpha = .66$; job control: $\alpha = .70$; job support: $\alpha = .71$). The scale distributions did not differ strongly from a normal distribution.

Results

Overall degree of burnout

The total sample mean value is 2.68 ($SD = 0.79$, Range = 1-5) in emotional exhaustion, and 1.82 ($SD = 0.58$, Range = 1-5) in depersonalization. A comparison with the norm sample of Büssing and Perrar (1992) indicates generally low burnout values for the total sample of psychotherapists. Also, compared to another large sample of nurses (Büssing & Glaser, 1999, 2000) the mean burnout values of the psychotherapists are relatively low.

A comparison of female and male psychotherapists indicated no significant sex differences in emotional exhaustion (women: $M = 2.69$, men: $M = 2.69$, $t = -0.05$, $p = .96$), and somewhat higher values in depersonalization for men (women: $M = 1.77$, men: $M = 1.98$, $t = -3.49$, $p = .01$).

Emotional exhaustion showed a significant decrease with age (< 40 years: $M = 2.81$, 41-50 years: $M = 2.74$, 51-60 years: $M = 2.63$, > 60 years: $M =$

2.37; $F = 2.63$, $p < .05$). No significant age effects were found in the amount of depersonalization.

Working conditions and burnout

As expected, most psychotherapists only work in private practice ($n = 253$, 55%), or in a mixed work setting including a small part of work in institutions ($n = 106$, 23%). Only 99 psychotherapists in our sample (22%) spend more than 50% of their total working time in institutions. In the latter group of psychotherapists, the weekly psychotherapeutic working time is higher ($M = 26.1$ hours/week) compared to the other two groups (mixed work setting: $M = 23.0$ hours/week, only private practice: $M = 16.8$; $F = 34.18$, $p < .001$).

Burnout rates among those psychotherapists working mainly in institutions are higher (EE: $M = 2.92$, DP: $M = 1.99$ compared to the other two work settings (mixed work setting: EE: $M = 2.91$, DP: $M = 1.94$; only private practice: EE: $M = 2.81$, DP: $M = 1.94$; $F = 4.38$, $p < .001$).

A significant correlation is observable between the psychotherapeutic working hours per week and emotional exhaustion (EE: $r = .17$, $p < .001$; DP: $r = .07$, n.s.).

The psychotherapists were asked to rate the proportion of their work with different patient groups. The following table shows the ratings in comparison between the work settings (table 1).

Table 1: Symptoms of the clients in different work settings

Symptoms of the clients	Private work setting ($n = 254$)	Mixed work setting ($n = 106$)	Mainly institutional setting ($n = 99$)
Clients with minimal symptoms (e.g., transient daily life problems)	12.5%	13.3%	10.2%
Clients with light, but enduring symptoms (e.g., light episode of depression)	40.9%	38.5%	38.3%
Clients with severe symptoms (e.g., suicidal thoughts, compulsion)	39.2%	39.6%	42.7%
Clients with very severe symptoms (e.g., hallucinations, self endangerment)	4.4%	6.8%	7.2%

Based on their own perceptions, psychotherapists typically work with clients showing a mixed 'middle' range of symptoms. Psychotherapists working mainly in institutions have a slightly higher percentage of clients with severe or very severe symptoms.

Important for the analysis presented here is the fact that there is only an insignificant correlation between the percentage of severe/very severe cases and the burnout scales (EE: $r = .06$, n.s.; DP: $r = .00$, n.s.). Therefore, with regard to burnout, as compared to the patient structure, the working hours per week seems to be the most important job demand on psychotherapists.

As expected for this type of human service work, the scale mean of the job control scale (M = 3.39, SD = .69, Range = 1-4) indicates strong subjective control perceptions regarding working conditions among psychotherapists. There is a significant negative correlation between job control and the burnout scales (EE: $r = -.27$, $p < .001$; DP: $r = -.19$, $p < .001$).

More than two thirds of the psychotherapists ($n = 315$, 69%) take part in regular clinical supervision of their work. Burnout rates do not differ significantly between psychotherapists with and without regular clinical supervision. ($F = 1.70$, $p = .17$). An interesting interaction is found between work settings, regular clinical supervision, and burnout: Those therapists working mainly in institutional settings *without* regular clinical supervision show significantly increased values of emotional exhaustion (Interaction: $F = 3.82$, $p = .02$). This result indicates that regular clinical supervision – as a measure of job support for psychotherapists – seems to be especially important as a burnout prevention measure in more intense work settings.

In general, the psychotherapists perceive sufficient support from their social environment (M = 3.51, SD = .64, Range = 1-4). There is a significant negative correlation observable between the amount of social support and the burnout scales (EE: $r = -.21$, $p < .001$; DP: $r = -.22$, $p < .001$).

Testing the demand-control-support model

In the final step of data analysis the demand-control-support model was tested. For each of the three predictors of burnout we selected those aspects showing a significant relation with burnout in the previous analyses. Those dimensions previously found as not relevant to burnout (such as the client symptom severity) and support dimensions (i.e., regular supervision) were not included in these analyses. Therefore job demands were measured in terms of working hours and a median split of the weekly working hours (up to 20 hours/week, more than 20 hours/week) was calculated. A median split based on the respective scales was calculated for both job control and support. Figure 1 shows mean values and standard errors for the two burnout scales separated for the demand-control-support combinations (cell sizes between $n = 42$ and $n = 130$).

Figure 1: Emotional exhaustion and depersonalization values separated for the demand-control-support conditions (mean values, standard errors)

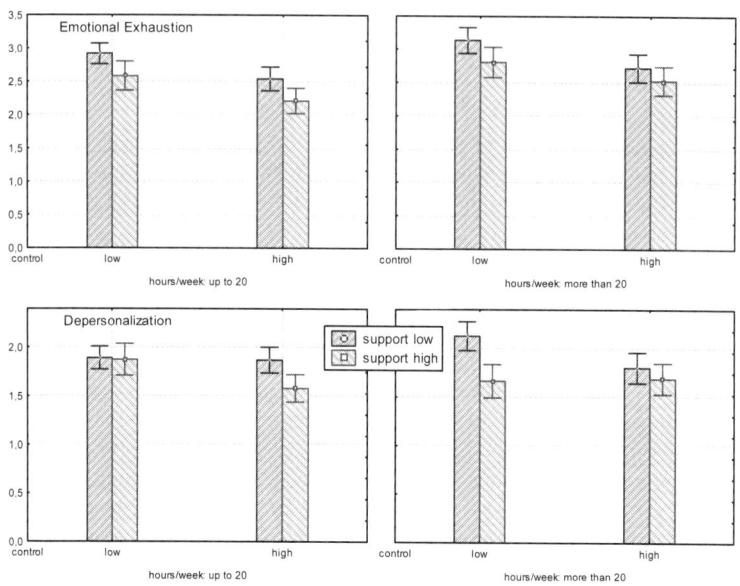

In terms of emotional exhaustion and depersonalization, the highest values are observable for the high demand – low control – low support condition. Table 2 shows the MANOVA main results.

Table 2: Burnout and demands-control-support: MANOVA results

Effect	F	p	η^2
Demand	6.55	.002	.03
Control	12.65	.000	.05
Support	11.16	.000	.05
D x C	0.02	.977	.00
D x S	1.61	.199	.00
C x S	0.13	.875	.00
D x C x S	4.82	.009	.02

The significant triple interaction confirms the demand-control-support model. ANOVAs separately calculated for the EE and DP scales reveal a significant triple interaction for depersonalization, only ($F = 2.61$, $p = .004$, $\eta^2 = .02$). Although the significant interaction may be interpreted as a confirmation of the demand-control-support model, it has to be noted that the effectual sizes are small.

Discussion

Burnout among psychotherapists was investigated in this study in a sample of Austrian psychotherapists. The general level of burnout, i.e., the frequency of perceived symptoms of emotional exhaustion and depersonalization, was relatively low. In accordance with the research literature, burnout was somewhat higher in less experienced and male psychotherapists. The number of working hours (hours of therapy) per week was confirmed as the most important job demand on psychotherapists, since the severity of client symptoms (i.e., the client structure of the psychotherapist) was not related to burnout. Both job control and social support – in their specific forms for this type of human service work – were confirmed as job resources. The importance of clinical supervision of the psychotherapeutic processes increases with the number of working hours. Supervision is of specific importance in institutional environments.

Based on a sample representative in socio-demographic variables, the data give a good picture of the general burnout situation among psychotherapists. Although, before discussing these results in more detail, the limits of this study have to be taken into consideration. It should be noted that 'burnout', as captured by the MBI scales, refers to burnout as a process, and not to a clinical diagnosis of burnout. Furthermore, causal relationships cannot be tested in this type of cross-sectional study. Since the most important job demand is the number of working hours per week, a relation between 'objective' demands and burnout could be tested. For job resources, higher correlations are to be expected because of the more subjective nature of these dimensions. In general, the data should be treated as empirically well-founded indications rather than as 'true' causal facts.

Regarding the relatively low general level of burnout in psychotherapists, our data are in line with the earlier research literature (e.g., Willutzki & Ambühl, 1997). These data indicate that psychotherapy is not only an important profession for a modern society, but at the same time a human service work with a beneficial profile with regard to task and characteristics (Kramen-Kahn & Downing Hansen, 1998). On the other hand, burnout ranges and standard deviations indicate at least a potential for higher burnout values, which has to be taken carefully into consideration.

Job demands

Since sample selection was based on membership in a professional organization (a voluntary membership), these data reflect well the job demands of psychotherapists with a strong job identification. The data show that the number of working hours per week is an important aspect of the specific job demands in psychotherapy. The working hours per week are not only an indicator of the amount of working time of highly demanding relationship work, they also correlate with the number of different clients confronting the psychotherapists with a wide range of personal issues and problems. A precondition of the (entrepreneurial) free-market setting of independent private practice work is the fact that control of working hours is affected at least partly by market conditions. Caseload uncertainty leading to working conditions that include too many or too few cases is one aspect of independent private practice work. From this point of view, burnout is at least partly affected by unfavorable free market conditions. On the other hand, significant higher burnout rates in psychotherapists working mainly in institutional settings may lead to the assumption of generally unfavorable working conditions in these settings. One may speculate therefore that a mixed (partly private and institutional) work setting offers the best conditions to prevent burnout among psychotherapists.

Psychotherapists typically see a wide range of clients, including a substantial number of clients with severe psychological and/or psychiatric disorders. An interesting fact in this context is the insignificant relation between the percentage of clients with severe disorders and burnout rates. The severity of patients´ disorders does not affect significantly the rate of burnout among psychotherapists. This could be due to the fact that the work may seem more meaningful when working successfully with patients with severe disorders. Combining the effects of working hours and client disorders, it seems to be that psychological demands (working hours) are more predictive for psychotherapists´ burnout than emotional demands (dealing with clients with severe disorders) (van Vegchel et al., 2004).

Higher burnout rates were observed in younger, less experienced psychotherapists. Professional job support especially for these psychotherapists is important, including information about burnout in psychotherapeutic training programs, regular and frequent case supervision, and help from colleagues to control their individual work load. The gender effect of increased depersonalization in male psychotherapists confirms the results of earlier studies.

Resources

In single private practice work job support is offered mainly by a private social network, i.e., from partners, friends, and family members. Institutional work settings may offer the possibility of social support through colleagues in the institution. As expected, job support is negatively related to burnout. One may recommend therefore that psychotherapists maintain a highly effective support network depending on their individual work settings. Boundaries between professional and nonprofessional life are a characteristic of work commitment among psychotherapists (Dlugos & Friedlander, 2001).

Regular and frequent clinical supervision is a basic recommendation for professional psychotherapeutic work. The importance of regular clinical supervision also for burnout prevention increases in highly demanding institutional work settings.

The isolated work setting of an independent one person psychotherapeutic practice also requires adequate forms of support. Besides regular clinical supervision, those psychotherapists working in such a setting should seek mutual supervision and a supportive network of colleagues. Psychotherapists working in institutions or with other colleagues in group practices generally have a better support structure for their work.

Job control was found as an important resource for burnout prevention. Job control in psychotherapy refers to the control of both the number and profile of clients. Again, a free market work setting may contradict control of client number and client structure for psychotherapists. In particular, younger and less experienced psychotherapists are more dependent on 'market supplies', and they also demonstrate higher burnout rates. This could be an effect of little control of their work setting. Again, occupational networks of psychotherapists and/or institutional work and working with other psychotherapists in group practices are ways to increase control over the working situation.

The D-C-S model

The study results may be seen as a confirmation of the job demand-control-support model with regard to burnout among psychotherapists. Those psychotherapists having low control of working conditions, low social support and high job demands show the highest burnout degree. Although a significant triple interaction could be found, the observed effect sizes are relatively low.

A generalized job demands-resources model (e.g., Bakker et al., 2003; Demerouti et al., 2001) is at least partly supported, as job demands (working hours) are only significantly related to emotional exhaustion. On the other hand resources (control and support) show significant relations both to emotional exhaustion and depersonalization (cynicism). The generalized job demands-resources model also can be a highly useful model for interaction work and it needs to be adapted for specific work settings and for analyzing objective and subjective demands/resources.

Recommendations for job structure

Based on our study the following recommendations for improving the job structure for psychotherapists and for carefully controlling burnout risk factors can be given:

Control over working hours, time management and choice of clientele is highly important. In contrast to other human service jobs, burnout regulation is mainly the sole responsibility of the therapist.

Social networks in private and job contexts play an important role as a resource to prevent job burnout.

Both a combination of institutional and private work settings and private group practices (centers of psychotherapy) rather than single practices are organizational settings which help prevent burnout.

Information about burnout prevention and job/organizational structure in the field of psychotherapy should be included in training programs.

References

Ackerley, G. D., Burnell, J., Holder, D. C. & Kurdek, L. A. (1988). Burnout among licensed psychologists. *Professional Psychology: Research and Practice, 19* (6), 624-631.

Bakker, A. B., Demerouti, E., Taris, T. W., Schaufeli, W. & Schreurs, P. J. G. (2003). A multigroup analysis of the job demands-resources model in four home care organizations. *International Journal of Stress Management, 10* (1), 16-38.

Bakker, A. B., Schaufeli, W., Sixma, H., Bosveld, W. & van Dierendonck, D. (2000). Patient demands, lack of reciprocity, and burnout: A five year longitudinal study among general practicioners. *Journal of Organizational Behavior, 21,* 425-441.

Brentup, M. (2002). Selbstsorge und self-care. Über den Zusammenhang zwischen Helfen, Gesundheit und Wirksamkeit von PsychotherapeutInnen. *Systema, 1,* 8-9.

Büssing, A. & Glaser, J. (1999). Work stressors in nursing in the course of redesign: Implications for burnout and interactional stress. *European Journal of Work and Organizational Psychology, 8* (3), 401-426.

Büssing, A. & Glaser, J. (2000). Four-stage process model of the core factors of burnout: The role of work stressors and work-related resources. *Work & Stress, 14* (4), 329-346.

Büssing, A. & Perrar, K. M. (1992). Messung von Burnout. Untersuchung einer deutschen Fassung des MBI. *Diagnostica, 38,* 328-353.

Coster, J. S. & Schwebel, M. (1997). Well-functioning in professional psychologists. *Professional Psychology: Research and Practice, 28* (1), 5-13.

Demerouti, E., Bakker, A. B., Nachreiner, F. & Schaufeli, W. (2001). The job demands-resources model of burnout. *Journal of Applied Psychology, 86* (3), 499-512.

Dlugos, R. F. & Friedlander, M. L. (2001). Passionately committed psychotherapists: A qualitative study of their experiences. *Professional Psychology: Research and Practice, 32* (3), 298-304.

Dupree, P. I. & Day, H. D. (1995). Psychotherapists' job satisfaction and job burnout as a function of work setting and percentage of managed care clients. *Psychotherapy in Private Practice, 14* (2), 77-93.

Elman, B. D. & Dowd, E. T. (1997). Correlates of burnout in inpatient substance abuse treatment therapists. *Journal of Addictions & Offender Counseling, 17* (2), 56-65.

Figley, C. R. (2002). Compassion fatigue: Psychotherapist´s chronic lack of self care. *Journal of Clinical Psychology, 58* (11), 1433-1441.

Gilroy, P. J., Carroll, L. & Murra, J. (2002). A preliminary survey of counseling psychologists´ personal experiences with depression and treatment. *Professional Psychology: Research and Practice, 33* (4), 402-407.

Guy, J. D., Poelstra, P. L. & Stark, M. J. (1989). Personal distress and therapeutic effectiveness: National survey of psychologists practicing psychotherapy. *Professional Psychology: Research and Practice, 20* (1), 48-50.

Karasek, R. A. (1979). Job demands, job decision latitude, and mental strain: Implications for job redesign. *Administrative Science Quarterly, 24*, 285-308.

Karasek, R. A. & Theorell, T. (1990). *Healthy work: Stress productivity and the reconstruction of working life.* New York: Basic books.

Kramen-Kahn, B. & Downing Hansen, N. (1998). Rafting the rapids: Occupational hazards, rewards, and coping strategies of psychotherapists. *Professional Psychology: Research and Practice, 29* (2), 130-134.

Malach Pines, A. (2002). A psychoanalytic-existential approach to burnout: Demonstrated in the cases of a nurse, a teacher, and a manager. *Psychotherapy: Theory/Research/Practice/Training, 39* (1), 103-113.

Maslach, C. & Jackson, S. E. (1986). *Maslach Burnout Inventory* (2nd ed.). Palo Alto, Ca: Consulting Psychologists Press.

Orlinsky, D., Ambühl, K. & Andreoli, A. (1989). Psychotherapy research in social contexts: A cross-national comparison of psychtherapy delivery systems. In *Proceedings of the 3rd European Conference of Psychotherapy Research*, Bern, Switzerland.

Raquepaw, J. M. & Miller, R. S. (1989). Psychotherapist burnout: A componential analysis. *Professional Psychology: Research and Practice, 20* (1), 32-36.

van Vegchel, N., de Jonge, J., Söderfeldt, M., Dormann, C. & Schaufeli, W. (2004). Quantitative versus emotional demands among Swedish human service employees: Moderating effects of job control and social support. International *Journal of Stress Management, 11* (1), 21-40.

Vredenburgh, L. D., Carlozzi, A. F. & Stein, L. B. (1999). Burnout in counseling psychologists: type of practice setting and pertinent demographics. *Counselling Psychology Quarterly, 12* (3), 293-302.

Willutzki, U. & Ambühl, H. (1997). Zufrieden oder ausgebrannt. Die berufliche Moral von PsychotherapeutInnen. In P. L. Janssen (Hrsg.), *Psychotherapie als Beruf* (S. 207-222). Göttingen: Vandenhoek & Ruprecht.

Burnout of nurses working in three different medical fields

Karin Proost[1]*, Karel De Witte[1], Hans De Witte[2] & Georges Evers[3]
[1] *Centre for Organizational and Personnel Psychology, University of Leuven, Belgium*
[2] *Research group for Stress, Health and Well-being, University of Leuven, Belgium*
[3] *Center for Research on Health Services and Nursing Management, University of Leuven, Belgium*

Since the late 1970s the concept of burnout has received a lot of attention, especially in human service professions, such as teaching (Koustelios, 2001) and nursing (Peeters & Le Blanc, 2001). The reason for this bulk of research on burnout is the finding that burnout has important dysfunctional consequences such as an increase in turnover, absenteeism and reduced productivity implying substantial costs for individuals, organizations and even society (Leiter & Maslach, 1988; Shirom, 1989). For example, Vlerick (1997) showed that burnout among nurses led to an increased number of health problems, slower organizational commitment and higher turnover intentions. Most studies have investigated the prevalence of burnout among nurses in general. However, nurses can be divided in different groups on the basis of the medical field in which they work, which can lead to differences in the prevalence of burnout. The few studies that have paid attention to this question until now, yielded inconsistent results.

For example, some studies (Stewart, Meyerowitz, Jackson, Yarkin & Harvey, 1982; Olkinuora, Asp, Juntunen, Kauttu, Strid & Äärimaa, 1990) showed a higher level of burnout for nurses working in oncology wards than for other wards while other studies (Papadatou, Anagnostopoulos & Monos, 1994) showed no significant difference in the degree of burnout experienced by nurses in oncology and those in general hospitals. Hurny (1988) suggested that the continuous confrontation with death, purging oncology nurses to acknowledge the limits of modern medicine, may cause them to feel incompetent and helpless, which might lead to feelings of reduced personal accomplishment.

Other studies found that working in intensive care wards is extremely stressful and that these nurses suffer significantly more from depersonalization than

* *Correspondence: Karin Proost, karin.proost@psy.kuleuven.ac.be*

other nurses (Zwerts, Schaufeli, Keijsers, Le Blanc & Reis, 1995), while other researchers (Pelosi, Caironi, Vecchione, Trudu, Malacrida & Tomamichel, 1999) found that the intensive care environment was not more stressful for nursing staff than general medicine units. On the contrary, in this study it was found that general medicine units caused a more severe burnout syndrome than intensive care units.

Apparently, instead of focusing purely on the medical field in which the nurses work, other factors are at play that cause nurses to feel burned out. In the literature, the job Demand-Control-Support model is often used in order to study antecedents of stress and psychological well-being. To a lesser extent, this model has also been applied to the study of burnout (Rafferty, Friend & Landsbergis, 2001).

The model, as originally proposed by Karasek (1979), identifies two major aspects in the work situation, job demands and job control, which impact on an individual's level of well-being (Sargent & Terry, 2000). Job demands refer to the workload, and have been operationalized mainly in terms of time pressure and role conflict (for a review, see Van der Doef & Maes, 1999). Job control, also named decision latitude, refers to the extent to which the employee can exert influence over tasks and includes two components: skill discretion and decision authority. A high strain job, leading to health complaints and decreased psychological well-being, is characterized by high demands and low control. In the 1980s, a social dimension was added to the model (Johnson & Hall, 1988) resulting in the Demand-Control-Support (JDCS) model. According to this model, an 'iso-strain' job, characterized by high job demands combined with both low levels of job control and high levels of social isolation, represents the most noxious work situation. On the other hand, social support is supposed to buffer for the negative consequences of a high strain job.

On the basis of inspection of the jobs and environmental contexts of nurses in different wards, we believe that the different wards can be situated at different positions on these dimensions, leading to different prevalence of burnout. For example, Whippen and Canellos (1991) identified a heavy workload as an important contributing factor to burnout for oncology nurses. Also Barrett and Yates (2002) found that workload is an important contributing factor to burnout for oncology nurses. In their study, 40% of the oncology nurses reported workloads they perceived excessive. As stated by Medland, Howard-Ruben and Whitaker (2004), oncology nursing is intensely demanding, both physically and emotionally. Also emotional exhaustion has been shown to be a very real concern. In the study of Barrett and Yates, over 70% of the sample experienced moderate to high levels. In order to cope with these high demands, social support might be an important issue. Medland, Howard-Ruben and Whitaker (2004) stated that the psychological impact of caring for patients with cancer and their families can prove overwhelming if the appropriate support system is not in place. Also Hinds, Quargnenti, Hickey and Mangum (1994) found among pediatric oncology nurses that a lack of social support from their coworkers made a significant contribution to leaving their positions prior to the twelfth month of employment. Also social support of the supervisor seems to be important. López-Castillo, Gurpegui, Ayuso-Mateos, Luna and Catalan (1999) found that oncology professionals asked for individual supervision more frequently than health care professionals serving HIV-infected patients and internal medicine professionals.

On the other hand, also nurses working on intensive care wards have contact with very sick patients and are regularly confronted with death. However, the nature of their relationship with the patient and family differs. First, where oncology nurses are intensely involved in the relationship with the patients and family, the relationship at the intensive care unit is more short-term. As soon as the patients start to feel better, they leave to another ward. Only patients with serious complications stay. Moreover, intensive care patients are often limited in their verbal communication possibilities and also contacts with families are limited to restricted visiting hours. This might make working at the intensive care unit less emotionally demanding as compared to the oncology unit. On the other hand, this aspect of the relationship might stimulate a more cynical attitude and feelings of depersonalization. The medical situation of the patient might prompt nurses to physically distance themselves in encounters with patients through lack of eye contact or minimal conversation, to spend less time with patients and more time talking and socializing with staff, to 'go by the book', rather than responding to a patient's uniqueness. On the contrary, the work in an intensive care unit is often regarded as physically demanding. It is generally believed that the more critically ill the patient, the more nurse time is needed to care for the patient, which might lead to higher workload for the intensive care nurses. However, Adomat and Hicks (2003) found that many mechanically ventilated critically ill patients needed less nursing care than patients who are self-ventilating and allocated a lower level of dependence. Lewandowski and Kositsky (1983) argued that the level of job control at intensive care wards is often insufficient to cope with the high demands, which may cause burnout.

For nurses working in a general surgery department, Ferrari, Accettella, De Angelis, Innamorati, Soccorsi and Tatarelli (1999) found that they were characterized by total absence of emotional exhaustion and that they were not influenced by any particular stressor.

In this study, we try to extend previous research in several ways. First, we investigate the different prevalence of emotional exhaustion, depersonalization and reduced personal accomplishment for nurses working in different wards, namely general surgery and internal medicine, oncology and intensive care. Second, we suggest that several aspects of the job that are typically bound with the medical field in which the nurses work could be held responsible for differences in the prevalence of burnout. In order to study the job dimensions that can lead to burnout for nurses in different work settings, the job Demand-Control-Support model is used. In this study, the following hypotheses will be tested:

Oncology nurses, working with cancer patients and their families, feel more emotionally exhausted than the other groups.

Intensive care nurses, often confronted with very-ill patients who have limited verbal communication possibilities, suffer more from depersonalization than oncology nurses and general surgery nurses.

Oncology nurses, because of the frequent confrontation with the limits of modern medicine, feel less personally accomplished than nurses working at an intensive care unit and a general surgery and internal medicine unit.

Not the wards itself, but the three dimensions of the job Demand-Control-Support model are responsible for these differences in burnout for the three groups of nurses, suggesting a mediated relationship between ward and burnout.

Both oncology and intensive care nurses are confronted with high demands. However, the consequences with respect to burnout differ for both groups. For oncology nurses, especially social support is supposed to be important to buffer for the negative consequences of the high demands. For the intensive care nurses, especially task autonomy is supposed to be an important buffer.

Method

Procedure

This study was introduced in all Flemish hospitals which had an intensive care ward and an oncology or radiotherapy ward, resulting in 27 hospitals of which 15 hospitals agreed to cooperate. The introduction was done by means of both written and oral communication, under the label of 'investigating work conditions of nurses'. The questionnaires were distributed to the senior nurses, who spread the questionnaires to all the nurses of the specific wards and also recollected the questionnaires at later times. After the deadline, one reminder was sent to all the nurses. This procedure led to a response ratio of 69.5% for oncology nurses, 74.7% for intensive care nurses and 69.1% for nurses in wards of general surgery and internal medicine.

Sample

Respondents were 2,075 Belgian nurses, divided over 15 hospitals, working in three different medical fields: oncology, intensive care, and general surgery and internal medicine. The spread over the three medical fields was respectively 21%, 25% and 54%. The mean age of the respondents was 35 with a standard deviation of 8.8 and 84% of the respondents were women. The average amount of work experience was 163 months with a standard deviation of 106.6. The average amount of work experience at the ward was 110 months with a standard deviation of 94. 58% of the participants worked full-time and 76% of the respondents followed an extra training during the last year.

Measures

Burnout

Burnout was measured by a Dutch translation of the Maslach Burnout Inventory, the Utrechtse Burnout Schaal or UBOS (Schaufeli & van Dierendonck, 2000). This scale measures the three dimensions of burnout on a Likert-type scale from 1 to 7. Emotional exhaustion and depersonalization were measured with seven items while personal accomplishment was measured with eight items. In this study, Cronbach's α for the three dimensions were 0.88 for emotional exhaustion, 0.78 for depersonalization and 0.81 for personal accomplishment.

Job Demands

Job demands were measured with three items, mainly referring to time pressure (e.g., 'Speed of work is too high'). Answers were given on a Likert-type scale, ranging from 1 (totally disagree) to 5 (totally agree). Cronbach's α for this scale was 0.90.

Job Control

Job control was measured with five items, measuring decision authority. Items were formulated in the negative sense (e.g., 'I have the feeling that I'm not consulted when important decisions have to be taken') and the scale was positively transformed afterwards. The same Likert-type scale was used as for job demands. Cronbach's α for this scale was 0.89.

Social Support

For the measurement of social support, a distinction was made between social support of colleagues and social support of the supervisor. The same Likert-type scale was used, consisting of 6 items to measure social support of colleagues (e.g., 'My colleagues pay attention to my feelings and problems') and 5 items to measure social support of supervisor (e.g., 'My supervisor pays attention to my feelings and problems'). Cronbach's α was 0.82 and 0.91 respectively.

The scales for job demands, job control and social support were taken from a study of Le Blanc, Van Heesch and Schaufeli (1998). However, in order to limit the number of questions in the questionnaire, only a limited number of items were taken from the original scales. The construct validity of the scales was well-supported by the results of a principal component analyses with varimax rotation. The total amount of variance explained with 4 factors was 67%.

Analyses

In order to test the different prevalence of burnout in the three different medical fields, a Manova was executed with ward as independent variable and each of the three dimensions of burnout as dependent variables.

In order to test for mediation, several regression analyses were executed, following the steps suggested by Baron and Kenny (1986). These authors recommend three steps in order to test for mediation, namely (1) regressing the mediator on the independent variable, (2) regressing the dependent variable on the independent variable and (3) regressing the dependent variable on both the independent variable and on the mediator.

In order to test the last hypothesis, moderated hierarchical regression analyses were executed. In the first step, the main effect terms of job demands, job control and social support of supervisor and colleagues were entered. In the second step, three interaction terms with job demands were entered.

Results

Tables 1, 2 and 4 show the means, standard deviations and Pearson correlations of the variables in this study, for each medical field separately. As can be seen in the tables, all the variables in the model were significantly related to the three dimensions of burnout, for each of the three medical fields.

With respect to the prevalence of burnout, a Manova revealed significant differences in emotional exhaustion ($F = 4.39$, $p = .013$) and personal job accomplishment ($F = 13.27$, $p = .000$). For depersonalization, the difference between the wards was only marginally significant ($F = 2.89$, $p = .056$).

Table 1: Descriptive statistics for and correlations between the variables in this study for general surgery and internal medicine

Variable	M	SD	2	3	4	5	6	7	8	9	10	11
1. Age	36.69	9.04	-.00	.94**	.65**	.08**	-.06	-.11**	-.04	.09**	.07*	-.15**
2. Gender	1.92	.28		.04	.04	-.01	.10**	.06	.03	-.03	-.07*	-.02
3. Tenure in general	178.1	111.8			.70**	.10**	-.07*	-.08**	-.04	.10**	.07*	-.15**
4. Tenure in this department	121.3	100.7				.08*	-.06	-.03	-.02	.05	.05	-.10**
5. Job demands	3.84	.91					-.37**	-.13**	-.16**	.45**	.29**	-.17**
6. Job control	3.33	.92						.21**	.32**	-.23**	-.19**	.11**
7. Social support of colleagues	3.54	.64							.51**	-.24**	-.19**	.26**
8. Social support of supervisor	3.20	.92								-.22**	-.19**	.23**
9. Emotional exhaustion	2.68	1.14									.62**	-.34**
10. Depersonalization	2.04	.79										-.44**
11. Personal accomplishment	5.14	.95										

** p < .05; ** p < .01

247

Burnout of nurses working in three different medical fields

Table 2: Descriptive statistics for and correlations between the variables in this study for intensive care

Variable	M	SD	2	3	4	5	6	7	8	9	10	11
1. Age	32.99	7.78	-.14**	.95**	.76**	-.01	.01	-.10*	-.00	.06	.04	-.10
2. Gender	1.71	.45		-.09*	-.03	.04	.04	.01	.02	-.07	-.20**	-.02
3. Tenure in general	133.2	90.82			.80**	-.02	.00	-.11*	.01	.05	.04	-.06
4. Tenure in this department	107.94	91.41				.00	-.02	-.05	.02	.03	.05	-.06
5. Job demands	3.44	1.01					-.38**	-.06	-.10*	.41**	.21**	-.12*
6. Job control	3.17	.91						.16**	.28**	-.13**	-.15**	.06
7. Social support of colleagues	3.49	.55							.50**	-.28**	-.23**	.37**
8. Social support of supervisor	3.13	.85								-.21**	-.24**	.27**
9. Emotional exhaustion	2.54	.98									.59**	-.46**
10. Depersonalization	2.12	.82										-.49**
11. Personal accomplishment	4.98	.93										

** p < .05; ** p < .01

Table 3: Descriptive statistics for and correlations between the variables in this study for oncology

Variable	M	SD	2	3	4	5	6	7	8	9	10	11
1. Age	35.37	8.69	-.12*	.95**	.57**	.00	-.09	-.21**	-.13**	.11*	.04	-.10*
2. Gender	1.81	.40		-.07	-.12*	.04	.04	.10*	.05	-.10*	-.20**	.06
3. Tenure in general	158.3	102.9			.60**	.00	-.07	-.22**	-.11*	.11*	.03	-.09
4. Tenure in this department	85.25	74.65				.03	.00	-.12*	-.07	.13**	.06	-.05
5. Job demands	3.72	.93					-.39**	-.09	-.07	.45**	.30**	-.15**
6. Job control	3.26	.90						.21**	.23**	-.25**	-.23**	.22**
7. Social support of colleagues	3.54	.55							.49**	-.26**	-.22**	.29**
8. Social support of supervisor	3.24	.92								-.23**	-.20**	.25**
9. Emotional exhaustion	2.75	1.04									.67**	-.42**
10. Depersonalization	2.02	.78										-.48**
11. Personal accomplishment	5.31	.90										

* p < .05; ** p < .01

In line with the first hypothesis, nurses working in oncology suffered significantly more from emotional exhaustion than nurses working in intensive care departments. Nurses working in general surgery and internal medicine units showed an intermediate level of emotional exhaustion.

In line with the second hypothesis, nurses working at intensive care units showed higher feelings of depersonalization than the other groups. Oncology nurses and nurses working in general surgery and internal medicine units showed the same, lower level of depersonalization. Contrary to the third hypothesis, nurses working in oncology reported the highest feeling of personal accomplishment, followed by nurses working in general surgery and internal medicine. The lowest values were reported by nurses working in intensive care units.

With respect to the mediating effects, no evidence was found for a mediating role of any of the three dimensions of the job Demand-Control-Support model for the relationship between working in oncology and two dimensions of burnout, namely emotional exhaustion and personal accomplishment. Four different regression analyses showed no effect of the dummy variable 'working in oncology' on job demands ($B = .001$, $p = .96$), job control ($B = -.01$, $p = .72$), social support of the supervisor ($B = .03$, $p = .17$) and social support of colleagues ($B = .01$, $p = .68$).

A second mediational analysis was done in order to test the mediating role of job demands, job control and social support on the relationship between the dummy variable 'working in intensive care' and depersonalization. In the first step, working in intensive care showed a significant effect on job demands ($B = -.16$, $p = .00$) and job control ($B = -.06$, $p = .01$) but not on social support from supervisor and social support of colleagues. The negative β-values indicated that nurses in intensive care units are confronted with lower job demands and less task autonomy. In the second step, a significant effect was found of working in intensive care on depersonalization ($B = .05$, $p = .02$). However, the third and final step showed no mediating effect of job demands and job control on the relationship between working in intensive care and depersonalization ($B = .09$, $p = .00$).

The results of the moderated hierarchical regression analysis are presented in table 4.

Table 4: Results of the moderated hierarchical regression analyses for personal accomplishment with oncology nurses and for depersonalization with intensive care nurses

Predictor	Depersonalization – intensive care		Personal accomplishment – oncology	
	Step 1	Step 2	Step 1	Step 2
Job demands	.15**	.14**	-.06	-.06
Job control	-.04	-.04	.12	.11
Supervisor support	-.20**	-.21**	.16*	.17**
Colleague support	-.10	-.10	.16*	.15*
Job demands* job control		.04		.00
Job demands* supervisor support		-.14*		-.14*
Job demands* colleague support		.07		.06
R² cumulative	.11	.12	.12	.14
R² adjusted	.10	.11	.11	.12
R² change	.11	.01	.12	.01
F change	12.13**	1.66	10.59**	1.50
Df1	4	3	4	3
Df2	399	396	298	295

All entries are standardized regression coefficients.

$* p < .05; ** p < .01$

In line with the last hypothesis, these results showed a significant interaction effect between job demands and social support of the supervisor for oncology nurses, but only on personal accomplishment ($B = -.14$, $p = .04$). However, this interaction effect does not represent the expected buffering effect (see figure 1). Especially when job demands are low, supervisor support can make a difference. Interaction effects with respect to emotional exhaustion and depersonalization were not significant.

Also no evidence was found for the suggested interaction effect between job demands and job control on burnout for intensive care nurses. However, also for this group, a significant interaction effect was found between job demands and supervisor support ($B = -.07$, $p = .02$). Figure 2 shows that supervisor support can buffer for the negative impact of high demands on feelings of depersonalization for intensive care nurses.

Figure 1: Interaction effect between job demands and supervisor support on personal accomplishment for oncology nurses

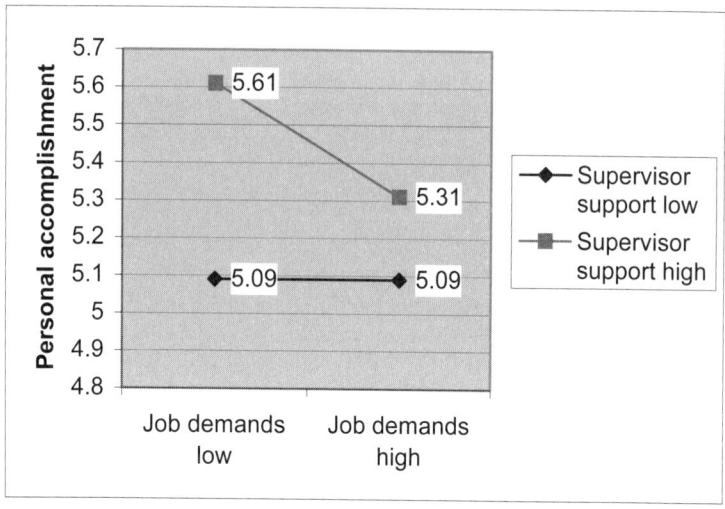

Figure 2: Interaction effect between job demands and supervisor support on depersonalization for intensive care nurses

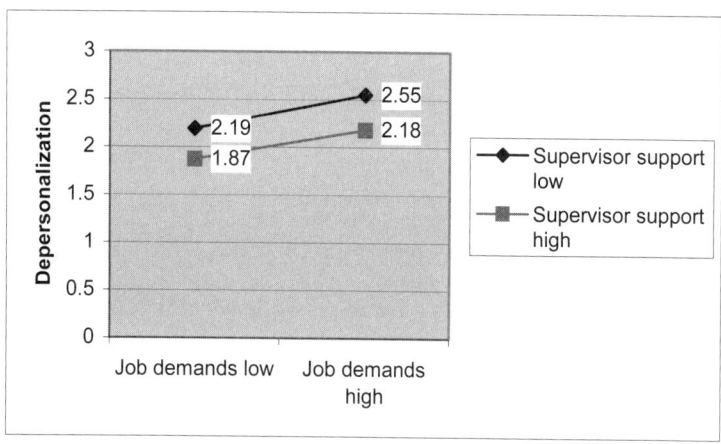

Discussion

In this study, it was suggested that nurses working in different medical fields suffered to different degrees from burnout. The results showed that for nurses working in oncology, emotional exhaustion might be an important concern. Higher levels of emotional exhaustion were found for this group of nurses as compared to nurses working at intensive care wards. But, on the other hand and contrary to our expectations, these nurses felt more personally accomplished than the other groups of nurses. For nurses working at intensive care wards, higher levels of depersonalization were found.

In this study, it was also suggested that not ward itself but characteristics of the job are responsible for the different prevalence of burnout. However, this hypothesis was not confirmed by our data. With respect to the mediating role of the job Demand-Control-Support model, no evidence was found to support it. Apparently, other factors within the work environment are at play, that cause oncology nurses to feel more emotionally exhausted and for intensive care nurses to feel more depersonalized.

For oncology nurses, caring for patients with cancer and their families might be psychologically so demanding, that these nurses suffer more from emotional exhaustion than other nurses. Therefore, in the case of oncology care providers, it might be extremely relevant to include additional job demands that refer specifically to the emotionally demanding aspects of interactions with patients. Until now, different types of job demands have rarely been incorporated in tests of the JDC model and, in turn, are not profoundly examined (Peeters & Le Blanc, 2001). The few studies (Söderfeldt, Söderfeldt, Muntaner, O'Campo, Warg & Ohlson, 1996; De Jonge, Mulder & Nijhuis, 1999) that have examined this, did find that different types of demands were important in predicting different aspects of health.

For intensive care nurses, as mentioned in the literature review, the short-term relationship with patients who are often unable to communicate, might cause intensive care nurses to distance themselves psychologically. Further research should take these relational variables into account. The lower level of personal accomplishment of intensive care nurses might be related to the highly complex technological environment in which these nurses work. For example, Alasad (2002) found in his study that the ability to manage technology was a main component of being a critical care nurse.

In the last part of this study, moderating effects are investigated. For oncology nurses, the lowest levels of personal accomplishment were found when supervisor support is low, independent of the level of workload. However, an increase in supervisor support led to higher levels of personal accomplishment, especially when the nurses have time to benefit from the support of the supervisor. On the contrary, when workload is so high that nurses are completely absorbed by daily tasks, the influence of supervisor support on personal accomplishment is more restricted. In practice, this might mean that it is important at an oncology ward to explicitly make time for supporting moments with the supervisor, for example by means of individual or collective consulting moments.

Also for intensive care nurses, evidence was found for the importance of social support of the supervisor. Higher levels of supervisor support led to lower levels of depersonalization, independent of the level of job demands. However, the effect of supervisor support was slightly more important when job demands were high. Therefore, especially when job demands are high, it seems important to guarantee good support from the supervisor in order to prevent intensive care nurses from developing a cynical attitude toward patients and families.

The most important strength of this study is that nurses are not considered as one homogeneous population. Explicit attention is paid to differences in prevalence and antecedents of burnout for nurses working in three different medical fields, showing different levels of burnout for different wards.

However, this study also suffers from some important weaknesses. The job Demand-Control-Support model was used in order to test antecedents of burnout for the different groups of nurses, but was not supported. Apparently, several other factors are at play in these different medical fields that were not incorporated in this study. As already mentioned, psychological demands might play an important role for oncology nurses but were not measured in this study. Also the nature of the relationship with patients for oncology nurses versus intensive care nurses might play an important role and was not measured. Other possible factors are: speed of development of new curing practices, amount of extra training that nurses are allowed to follow, technological developments, etc.

Another important topic that starts to receive some attention with respect to burnout, is work-life conflict. Especially employees working long or inflexible hours, as is the case for nurses, are suffering from heightened conflicts between work and home roles (Burke, Weir & Duwors, 1980; Pleck, Staines & Lang, 1980). Nurses working in different wards could suffer to different degrees from work-life conflict. Consequently, work-life conflict could lead to burnout in different gradations for nurses working in different medical fields. Future studies could incorporate this variable in their study of antecedents of burnout as well.

References

Adomat, R. & Hicks, C. (2003). Measuring nursing workload in intensive care: an observational study using closed circuit video cameras. *Journal of advanced nursing, 42*(4), 402-412.

Alasad, J. (2002). Managing technology in the intensive care unit: The nurses' experience. *International journal of nursing studies, 39*(4), 407-413.

Baron, R. M. & Kenny, D. A. (1986). The moderator-mediator variable distinction in social psychological research: Conceptual, strategic, and statistical considerations. *Journal of personality and social psychology, 51*(6), 1173-1182.

Barrett, L. & Yates, P. (2002). Oncology/haematology nurses: a study of job satisfaction, burnout, and intention to leave the specialty. *Australian health review, 25*(3), 109-121.

Burke, R. J., Weir, T. & Duwors, R. (1980). Work demands on administrators and spouse well-being. *Human Relations, 33*, 253-278.

De Jonge, J., Mulder, M. J. & Nijhuis, F. J. (1999). The incorporation of different demand concepts in the job demand-control model: effects on health care professionals. *Social science and medicine, 48*, 1149-1160.

Ferrari, V., Accettella, U., De Angelis, R., Innamorati, M., Soccorsi, R. & Tatarelli, R. (1999). The burn-out syndrome: Comparison between an emergency unit vs a general surgery department. *European journal of psychiatry, 13*(1), 19-31.

Hinds, P. S., Quargnenti, A. G., Hickey, S. S. & Mangum, G. H. (1994). A comparison of the stress-response sequence in new and experienced pediatric oncology nurses. *Cancer nursing, 17*, 61-71.

Hurny, C. (1988). Psychosocial support of cancer patients: a training program for oncology staff. *Recent results in cancer research, 108*, 295-300.

Johnson, J. V. & Hall, E. M. (1988). Job strain, workplace social support and cardiovascular disease: A cross-sectional study of a random sample of the Swedish working population. *American journal of public health, 78*, 1336-1342.

Karasek, R. A. (1979). Job demands, job control and mental strain: Implications for job redesign. *Administrative Science Quarterly, 24*, 285-308.

Koustelios, A. (2001). Organizational factors as predictors of teachers' burnout. *Psychological Reports, 88*, 627-634.

Le Blanc, P. M., Van Heesch, N. & Schaufeli, W. (1998). Rapportage werkbeleving zorgverleners oncologie. Utrecht: Universiteit Utrecht.

Leiter, M. P. & Maslach, C. (1988). The impact of interpersonal environment on burnout and organizational commitment. *Journal of organizational behavior, 9*(4), 297-308.

Lewandowski, L. A. & Kositsky, A. M. (1983). Research priorities for critical care nursing: A study by the American Association of Critical-Care Nurses. *Heart and Lung, 12*, 35-44.

López-Castillo, J., Gurpegui, M., Ayuso-Mateos, J. L., Luna, J. D. & Catalan, J. (1999). Emotional distress and occupational burnout in health care professionals serving HIV-infected patients: A comparison with oncology and internal medicine services. *Psychotherapy and psychosomatics, 68*, 348-356.

Medland, J., Howard-Ruben, J. & Whitaker, E. (2004). Fostering psychosocial wellness in oncology nurses: Addressing burnout and social support in the workplace. *Oncology nursing forum, 31*(1), 47-54.

Olkinuora, M., Asp, S., Juntunen, J., Kauttu, K., Strid, L. & Äärimaa, M. (1990). Stress symptoms, burnout and suicidal thoughts in Finnish physicians. *Social psychiatry and psychiatric epidemiology, 25*, 81-86.

Papadatou, D., Anagnostopoulos, F. & Monos, D. (1994). Factors contributing to the development of burnout in oncology nursing. *British journal of medical psychology, 67*(2), 187-199.

Peeters, M. C. W. & Le Blanc, P. M. (2001). Towards a match between job demands and sources of social support: A study among oncology care providers. *European Journal of Work and Organizational Psychology, 10*(1), 53-72.

Pelosi, P., Caironi, P., Vecchione, A., Trudu, G., Malacrida, R. & Tomamichel, M. (1999). Ansia e stress del personale infermieristico. Analisi comparata tra Terapia Intensiva e reparti di base. *Minerva Anestesiologica, 65*(5 Suppl 1), 108-115.

Pleck, J., Staines, G. & Lang, L. (1980). Conflicts between work and family life. *Monthly Labor Review, 103*(3), 29-32.

Rafferty, Y., Friend, R. & Landsbergis, P. A. (2001). The association between job skill discretion, decision authority and burnout. *Work & Stress, 15*(1), 73-85.

Sargent, L. D. & Terry, D. J. (2000). The moderating role of social support in Karasek's job strain model. *Work & Stress, 14*(3), 245-261.

Schaufeli, W. B. & van Dierendonck, D. (2000). *UBOS: De Utrechtse Burnout Schaal. Handleiding* [UBOS: The Utrecht Burnout Scale, Manual]. Lisse, the Netherlands: Swets & Zeitlinger.

Shirom, A. (1989). Burnout in work organizations. In C. L. Cooper & I. Robertson (Eds.), *International review of industrial and organizational psychology* (pp. 25-48). New York: Wiley.

Söderfeldt, B., Söderfeldt, M., Muntaner, C., O'Campo, P., Warg, L. & Ohlson, C. (1996). Psychosocial work environment in human service organizations: A conceptual analysis and development of the demand-control model. *Social science and medicine, 42*, 1217-1225.

Stewart, B. E., Meyerowitz, B. A., Jackson, L. E., Yarkin, K. L., & Harvey, J. H. (1982). Psychological stress associated with outpatient oncology nursing. *Cancer nursing, 5*, 393-387.

Van der Doef, M. & Maes, S. (1999). The Job Demand-Control(-Support) Model and psychological well-being: a review of 20 years of empirical research. *Work & Stress, 13*(2), 87-114.

Vlerick, P. (1997). Economisch-psychologische gevolgen van burnout. In Verslagboek van de Tweede (Ed.), *Arbeidsmarktonderzoekersdag* (pp. 87-102). Brussel: Steunpunt Werkgelegenheid, Arbeid en Vorming (K.U.Leuven).

Whippen, D. A. & Canellos, G. P. (1991). Burnout syndrome in the practice of oncology: results of a random survey of 1000 oncologists. *Journal of clinical oncology, 9*(10), 1916-1920.

Zwerts, C., Schaufeli, W., Keijsers, G., Le Blanc, P. & Reis, D. (1995). Burnout en prestatie in intensive care units. *Tijdschrift Sociologische Gezondheidszorg, 73*, 382-389.

Performance obstacles and facilitators of healthcare providers

Pascale Carayon[1,2], Ayse P. Gurses[1,2], Ann Schoofs Hundt[1], Phillip Ayoub[3], and Carla J. Alvarado[1]*

[1] *Center for Quality and Productivity Improvement, University of Wisconsin-Madison, USA*
[2] *Department of Industrial Engineering, University of Wisconsin-Madison, USA*
[3] *The Harold & Inge Marcus Department of Industrial & Manufacturing Engineering, Pennsylvania State University, USA*

Much research has been done to characterize the job characteristics and stressors of healthcare providers (Crickmore, 1987; Gray-Toft & Anderson, 1981; Keijsers, Schaufeli, LeBlanc, Carmen & Miranda, 1995; Linzer et al., 2000; Oates & Oates, 1995). While this information is important, we believe that it provides limited information on how to redesign and improve work in healthcare. Many important characteristics and stressors of healthcare jobs are inherent to the jobs themselves and cannot be changed. Therefore, we are proposing a more 'micro' approach that examines the factors in one's immediate work system that might hinder or facilitate performance in particular situations. This concept of performance obstacles has been studied only in manufacturing settings. In this paper, we present data on performance obstacles from two groups of healthcare providers: one group of healthcare staff in five outpatient surgery centers, and a group of ICU nurses.

Performance obstacles

In this paper, we use the term of 'performance obstacles'. Performance obstacles have also been called 'situational constraints'. Peters and O'Connor

* *Correspondence: Pascale Carayon, carayon@engr.wisc.edu*

NOTE: Phillip Ayoub contributed to this work as a research intern at the Center for Quality and Productivity Improvement of the University of Wisconsin-Madison from January to August 2003.

This research is funded by AHRQ Grant # P20 HS11561-01 (PI: Pascale Carayon). We are indebted to the five outpatient surgery centers' administration and staff for their willingness to cooperate in this research, and to the intensive care unit nurses, their supervisor and the director of the unit for their help and support in this research

(1980) define situational factors as factors that interfere with the translation of individual ability and motivation into effective performance. Brown and Mitchell (1991) define performance obstacles as factors in the work environment that restrict productivity by inhibiting employees in the execution of task responsibilities. Both of these definitions[1] emphasize the importance of work factors that may impede performance or one's ability to optimally perform one's job. Both definitions emphasize the local context (or situation) in which these obstacles or constraints occur and impede performance. We put special emphasis on this conceptual characteristic of performance obstacles: one can identify work situations that impede one's capacity to perform, and therefore restrict or limit performance, but also create feelings of frustration and discouragement among affected workers who cannot produce at their optimal level. We believe that this approach is particularly appropriate if one is interested in redesigning work in order to improve performance *and* quality of working life. This approach emphasizes the important local or situational factors that can be changed in order to improve performance and quality of working life.

In a review of research on performance obstacles Peters, O'Connor and Eulberg (1985) identified 11 categories of performance obstacles (see table 1). These categories of performance obstacles have been examined in a range of field and laboratory studies. Peters and colleagues argue that this taxonomy is sufficiently generalizable to apply to a range of jobs and organizations. At least, it can provide a good basis for identifying the performance obstacles in a specific organization or job. This taxonomy of performance obstacles can be mapped onto the work system model developed by Smith and Carayon (Carayon & Smith, 2000; Smith & Carayon-Sainfort, 1989). The work system model recognizes that *workers* perform *tasks* utilizing *tools and technology* in a given *environment* within an *organization*. Table 1 shows how the 11 categories of performance obstacles cover all the elements of the work system model.

---

[1] In the rest of the paper, we will use the term 'performance obstacles'.

Table 1: Categories of performance obstacles (Peters et al., 1985)

Categories of perform-ance obstacles	Definitions	Elements of the work system model*
Job-related information	Information from various sources needed to do the job assigned	TASK ORGANIZATION
Tools and equipment	Specific tools, equipment and machinery needed to do the job	TOOLS & TECHNOLOGY
Materials and supplies	Materials and supplies needed to do the job assigned	TOOLS & TECHNOLOGY
Budgetary support	Financial resources needed to do the job assigned	ORGANIZATION
Required services and help from others	Services and help from others needed to do the job assigned	ORGANIZATION
Task preparation	Preparation through education, training and experience	WORKER
Time availability	Availability of time to do job assigned, taking into consid-eration time limits, interrup-tions, unnecessary meetings, nonjob related distractions, etc…	TASK ORGANIZATION
Work environment	Physical aspects that affect ability to do the job assigned	ENVIRONMENT
Scheduling of activities	Arrangement of work schedule for best utilization of re-sources	ORGANIZATION
Transportation	Transportation needed to get to and complete job	ORGANIZATION
Job-relevant authority	Authority needed to do the job as assigned	ORGANIZATION

* Carayon and Smith, 2000; Smith and Carayon-Sainfort, 1989

The field research on performance obstacles has been performed in the manu-facturing sector. Brown and Mitchell (1988) compared performance obstacles reported by engineers versus assemblers in 12 American electronics compa-nies. For the manufacturing engineers, information, schedules and distractions were the most important obstacles. For assemblers, parts and drawings were the most important obstacles. In a study comparing performance obstacles produced by different technologies, Brown and Mitchell (1991) found that workers in a Just-In-Time (JIT) manufacturing system experienced fewer obstacles caused by parts and job-related information, but more obstacles due to computer system use, training, scheduling and reliance on co-workers.

To our knowledge, the concept of performance obstacles has not been applied to healthcare. We argue that this concept can provide a useful approach to the identification of work factors of need of redesign in healthcare. The literature on performance obstacles emphasizes the negative work factors that hinder performance. We extend this concept to include not only negative factors, but also positive factors that can facilitate performance, i.e., performance facilitators[2]. This approach of including both negative and positive work factors is in line with current job stress research (i.e., job stressors and resources) (e.g., Karasek & Theorell, 1990; Siegrist, 1996). In applying the concept of performance obstacles to healthcare, we are interested in how performance obstacles and facilitators can affect quality of working life of the 'workers', i.e., healthcare providers, and their performance, i.e., the quality and safety of care they provide.

The goal of our research is to examine the applicability of the concept of performance obstacles (and facilitators) in healthcare work environments. In this paper, we report data from two studies of healthcare providers on performance obstacles and facilitators. The first study includes staff of five outpatient surgery centers, and the second study focuses on nurses in an intensive care unit.

Methods

Study of five outpatient surgery centers

Brief description of larger project and its objectives

In the context of a larger project examining the impact of a work system intervention on worker and patient outcomes[3], we conducted a study to identify performance obstacles perceived by the staff of five outpatient surgery

---

[2] We are indebted to Professor Wolfgang Friesdorf of the Technical University of Berlin, Germany, for suggesting to extend our concept of performance obstacles to include performance facilitators.

[3] This is part of the AHRQ-funded SEIPS (Systems Engineering Initiative for Patient Safety) project (Carayon, Alvarado, Brennan, Gurses, Hundt, Karsh & Smith 2003). The SEIPS pilot study is one of the first known studies of its type addressing patient safety in outpatient surgery.

centers. Because we intended to make improvements in light of the work system model, it became apparent in the early stages of our project that we would benefit by utilizing past research on performance obstacles.

Data collection method (questionnaire) and procedures

In order to collect information on performance obstacles and facilitators from the staff, we developed a questionnaire with 3 open-ended questions. Two questions asked about performance obstacles and facilitators, and a third question asked about quality and safety of patient care issues. This latter question (which we are not discussing in this paper) asked staff to identify quality of care and patient safety issues they believe patients incur at specific stages of the outpatient surgery process – from the work-up (prior to presenting for surgery) to patient follow-up at home (Carayon, Alvarado, Hundt & Springman, 2003). The question on performance obstacles asked staff to identify 'instances when your performance was challenged or below par' and the question on facilitators asked staff to describe 'instances when you were able to perform your job very well'. The questions are similar to the critical incident approach where people are asked to remember specific incidents and the context surrounding those incidents (Flanagan, 1954). The format of the questionnaire included one blank page per question. The question was written and clarified by providing examples listed at the top of the page: 'your work-space or environment; resources needed to accomplish your job, such as equipment, other workers, or time available; information needed to do your work; your work schedule; the training provided to you; policies and procedures related to your work; goals and expectations given to you; or some other reason'. This was done so staff could understand the number and magnitude of issues they could consider and include in their responses.

While attending staff meetings at each of the five participating outpatient surgery centers, we introduced and explained our research project and then distributed questionnaires to all staff present. Because attendance was taken at each of the sites' meetings, questionnaires were later distributed by supervisory staff to those not present at the meeting. The presentations were well received and staff expressed interest and willingness to participate in the study. We attached IRB-required cover sheets (in lieu of obtaining subjects' written consent) to all of the questionnaires to ensure that staff fully understood the intent and consequences of participation. We also offered staff the option of completing paper or electronic versions of the questionnaire, including a web format or entry on an rtf-formatted diskette. Seventy-seven of the seventy-nine responses received were completed on the paper version and two respondents utilized the web format. Completed paper surveys were deposited in locked mailboxes at each site to assure confidentiality. Research staff collected the surveys twice a week for the three weeks during which the surveys could be completed and returned.

Sample

We enrolled five outpatient surgery centers (sites) in the city of Madison, Wisconsin to participate in the study. All of the sites are members of the Madison Patient Safety Collaborative, a group of local providers collectively committed to improving patient safety in the community who have also agreed to not use patient safety to their competitive advantage (Carayon, Bogsdorf, Hundt & Alvarado, 2003). A total of 79 responses were received (estimated response rate: 35%). Although we had no intention of identifying the respondents personally, or by type of caregiver (nurse, surgeon, anesthesiologist), it was apparent by the nature of the responses received that the vast majority of those completing the survey were nurses. We were not surprised by this because the open-ended nature of the survey affected the attitude and willingness of physicians to participate. Physicians overtly stated to both the researchers and their center staff that they did not 'have time' to complete this type of data collection instrument.

Data analysis

We performed content analysis on responses to the two questions of the surveys. This was done after initially reading all of the responses, and then entering them in an Excel spreadsheet to group similar responses and ultimately determine categories. In order to distinguish between responses to the facilitator versus obstacle questions, we were careful to associate each response to one of the two questions. To achieve this we had separate columns in the spreadsheet for each question. For example, the category 'communication from referring physician' had negative responses (e.g., 'not having a complete history and physical delays our ability to proceed safely with surgery'), as well as positive responses (e.g., 'thorough history and physicals streamline pre-op assessments'). Both of these examples were assigned to the same category however one was obviously noted as a facilitator and the other an obstacle. Once we completed this initial process, we then recoded the responses by entering each of the questionnaires into a unique Microsoft Word document and then using NVivo© software to perform a more detailed systematic content analysis. We used the NVivo© (QSR International Pty. Ltd., 1999-2000) qualitative data analysis software to code our data. NVivo© allows the researcher to code each category and subcategory as a node and sub-node, respectively; hence forming a node tree. The node structure developed initially was entered into NVivo© and several rounds of modification to the node structure were made through input and discussion of the researchers.

Study of intensive care unit nurses

Brief description of larger study and its objectives

We are conducting a study on nursing workload in intensive care units (ICUs) and its impact on nurses' perceived quality of care (i.e., performance) and quality of working life. One aim of this study is to identify the performance obstacles and facilitators among ICU nurses. Research has identified high workload as a key stressor for ICU nurses (Keijsers et al., 1995), and also as an important root cause of medical errors and suboptimal quality of care (Pronovost et al., 1999). In this study, we are interested in identifying the local or situational causes of nursing workload. We believe that such an approach can help in efforts for redesigning and improving the work of ICU nurses.

Data collection method (interviews) and procedures

We used individual, semi-structured interviews to collect data on performance obstacles and facilitators from a group of 15 ICU nurses. During the interviews, nurses were asked two open-ended questions. First, they were asked to think of instances when they had a high workload, or when they felt stressed and unsatisfied with their job, or when their performance was below the optimum level, and then to recall situations in the work environment that were present at that time. Second, they were asked to think of instances when their workload was reasonable, or when they were not stressed and satisfied with their job, or when their performance was good, and then again to recall situations in the work environment that were present at that time.

Participation in the interviews was voluntary. We distributed an information sheet for participation in interviews to all nurses in the participating ICU and asked them if they were willing to participate. The first 15 nurses who agreed to participate to the study were recruited. We conducted the interviews in a private quiet room.

The interviews took place during the work hours of the nurses. Both day- and night-shift nurses participated in the study. Seven of the 15 interviews took place during the night shift and eight during the day shift. Seven of the interviews took place during weekend and eight during weekdays. It was important to collect data on different shifts (day versus night, and weekend versus weekday) because performance obstacles and facilitators are likely to vary depending on the shift. For example, during the interviews, eight nurses noted that not seeing physician orders in a timely fashion was a problem during the day shift, but not during the night shift. The average duration of the interviews was 29 minutes, ranging from 14 minutes to 64 minutes. All the interviews were audio taped, and tapes were transcribed.

Sample

A total of 15 nurses working in a medical/surgical ICU at an academic hospital in the city of Madison, Wisconsin participated in this study.

Data analysis

We performed content analysis on the interview data to identify common themes and categories of performance obstacles and facilitators. The first step in our content analysis was to code the data into common themes. This was done using the NVivo© software. One researcher performed the bulk of the coding. Another researcher reviewed the coding scheme and the text coded. She suggested changes to the coding scheme, which were discussed by the researchers who then came up to a consensus about changes to make to the coding scheme. This iterative process yielded a five-dimensional node structure.

Results

Study of outpatient surgery centers

Each piece of text was coded under at least one coding node. Text was coded in more than one category if comments inferred multiple issues or if comments were too general to determine a single identifiable category. The coding process resulted in a total of 51 nodes grouped into 6 categories of performance obstacles and facilitators. The same generic categories were applied to both obstacles and facilitators. Table 2 shows the six categories of performance obstacles and facilitators identified in the questionnaire data. For each category, we also report the number of pieces of text coded either as a performance obstacle or as facilitator. A preliminary analysis of this data was presented at the 2003 conference of the Human Factors and Ergonomics Society (Hundt, Carayon, Ayoub & Alvarado, 2003).

Table 2: Performance obstacles and facilitators among outpatient surgery center staff

Categories	Performance obstacles	Performance facilitators
Communication:	8	4
• To patient		
• To caretaker		
• Timing of instructions and information		
• Inconsistencies between providers		
Coordination:	8	8
• Caretaker		
• Reports and forms		
Time issues:	32	9
• Patient flow		
• Patient and staff time pressures		
• Physician availability		
• Staff tasks		
Equipment and supplies:	33	18
• Availability		
• Quality		
Environment:	56	7
• Work space		
• Noise		
• Cleanliness		
• General		
Organization:	65	87
• Quality and safety of care		
• Case scheduling		
• Staff		
• Teamwork		

Note: The numbers represent the number of times a piece of text was coded under one of the categories.

The most frequently cited performance obstacles were related to the organization and the environment, followed by time issues and equipment and supplies (see Table 2). By far the most frequently cited category of performance facilitators was organization (65 comments). A range of organizational factors were identified as performance obstacles: conflict among nurses and between physicians and nurses, lack of staffing, lack of staff training, and poor work schedules. The following quote illustrates some of the organizational factors identified as performance obstacles.

"We do not get float staff, so if someone calls in sick, it is quite often that someone is pulled from secondary recovery to float to PACU or up front with the secretary's and secondary recovery is expected to fend for itself, which can be frustrating because we're usually quite busy. It is difficult getting to use your comp-time back which has been earned by staying overtime because there doesn't seem to be adequate staffing."

Environmental issues included the physical layout, noise, lighting, crowded and messy workspaces, and lack of staff availability to help with immediate clean up of the environment or equipment. The noise, the housekeeping, the level of constant activity, the size of the rooms or physicians' and nurses' personal space (if any), patients/staff coming and going, crowds of people waiting to get a moment of the physician's or the nurse's time and attention may all make the physical environment more difficult to carry out tasks. The following quote illustrates some of the environmental issues.

"The physical layout is not conducive to maintaining patient privacy. The step-down rooms on the B-side are small, cramped with equipment and noisy. The nursing area in step down does not provide for patient privacy, when there is a constant stream of patients and visitors walking through there."

In the time issues categories, time constraints of outpatient surgery that may prevent or hinder patient safety, and lack of time for assuming safe or unsafe behavior by the health care professional based on task and the time allotted for that task were mentioned. The following quote is an example of those time issues.

"When the pre-op workup isn't done before the day of surgery, it creates a hurried, less than perfect workup the day of surgery. Patients still present without completed workups and the doctors try and scramble to get them done quickly. This leads to something important being missed or normally required tests, labs etc. by-passed because the operating room is waiting."

Several aspects of equipment and supplies were identified as performance obstacles: availability of needed supplies, the type of supplies, tools, technology desired, the working condition of the equipment, and the new technology available or unavailable. The following quote shows how equipment and supplies can be obstacles to optimal performance.

"We were performing a tubal banding when one of the fallopian tubes was lacerated and needed to be cauterized. We had a cautery instrument available to our room earlier, but another room needed to use it for their case, and it then wasn't available when we needed it. By the time another instrument was sterilized and available to our room; our patient was in the OR an extra 25 minutes."

There is also a range of organizational factors that were mentioned as performance facilitators (87 comments; see Table 2). The following quotes illustrate how organizational factors can act as performance facilitators.

"When we have adequate staffing we are able to provide a high standard of care."

"I appreciate the early hours that I work and the flexibility of our staff. They are willing to change hours when needed to cover busy days. Part-time nurses are willing to pick up hours when needed."

Study of intensive care nurses

Our coding process for the study of ICU nurses was as follows. First, we coded the data either under the 'obstacles' category or the 'facilitators' category. Since each obstacle or facilitator may involve or be affected by specific people *(most frequently cited: nurses and physicians)*, occur at a specific location *(most frequently cited: patient rooms)*, or at a specific time *(most frequently cited: night shift, shift change and day shift)*, or result in a specific output *(workload, quality of working life, perceived quality and safety of care)*, these four dimensions were added to the node structure. In other words, a specific piece of text was first coded either under the obstacles or facilitators node. Then, the same text was coded under people, location, time, or output nodes whenever appropriate. Although each piece of text had to be coded either as an obstacle or facilitator, it did not necessarily have to be coded under the people, location, time, or output nodes. Ultimately, we developed a five dimensional node structure to code the interview data. Each of the five dimensions or primary nodes was further subdivided into sub-nodes.

Table 3: Performance obstacles and facilitators among intensive care nurses

Categories and dimensions of performance Obstacles and facilitators	Frequency
Performance obstacles:	531
- physical environment (workspace, environment)	31
- tools and equipment (poor condition, wrong location, unavailability)	77
- materials and supplies (wrong location, unavailability, locked)	42
- inter-provider communication (ineffective, ineffective medical rounds, time consuming)	49
- information (hard to access, poor structure)	13
- intra-hospital transport of patients or 'road trips'	41
- patient requirements	115
- family relations	26
- unavailability of beds	3
- training (inadequate, inconvenient)	12
- lack of authority	2
- inadequate staffing	106
- teaching institution	4
- paperwork	2
- medical procedures	8
	243

Performance facilitators:	10
- physical environment (good layout, good environment)	25
- tools and equipment (available, good condition)	21
- materials and supplies (available, located in close proximity)	25
- inter-provider communication (able to make suggestions, effective)	11
- information (easy access)	17
- intra-hospital transport of patients or 'road trips'	8
- patient-related factors	4
- family relations	21
- training	10
- adequate authority	88
- help from others (available, adequate, skilled)	1
- continuity of care	1
- teaching institution	1
- medical procedures	
People involved in the obstacles and facilitators:	339
- nurses	162
- physicians	98
- respiratory therapist	5
- pharmacy	14
- unit clerk	11
- central supply	18
- radiology department	6
- other people (dietician, social workers, escort, admitting personnel)	25
Location involved in the obstacles and facilitators:	49
- peer workspace	6
- patient rooms	21
- unit	10
- other (central stock area, outside patient rooms, unit clerk's desk, call room, general floor)	12
Time of the obstacles and facilitators:	131
- day shift	23
- night shift	66
- weekend	9
- shift change	28
- other (24 hours, summer)	5
Output of the obstacles and facilitators:	298
- workload and time availability (negative such as time pressure, positive such as time available)	125
- quality of working life (negative such as frustrated, positive such as interesting job)	77
- quality of care (negative such as medical errors, positive such as knowledge about patient)	66
- quality of relations with family	9
- preference for working at night	17
- preference for working during day	4

Note: The numbers represent the number of times a piece of text was coded under one of the categories.

The coding process resulted in a total of 483 nodes (including all sub-nodes), of which 302 nodes represented the performance obstacles and facilitators. Table 3 shows a summary of the interview data. Each dimension of the coding structure with its specific categories and the number of pieces of text coded in each category are shown in table 3. The most frequently cited obstacles were patient requirements and inadequate staffing (performance, skills, number), followed by inappropriate tools and equipment, ineffective inter-provider communication, materials and supplies, and 'road trips' (intra-hospital patient transport). The most frequently cited facilitators were quality and performance of staff, followed by appropriate tools and equipment, availability of materials and supplies, effective inter-provider communication, and training.

Patient requirements that were identified as performance obstacles related to the patient acuity, new admissions, patient needs, and patient assignment. The following quote addresses patient acuity.

"Sometimes acuity is so high that you feel like you are pulled in so many directions."

Inadequate staffing was identified as a major performance obstacle as demonstrated in the following quote.

"It's just like they don't staff comfortably so that we have a nice working environment. They staff so we can get by. And that's not how to provide the highest quality of care, just to get by."

Various aspects of tools and equipment can be performance obstacles such as unavailability of tools and equipment. The following quote shows how this performance obstacle can be a source of frustration.

"looking for equipment that you don't have or that isn't working, that is frustrating."

Ineffective inter-provider communication was also identified by the ICU nurses as a performance obstacle. The following quote shows how this performance obstacle occurs during the night shift.

"If you call for an order or a concern at night, they [cross-covering physicians] say, 'I'm just cross covering, I'm not going to deal with that,' that's probably the major communication problem. The cross covering team is not familiar enough with the patient to make the decisions and they don't want to take the time to get to know the patient to make the decisions, so they let it go until morning."

Inadequate materials and supplies can also represent a major performance obstacle.

"There are many times you'll reach to go get something and it just doesn't happen to be resupplied in the room and you may have to go to another room and take a supply from that room. When we're very busy, we run out of sheets and blankets to change the beds and that kind of thing, and so you're constantly wandering from room to room looking for sheets and that kind of thing."

Intra-hospital patient transport or 'taking patients on the road' for an exam, such as a radiological procedure, may create all kinds of problems in the unit, including problems for the patients who are 'left behind' in the unit.

"When the patient leaves the unit, is usually more difficult such as road trips because the nurse has another critical care patient."

With regard to performance facilitators, the quality and performance of staff was frequently cited by the ICU nurses.

"the good things are the team work that we have at night. We help each other so much."

Certain aspects of the tools and equipment were identified as performance facilitators.

"The fact that we have the central monitors, so that there is a monitor in each room and then feeds as hardwired into the monitor in the middle so that you can be charting at the desk and still watching your patients rhythm and blood pressure. That's real helpful."

Effective inter-provider communication can help achieve better performance. The following quote shows how communication between nurses and physicians may lead to better care for ICU patients.

"A lot of the nurses have a great deal of input as far as, we don't necessarily agree with the doctors, we give our suggestions out to the doctors or to the resident on that day."

Discussion

When asked about factors in their work environment that affect their ability to perform and provide care of high quality and safety, healthcare providers in outpatient surgery centers and intensive care nurses are able to identify a very large number of factors. In the outpatient surgery center, a total of 51 nodes characterizing 6 categories of performance obstacles and facilitators were identified. In the study of intensive care nurses, we defined a five-dimension node structure with 15 categories of performance obstacles and facilitators that represented a total of 302 nodes.

It is important to recognize that the data reported in this paper is part of two larger studies: one study on the effectiveness of a work system intervention in outpatient surgery centers and the other study on ICU nursing workload. In addition, different data collection tools and procedures were used, probably leading to different data characteristics. For instance, in the outpatient surgery study, we collected data from a total of 79 respondents using a questionnaire survey. On the other hand, the 15 intensive care nurses were interviewed, therefore producing richer and more detailed data than data produced by the 79 questionnaires collected in the outpatient surgery study. This difference in the data collection tool (questionnaire versus interview) can probably explain the difference in the overall structure of the coding. In the outpatient surgery study, the respondents provided short pieces of text and sentences that tended to be relatively easily coded under one category. In the study of ICU nurses, the interviewer was able to probe the interviewees and ask follow-up questions. The interview method provided flexibility so that the interviewer could ask questions to clarify a point or obtain more detailed information. This produced more detailed, complex data that was not easily coded under a single code; therefore leading to a multi-dimensional coding structure (five dimensions, including obstacles and facilitators, people, location, time and output).

The participants in the two studies tended to identify a greater number of performance obstacles than facilitators. In the outpatient surgery study a total of 202 pieces of text were coded as performance obstacles, and a total of 133 pieces of text were coded as performance facilitators (see Table 2). In the ICU nurses study, 531 pieces of text were coded as performance obstacles and 243 pieces of text were coded as performance facilitators (see Table 3). Interestingly, some of the same categories can be sources of both obstacles and facilitators. The following two quotes from respondents in the outpatient surgery study represent cases where both performance obstacles and performance facilitators were coded under the same category of time issues. The first quote suggests the addition of computerized log books as beneficial for workload and safety. The second quote notes that computer orders have slowed overall processing times.

"Putting the log book in the computer has helped make workload and quality assurance easier to access."

"Ordering X-rays and labs through the computer takes too long. Sometimes paper is a lot faster."

We found some categories of performance obstacles and facilitators that were similar in both samples. Staff of the outpatient surgery centers and the intensive care units both identified time issues, equipment and supplies, the physical environment and staffing as categories of performance obstacles and facilitators. As expected, there were categories specific to the two groups. In the outpatient surgery study, the staff identified coordination and case scheduling as key performance obstacles. The intensive care unit nurses identified patient-related factors and intra-hospital transport of patients (so called 'road trips') as important obstacles.

Table 1 lists eleven categories of work-related obstacles (job-related information, tools and equipment, materials and supplies, budgetary support, required services and help from others, task preparation, time availability, work environment, scheduling of activities, transportation and job-relevant authority) that have been found to impair performance (Peters et al., 1985). Additionally, table 1 classifies these eleven factors into the five elements of the work system model (Carayon & Smith, 2000). When comparing the eleven factors to the performance obstacles reported among the outpatient surgery center staff (see Table 2) and the intensive care nurses (Table 3), only two response areas were not common to the literature (see Table 1) and the healthcare professionals' responses. In neither location, outpatient surgery nor the ICU, did the respondents mention the factor of budgetary support as a performance obstacle. It could be inferred that surgery staff and ICU nurses responses regarding, for instance, a lack of availability or quality of equipment and supplies could have a direct relationship to lack of budgetary support but the responses do not directly mention the factor. On the other hand, some of the performance obstacles uncovered in our two studies have not been addressed in the performance obstacles literature (Table 1). The ICU nurses mention patient transportation or the so-called 'road trips' as a frequent performance obstacle. The eleven performance obstacles in Table 1 do include 'transportation' but only as it refers to the worker needing to get to a job not the 'patient transportation' as a performance obstacle. As suggested by Peters and his colleagues, their taxonomy provided a good start for us to examine performance obstacles in healthcare.

The results of the present research paint a fairly consistent picture. As expected time availability, the work environment, the organization involved, equipment and supplies, communication of information, all play heavily as performance obstacles in both respondent groups and involve a variety of interrelated elements of the work system model (Carayon & Smith, 2000; Smith & Carayon-Sainfort, 1989).

The data from the two studies demonstrate how a variety of work factors can affect performance either negatively (performance obstacles) or positively (performance facilitators). Some of the performance obstacles identified in the two studies may not be changed. For instance, the intensive care nurses discuss various patient-related factors as sources of performance obstacles. One ICU nurse says: *"I think time is always gonna be a problem if you have an unstable critical patient. You're just gonna be stressed for time. But it just very much depends on the patient."* Because of the characteristics of the intensive care setting, it is not possible to address performance obstacles related to patient-related factors. On the other hand, many of the work factors can be changed leading to work redesign that potentially can help workers and improve performance. For instance, in the outpatient surgery study a large numbers of responses fell in the area of 'coordination'. Because all of the sites rely heavily on outside physicians to evaluate and then communicate patients' clinical status, the coordination of this information (or lack of it) not only created additional employee tasks (e.g., follow-up to ensure complete information), it also created systems to ensure the information was available. By developing a process to ensure adequate and timely receipt of the necessary information at a site, work processes related to follow-up systems can be simplified. One of the performance obstacles identified by the ICU nurses is the unavailability of patient escort for road trips in a timely fashion, mostly because of the inadequate system to request an escort. Redesigning the system to request an escort may help address this particular performance obstacle, therefore improving performance of the ICU nurses, reducing their frustration and improving their satisfaction.

We argue that this approach of looking at the situational specific work-related factors that affect the performance of workers can provide very useful information for work redesign. Redesigning healthcare jobs has been shown particularly challenging because of the intrinsic stressful characteristics of these jobs. A successful intervention process would first identify the sources of performance obstacles and facilitators. This identification could use our data to construct a checklist of performance obstacles and facilitators. Using the checklist, one could specify the performance obstacles and facilitators present in a particular healthcare work environment. This information could then be used to identify and select redesign solutions aimed at eliminating performance obstacles and building up facilitators. This approach is similar to the clinical micro-system concept (Mohr & Batalden, 2002).

Clinical microsystems have been defined as small organized groups of providers and staff caring for a defined population of patients (Mohr & Batalden, 2002). They are comprised of the following elements: core team of health professionals, a defined population of patients they care for, an information environment to support actions of caregivers and patients, and support staff, equipment, and office environment (Nelson, Batalden, Mohr & Plume, 1998). Our focus on performance obstacles and facilitators in the local healthcare environment is similar to the focus on clinical microsystems advocated by Batalden, Mohr, Nelson, Barach and colleagues (Batalden & Splaine, 2002; Mohr, Abelson & Barach, 2002; Mohr & Batalden, 2002; Nelson et al., 1998). The performance obstacles and facilitators are experienced by the health professionals and originate from various aspects of the microsystem's environment (e.g., information environment, equipment, and support staff).

A total of five outpatient surgery centers representing different structures (e.g., stand-alone versus attached to a hospital), and different status (e.g., private versus academic) participated in the study. Preliminary comparison of the data across the five sites showed the emergence of common performance obstacles (Hundt et al., 2003), therefore leading some confidence as to the generalizability of the categories of performance obstacles and facilitators among outpatient surgery staff. The intensive care nurses' study was conducted in only one ICU at an academic hospital. Future research is needed to identify work obstacles and facilitators among nurses working in other kinds of ICUs, especially ICUs of non-academic hospitals.

Future research in this area includes the need for more in-depth research on specific performance obstacles, such as patient transport in ICU's and inter-provider communication. We also need to assess the impact of performance obstacles and facilitators on both quality of working of life and performance of healthcare providers. In particular, given the heightened attention on medical errors and patient safety (Institute of Medicine Committee on Quality of Health Care in America, 2001; Kohn, Corrigan & Donaldson, 1999), studying how performance obstacles may affect the quality and safety of care is important. The most recent report by the Institute of Medicine emphasizes the work environment as a contributor to (lack of) patient safety (Institute of Medicine Committee on the Work Environment for Nurses and Patient Safety, 2004). Our approach emphasizes the local work environment and its various situations as potential contributors to poor performance, i.e., poor quality and safety of care. The most important area of research is to explore the main thrust of this paper, i.e., looking into performance obstacles and facilitators can be more fruitful for redesigning healthcare work and improving both quality of working life and performance.

Conclusion

In this paper, we have presented data on performance obstacles and facilitators experienced by healthcare providers in two care settings: intensive care and outpatient surgery. In this exploratory study the healthcare providers identified a wide range of situations as barriers to their performance, and sources of frustration and additional workload. In the outpatient surgery study, the most frequently cited performance obstacles were related to the organization and the environment. In the study of intensive care nurses, the most frequently cited performance obstacles related to patient requirements and inadequate staffing. Participants in the two studies also identified factors in their local work environment that facilitated their performance. In the outpatient surgery study, the most frequently cited performance facilitator related to various organizational factors, whereas in the study of ICU nurses, the most frequently cited performance facilitators included quality and staff of performance. This information on performance obstacles and facilitators can be used to focus efforts aimed at redesigning the work system of healthcare providers. This can be achieved in the context of a work redesign process, such as the one proposed by Parker and Wall (1998). It is very likely that different performance obstacles and facilitators may be found in different health care settings. Therefore, implementing a work redesign process that identifies the performance obstacles and facilitators present in a particular care setting is necessary to adapt the work redesign to that particular care setting.

References

Batalden, P. & Splaine, M. (2002). What will it take to lead the continual improvement and innovation of health care in the twenty-first century? *Quality Management in Health Care, 11*(1), 45-54.

Brown, K. A. & Mitchell, T. R. (1988). Performance obstacles for direct and indirect labour in high technology manufacturing. *International Journal of Production Research, 26*(11), 1819-1832.

Brown, K. Q. & Mitchell, T. R. (1991). A comparison of Just-In-Time and batch manufacturing: The role of performance obstacles. *Academy of Management Journal, 34*(4), 906-917.

Carayon, P. & Smith, M. J. (2000). Work organization and ergonomics. *Applied Ergonomics, 31*, 649-662.

Carayon, P., Bogsdorf, A., Hundt, A. S. & Alvarado, C. J. (2003). *Making a community safer for patients: The development of the Madison Patient Safety Collaborative.* Paper presented at the International Ergonomics Association Conference, Seoul, Korea, August 24-29.

Carayon, P., Alvarado, C. J., Brennan, P., Gurses, A., Hundt, A., Karsh, B.-T. & Smith, M. (2003). Work system and patient safety. In H. Luczak & K. J. Zink (Eds.), *Human Factors in Organizational Design and Management-VII* (pp. 583-589). Santa Monica, CA: IEA Press.

Crickmore, R. (1987). A review of stress in the intensive care unit. *Intensive Care Nursing, 3*, 19-27.

Flanagan, J. C. (1954). The critical incident technique. *Psychological Bulletin, 51*(4), 327-358.

Gray-Toft, P. & Anderson, J. G. (1981). The Nursing Stress scale: Development of an instrument. *Journal of Behavioral Assessment, 3*(1), 11-23.

Hundt, A. S., Carayon, P., Ayoub, P. & Alvarado, C. J. (2003). Collecting workers' perceptions of performance obstacles in outpatient surgery. In The Human Factors and Ergonomics Society (Ed.), *Proceedings of the Human Factors and Ergonomics Society 47th*

Annual Meeting (pp. 1424-1428). Santa Monica, CA: The Human Factors and Ergonomics Society.

Institute of Medicine Committee on Quality of Health Care in America (2001). *Crossing the Quality Chasm: A New Health System for the 21st.* Washington, DC: National Academy Press.

Institute of Medicine Committee on the Work Environment for Nurses and Patient Safety (2004). *Keeping Patients Safe: Transforming the Work Environment of Nurses.* Washington, D.C.: The National Academies Press.

Karasek, R. A. & Theorell, T. (1990). *Healthy Work: Stress, Productivity and the Reconstruction of Working Life.* New York: Basic Books.

Keijsers, G. J., Schaufeli, W. B., LeBlanc, P. M., Carmen, Z., & Miranda, D. R. (1995). Performance and burnout in intensive care units. *Work & Stress, 9,* 513-527.

Kohn, L. T., Corrigan, J. M. & Donaldson, M. S. (Eds.) (1999). *To Err is Human: Building a Safer Health System.* Washington, D.C.: National Academy Press.

Linzer, M., Konrad, T. R., Douglas, J., McMurray, J. E., Pathman, D. E., Williams, E. S., Schwartz, M. D., Gerrity, M., Scheckler, W., Bigby, JA. & Rhodes, E. (2000). Managed care, time pressure, and physician job satisfaction: Results from the Physician Worklife study. *Journal of General Internal Medicine, 15*(7), 441-450.

Mohr, J. J. & Batalden, P. B. (2002). Improving safety on the front lines: The role of clinical microsystems. *Quality & Safety in Health Care, 11*(1), 45-50.

Mohr, J. J., Abelson, H. T. & Barach, P. (2002). Creating effective leadership for improving patient safety. *Quality Management in Health Care, 11*(1), 69-78.

Nelson, E. C., Batalden, P. B., Mohr, J. J. & Plume, S. K. (1998). Building a quality future. *Frontiers of Health Services Management, 15*(1), 3-32.

Oates, R. K. & Oates, P. (1995). Stress and mental health in neonatal intensive care units. Archives of Disease in Childhood, 72, F107-F110.

Parker, S. & Wall, T. (1998*). Job and Work Design.* Thousand Oaks, CA: Sage Publications.

Peters, L. H. & O'Connor, E. J. (1980). Situational constraints and work outcomes: The influences of a frequently overlooked construct. *Academy of Management Review, 5*(3), 391-397.

Peters, L. H., O'Connor, E. J. & Eulberg, J. R. (1985). Situational constraints: Sources, consequences, and future considerations. *Research in Personnel and Human Resources Management, 3,* 79-114.

Pronovost, P. J., Jenckes, M. W., Dorman, T., Garrett, E., Breslow, M. J., Rosenfeld, B. A., Lipsett, P. A. & Bass, E. (1999). Organizational characteristics of intensive care units related to outcomes of abdominal aortic surgery. *Journal of the American Medical Association, 281*(14), 1310-1317.

QSR International Pty. Ltd. (1999-2000). *NVivo* (Version 1.2.142).

Siegrist, J. (1996). Adverse health effects of high-effort/low-reward conditions. *Journal of Occupational Health Psychology, 1*(1), 27-41.

Smith, M. J. & Carayon-Sainfort, P. (1989). A balance theory of job design for stress reduction. *International Journal of Industrial Ergonomics, 4,* 67-79.

Promoting healthy work: Self-reported minor injuries, work characteristics, and safety behaviour

*Nik Chmiel**
School of Psychology, Queen's University Belfast, UK

The health sector can be conceived in broad terms to include treatment of health-related problems, and health promotion activity designed to prevent problems or enhance well-being, by personnel in specialised units, such as hospitals, or elsewhere. Both functional aspects relate, not just to hospitals and public health agencies, but to the workplace, and in particular the work setting discussed in this chapter. The setting is a chemical processing plant in the UK which employs the services of a medical doctor and nurse in its on-site medical facility. A prime function for the facility is in treating injuries that arise through the activities of employees in carrying out their jobs, and in addressing concerns over employee stress. The medical facility is not limited to treatment, but also works with the organisation more widely in auditing health and safety issues, and promoting health at work.

In the UK workplace health care legislation is largely based on prevention of physical harm to employees (and contractors), and treatment after an injurious event. Mental harm through work-based stress is gaining increasing attention, and the Health & Safety Executive (HSE) has introduced management standards relating to stress in 2004, but legislation is not yet as advanced.

In relation to workplace health promotion Griffiths and Munir (2003) describe a number of stakeholder perspectives. First, from a public health point of view the workplace can be seen as a convenient access point to a majority of the adult population which can be taken advantage of by public health agencies to tackle major risks to public health. Second, from a human resource management perspective ill-health at work carries a personnel and financial cost, where effective health promotion can increase fitness and availability for work, and hence reduce health-related costs. Finally, from the perspective of safety managers and occupational health psychologists, workplaces themselves are seen as a source of danger and ill-health that require understanding in order to protect and promote individual and organizational health. The study reported in this chapter is concerned with the latter perspective.

---

* *Correspondence: Nik Chmiel, n.chmiel@qub.ac.uk*

Griffiths and Munir point out that workplace health promotion has "traditionally focused on the prevention of ill-health rather than on the promotion of positive well-being, and on the prevention of physical ill health rather than mental or social ill health" (2003, p. 319). Ill health is framed as "abnormal, unwanted, or incapacitating". Griffiths and Munir (2003) suggest organisational goals for health promotion include reducing absence, turnover and healthcare costs and increasing job satisfaction or productivity. It is clear these goals can be met in part by preventing injury at work, thus health promotion initiatives at work should include targeting the way a person behaves in relation to workplace hazards. Prevention of harm, and hence ill-health, is the desired outcome, and one that can be addressed through understanding the behavioural and psychological antecedents to injury at work, since meaningful health promotion interventions designed to reduce injury depend on such understanding. This chapter is concerned with exploring two indices of safety behaviour, some important work-based characteristics, and the relationship between them and injuries.

Given reducing injury is a goal in workplace health promotion initiatives the most desirable outcome measure is a complete and accurate accident record that can be related to antecedents. However such records are often problematic. Thompson, Hilton and Witt (1998) argue that accidents are normally rare events, and thus accident frequency rate can be statistically unreliable due to restriction of variance. Further, accidents are not always under the control of job incumbents, thus no matter how compliant they are with safety procedures other events can cause or contribute to accidents. A major problem is that accidents are not always consistently recorded, incentives can exist for both over and under reporting; and less severe accidents may not be recorded at all.

The potential inaccuracy of accident records can be illustrated by considering national accident statistics. Most European countries have legal requirements governing the reporting accidents at work. In the UK this system is called RIDDOR (Reporting of Injuries, Diseases and Dangerous Occurrence Regulations). Under this system injuries leading to more than 3 days absence from work become reportable. In the UK information on accidents at work is also collected through the Labour Force Survey (LFS) which includes questions to employees on work-related injury, and these two systems form the two main sources of workplace injury information. Analysis of the LFS data suggests that employers report about 44% of the non-fatal injuries that they should report under the RIDDOR system. In other words at a national level there are considerable numbers of > 3 days lost time injuries that go unreported. Minor injuries are not reported at all. It is not clear therefore that attempts to reduce injury through national health promotion initiatives in the workplace can be properly evaluated given that there is an incomplete picture of reportable injury, and no systematic collection of data on more minor injury.

The most recent available LFS analysis for 1999/2000 showed that about 1.03 million workers suffered a work-related injury, and there were 387,000 injuries reportable, an increase of 2% compared to 1998/1999. In the past the HSE has suggested that the ratio of fatalities to > 3 days lost time accidents to more minor injuries could be approximately 1:2:189. Of course the ratios are likely to alter year on year, but such ratios point up that minor injuries are much more likely than other, more major, injuries and fatalities.

An alternative approach to considering national accident records is to focus at the level of individual organisations in order to investigate the antecedents of injury in the workplace.

Brown (1990) suggests reporting accidents is the only practical way of evaluating system safety under real operating conditions, and of identifying factors which may be contributing to accident causation. He distinguished between the antecedents of an accident and its outcome. In other words an employee could be behaving in an unsafe manner and yet may or may not be injured, and it is thus important to get data on antecedents as well as injury events.

A fruitful approach considered the differences between companies with a good accident record and those with a poor record. Zohar (1980) showed companies across four industrial sectors with good accident records had several features: managements demonstrated a commitment to safety (for example, top management were involved in routine safety activities, safety was given high priority at company meetings and in production scheduling); Safety training was given importance; Open communication and frequent contact between management and workers was higher; and there was good house-keeping, for instance through orderly plant operations and use of safety devices. These observations led Zohar to suggest that an organisation could be deemed to have a safety climate, and he showed it could be measured via workforce perceptions. Zohar proposed safety climate had 8 dimensions: importance of safety training programmes; management attitudes to safety; effects of safe conduct on promotion; level of risk in the workplace; pace of work demands related to safety; status of the safety officer; the effects of safe conduct on social status; status of the safety committee. Subsequent research has sought to clarify the number and nature of safety climate dimensions, but in essence the importance of safety climate has been confirmed, and in particular the perception that management are committed to safety (see e.g., Flin, Mearns, O'Connor & Bryden, 2000).

Zohar (2000) suggested studying micro-accidents had several methodological advantages, thus addressing some of the concerns identified by Thompson, Hilton and Witt (1998). Micro-accidents were defined as on-the-job behaviour-dependent minor injuries requiring medical attention that do not incur lost workdays. First, micro-accidents occur much more frequently than lost-workday accidents, resulting in a homogeneous distribution as a function of time, as opposed to the highly skewed distribution characteristic of accident data in a single organization. Second, they provide an objective measure of behavioural safety, unaffected by sources of bias associated with self-report or other forms of rating, and third, in his study; they were strongly associated with lost-days accidents.

In his study Zohar (2000) took a multi-level approach to safety climate. He distinguished management approaches to safety from those related to supervisors. Top managers are concerned with policy making and the establishment of procedures to facilitate policy implementation, whereas supervisors execute procedures by turning them into predictable situation-specific action directives.

Zohar (2000) developed a scale of perceptions of supervisors' approach to safety with two subscales: action and expectation, and used it in a study of production workers in a metal processing plant. His results showed that at a group level both subscales predicted micro-accident rate. At an individual level the action subscale provided incremental prediction over workload (measured by the NASA TLX).

However micro-accidents are potentially subject to reporting bias, in the way more major injuries have been shown to be. An advantage of the UK system, in collecting reported injury data through RIDDOR, and questioning employees through the Labour Force Survey, is that the comparison between the two ways of collecting information highlights a discrepancy between them that raises questions about the accuracy of accident data. The study reported in this chapter demonstrates a case where there is a considerable discrepancy between minor injury data from one organisation's site medical facility and employees' reports on their own injuries.

In view of the problems with accident data, Thompson, Hilton and Witt (1998) went so far as to propose that:

"...perceptual data (i.e., self reports) might be the preferred criteria for safety research. Minor workplace accidents often go unreported yet those unreported events may be best indicator of improving or worsening safety conditions...

Members of the workforce out on the shop floor are likely to be sensitive to the type and frequency of accidents that go under-reported. Their perceived sense of workplace safety conditions might, therefore, be a better indicator of safety risk..." (1998, p. 21).

The quote above is ambiguous as to which type of self-report is to be preferred: self-reported accidents, perception of safety conditions, or some other measure. Recent research has used self-reported safety behaviours as alternative indices. One advantage is that such behavioural indices are easy to collect,

The Thompson, Hilton and Witt study was conducted at the Federal Aviation Administration's Logistic Centre that included warehousing, manufacturing and administrative units. The results showed that perceived management support for safety predicted perceptions of safety conditions, and that perceived supervisor support for safety predicted reported general compliance with safety rules.

Parker, Axtell and Turner (2001) used a 3 item measure of safety behaviour in two sites of a large UK glass manufacturing company over two time periods, and showed that the safety behaviour scale correlated significantly with team leaders ratings of safety compliance and safety-related consciousness, although its reliability was not very good (Cronbach's $\alpha = .57$). In addition the results showed no effect of role overload, a lagged effect of supervisory support (not safety specific) on safe working, and that cross-sectional predictors of safety behaviour were job autonomy and communication quality.

However, using safety behaviour as a primary index is not without its pitfalls. First the relationship between safety behaviour and accidents, whether self-reported or not, is not well established. Second safety behaviour is at a remove from accidents per se. Further the relationship between measures of safety behaviour and severity of accident is unclear. There is an important and interesting question whether self-report safety behaviour can be treated as an equally suitable index of safety as self-reported injury.

The study presented in this chapter focuses on minor injury, and in particular self-reported minor injury. Some of the advantages of using self-reported minor injuries are that the measure is nearer the accident problem than self-reported safety behaviours, and may be less subject to social desirability and other factors than reported safety behaviours.

A question then is what relationships, if any, there are between self-reported minor injuries, safety behaviour, and the important perceptions of organisational and work characteristics introduced above.

The approach taken to answer this question is to include measures of safety behaviour, and measures shown to impact self-reported safety behaviour, namely safety climate, workload, and job control, and consider first the relationship between safety behaviour and minor injuries, and then whether the other variables add to minor injury prediction.

Study

The organisation in which the study was conducted was a UK chemical manufacturing plant employing approximately 241 employees. A survey method was used. Questionnaires were given out over a period of 4 days, completed in an on-site training facility.

212 people responded, giving a response rate of approximately 88%. Respondents ages ranged from 18 - 64 years ($M = 41.7$, $SD = 9.5$), with a length of service ranging from 1 month - 43 years ($M = 16.5$, $SD = 10.9$). Approximately 86% of respondents were male.

The Questionnaire was broad ranging, and contained the following measures reported here:

Injury checklist: Respondents were asked to indicate how frequently in the previous 12 months they had sustained a number of major and minor work-related injuries such as a fractured bone or strained or sprained muscle. Response categories were: Not in the past 12 months, once, 2-3 times, 4-5 times, more than 5 times.

Other measures: All items were responded to on 5 point likert type scales (strongly disagree, disagree, neither agree/disagree, agree, strongly agree)

Safety behaviour: Principle components of 13 items produced two usable factors: 'working safely' and 'bending rules'. The working safely scale contained items such as "I always carry out my work in a safe manner" and "I always use safety equipment, even when it's not easily available". The bending rules scale contained items such as "I sometimes cut corners if it makes the task easier" and "When my boss is not around I can be more flexible with which procedures I follow". The appendix gives a complete list of items for the two scales.

Cronbach's α for the working safely scale was .72, and for the bending rules scale it was .82. Two items in the bending rules scale were identical to those in the 3 item 'safe working' scale validated against supervisors ratings in Parker, Axtell and Turner (2001) mentioned in the introduction. However α in their study was low (.57, or .68 for the two items included in the current scale)

Safety climate: The items used were based on Zohar (1980) and subsequent development.

Management safety climate: Principle components of 13 items produced 1 factor, containing such items as "management has a positive attitude towards safety" and "I am happy with the level of safety training for my job". The appendix gives a complete list of items for the scale. Cronbach's α was .93.

Supervisors safety climate: The two scales, supervisory action and expectation, were taken from Zohar (2000). Cronbach's α for the action scale was .76 and for the expectation scale was .92.

Workload and job characteristics measures: Scales for timing and method control, monitoring demand, problem solving demand, specially designed for production environments, were drawn from Jackson, Wall, Martin and Davids, (1993) and Wall, Jackson and Mullarky, (1995).

Job control: The timing and method control scales correlated highly (.74) and were therefore combined into one 10 item scale. (following the same procedure reported by Parker, Chmiel & Wall, 1997). Cronbach's α for the combined job control scale was .91

Workload: Cronbach's α for the monitoring demand scale was .69 (with one item dropped), and α for the problem solving demand scale was .74 (with one item dropped)

6 cases were dropped from analysis because their company tenure was less than 12 months, and the injury scale refers to last 12 months. 3 cases had missing values on 3 different variables and were therefore deleted. Finally management and accountant grades were excluded from analysis leaving a total of 162 respondents.

Results

The injuries checklist showed that the number of major injuries reported (fractures, serious back problems, concussion, hernia, others) was 20. This figure was calculated using the lowest figures attached to the scale response categories, for example if a respondent checked the 2-3 times box the figure was counted as 2. Thus this method is conservative.

The number of minor injuries reported was 344. Taking out the most minor of injuries (scratches, sprains, bruises, trip and hurts) thus leaving chemical burns, open wounds, burns, the number of minor injuries reported was 82.

Therefore the checklist produced good discrimination between major and minor injuries in the expected direction.

Recorded minor injuries at the site medical facility in the year prior to survey numbered 26, and the average recorded over the previous 3 years was approximately 30. In contrast, self-reported minor injuries in the survey period was 344, and even considering only chemical burns, open wounds, and burns, all of which should be treated at the site medical facility, self-reported injuries were 82, that is still over two and a half times the average recorded officially. Thus in this organisation there was a large discrepancy between self-reported and official recorded injury data. The official recorded figures are likely to be a considerable under-estimate of actual injuries. Potential reasons for the discrepancy are considered in the discussion below. Due to the manner in which reported injury data are treated by the company it was not possible to link actual injury with self-reported injury.

The injury checklist self-reports produced a very skewed picture. Most respondents reported either no or one injury, with only a few respondents reporting more. It was decided therefore to categorise respondents has either reporting an injury or not. The numbers in each category were roughly equal, with slightly more respondents reporting no injury.

Thus a sequential logistic regression using injury/no injury as the outcome was carried out (table 1).

Table 1: results for sequential logistic regression in predicting the likelihood of being in the injured group or not

	Variables entered	Nagelkerke r^2	Significance of change in r^2
Step 1	Working safely bending rules	.14	p<.001
Step 2	Monitoring demand problem-solving demand	.16	ns
Step 3	Job control	.22	p<.01
Step 4	Management safety climate	.24	p<.05
Step 5	Supervisor safety climate: action expectancy	.25	ns

The full sequential model is the same as a standard logistic regression with all variables entered at once. A test of the full model with all predictors, against a constant only model was statistically reliable s_x- (8) = 33.05, p<.0001 indicating that the predictors, as a set, reliably distinguished between those reporting injury or not. The logistical regression equivalent of variance accounted for was reasonable, with Nagelkerke r^2 = .25.

The prediction success of the full model was 69% of those reporting minor injury, and 72% of those reporting no injury, giving an overall success rate of 70% (for contribution of individual predictors see table 2).

Table 2: Significant predictors in full regression equation

Variable	Wald	Significance level	Exp(B)
Bending rules	5.71	.017	.51
Job Control	6.46	.011	.53
Safety Climate	3.72	.054	.44

A model run with the above predictors omitted was not reliably different from a constant plus remaining predictors model, indicating the above predictors reliably predict self-reported minor injury outcome as a set.

The results can be interpreted to mean that the likelihood (odds ratio) of being in the injured category is: 2 times less for each unit increase in safety behaviour (i.e., not bending rules); 1.9 times less for each unit increase in job control; and 2.3 times less for each unit increase in managerial safety climate.

Discussion

An interesting outcome of the study presented here is that not all types of self-reported safety behaviour predict self-reported injury. The key aspect is the construct to do with bending rules. This construct is related to whether safety procedures are ignored under high workload conditions, for example under pressure to produce rather than act safely. The trade-off between production pressure and safety is becoming recognised as an emergent theme in safety climate research (Flin et al., 2000).

In line with much past research perceived managerial safety climate has been confirmed once again as important in considering safety at work. Here safety climate predicted minor injury after safety behaviour, job control and workload were accounted for.

Another interesting outcome is that related to job control. Parker, Axtell and Turner (2001) found job control predicted safety behaviour, here it predicts minor injury after safety behaviour is accounted for. It is clear from the results therefore that it would be unwise to treat self-reported minor injury as equivalent to self-reported safety behaviour in using such approaches to assessing the efficacy of health promotion initiatives through work redesign.

The analysis does not show a significant effect of supervisor safety climate scales or workload in predicting minor injury. This result is in contrast to their effects found by Zohar (2000) when predicting actual micro-accidents. There are at least three possible reasons for these contrasting results. First, the injury checklist was subject to self-report biases that distort an accurate picture.

Second, the injury checklist includes injuries that would not be reported as micro-accidents requiring medical attention, so the two sets of data measure different things, and third the micro-accident data in Zohar's study are themselves not reported accurately, and may only be reported as a function of perceived supervisor climate. Whatever the case there is a question over whether recorded and self-reported injury can be treated as equivalent when exploring their relationships with other factors. Some commentators (e.g., see Wallace & Vodanovich, 2003) point to high correlations between actual and self-report data as evidence that one can reasonably substitute for the other without compromising the validity of findings unduly. The present study results suggest we should be cautious in this area, and highlights the value of collecting both types of data if possible.

In this study recorded minor injuries at the site medical facility until year prior to survey was 26, and the average recorded over the previous 3 years was approximately 30. In contrast, self-reported minor injuries in the survey period were 344 on a conservative tally. What reasons lie behind such a large discrepancy? In this company safety is linked to the bonus system. Interviews in one part of the site (the maintenance function) suggested strongly that many injuries were not reported, often because of a perception that the bonus could be affected, and that peers would blame the person for losing the bonus for the site. Thus there is a clear reason that recorded injury data may not give a complete picture in this company. It is also clear that biases in reporting can be due to a number of reasons despite organisations having a good framework for such reports (Van der Schaaf & Kanse, 2004).

The study here raises the possibility that recorded micro-accidents do not have the same antecedents as self-reported minor injuries at work. An outstanding issue concerns the relationship of minor injuries to more major accidents in general. The relationship is poorly theorised and understood, and minor injury antecedents may differ in significant and important ways from major accidents and deaths, and thus the results here cannot be generalised beyond the present study measures. A further point is that the relationships between different measures of safety behaviour and minor injuries need more investigation. Self-reported safety behaviour and minor injury cannot be treated as equivalent indices at this point. Further research will allow exploration of these issues.

Griffiths and Munir (2003) suggest evaluation of workplace health promotion programmes could take place on at least four different levels, ranging from their impact on the socio-economic environment, through the function and productivity of organisations and the working group to the effects on individual perceptions, belief, and values and their health-related behaviour and health status. The study reported here fits into the latter evaluative category. Interestingly the study reported above suggests that health promotion initiatives involving job redesign aimed at increasing perceived job control and hence reducing work stress may also be relevant to minor injury at work. Whether this is actually the case remains to be seen.

References

Brown, I. (1990). Accident Reporting and Analysis. In J.R. Wilson & E.N. Corlett (Eds.), *Evaluation of Human Work*. London: Taylor & Francis.

Flin, R., Mearns, K., O'Connor, P. & Bryden, R. (2000). Measuring safety climate: identifying the common features. *Safety Science, 34*, 177-192.

Griffiths, A. & Munir, F. (2003). Workplace Health Promotion. In D. Hofmann & L. Tetrick (Eds.), *Health and Safety in Organizations. A multilevel perspective.* San Francisco: Josey-Bass

Jackson, P., Wall, T., Martin, R. & Davids, K. (1993). New measures of job control, cognitive demand, and production responsibility. *Journal of Applied Psychology, 78*, 753-762.

Parker, S., Axtell, C. & Turner, N. (2001). Designing a safer workplace: Importance of job autonomy, communication quality, and supportive supervisors. *Journal of Occupational Health Psychology, 6,* 211-228.

Parker, S., Chmiel, N. & Wall, T. (1997). Work characteristics and employee well-being within a context of strategic downsizing. *Journal of Occupational Health Psychology, 2,* 289-303.

Thompson, R., Hilton, T. & Witt, L. (1998). Where the safety rubber meets the shop floor: A confirmatory model of management influence on workplace safety. *Journal of Safety Research, 29*, 15-24.

Van der Schaaf, T. & Kanse, L. (2004). Biases in incident reporting databases: an empirical study in the chemical process industry. *Safety Science, 42*, 57-67.

Wallace, J. C. & Vodanovich, S. J. (2003). Workplace safety performance: Conscientiousness, cognitive failure, and their interaction. *Journal of Occupational Health Psychology, 8,* 316-327.

Wall, T., Jackson, P. & Mullarky, S. (1995). Further evidence on some new measures of job control, cognitive demand, and production responsibility. *Journal of Organisational Behaviour, 16,* 431-455.

Zohar, D. (1980). Safety climate in industrial organisations: Theoretical and applied implications. *Journal of Applied Psychology, 65,* 96-102.

Zohar, D. (2000). A group-level model of safety climate: Testing the effect of group climate on microaccidents in manufacturing jobs. *Journal of Applied Psychology, 85,* 587-596.

Appendix

'working safely' scale items:

I always carry out my work in a safe manner.

I always report all safety-related incidents.

I always wear protective clothing, even when it's inconvenient and uncomfortable.

I never find following safety procedures a hassle.

I always report my colleagues if they break any safety rules.

I always use safety equipment, even when it's not easily available.

'bending rules' scale items

I sometimes cut corners if it makes the task easier.

Production pressures mean that I sometimes bend the rules.

Occasionally I bend the rules when I know it is safe to do so.

When my boss is not around I can be more flexible with which procedures I follow.

'management safety climate' scale items:

Management have a positive attitude towards safety.

Due recognition is given by management to employees who practice good safety habits.

Safe procedures at work are given enough publicity.

I am happy with the level of safety training for my job.

The company encourages employees to attend safety meetings and/or safety training.

The company is quick to respond to the safety concerns of their employees.

The company takes the safety ideas of employees seriously.

Safety is given a high priority in company meetings and planned activities.

Senior management are actively involved in safety programmes.

Managers take action on employees' non-compliance with safety rules or procedures.

Action is taken by senior management on reports of potential hazards.

The company encourages employees to voice their concerns about safety.

Violations to safety procedures, even when no damage has resulted, are taken seriously by management.

Working together in the operating theatre: Determinants of trust-based decisions

Cornelia Kleindienst & *Markus Schöbel*
Department of Work and Organizational Psychology, TU Berlin, Germany

There is a growing interest in the medical field for social and psychological dimensions of work processes. The increasing relevance of patient safety and quality management strategies makes it necessary to focus on the outputs of organizational performance, especially in the operating theatre. The treatment of patients requires a well coordinated collaborative action of different professional teams, converging in the specific therapy of each patient. The operating theatre is a point of intersection for multiple teams with their own agendas and requirements. It contains four identifiable teams during preoperative, operative and postoperative periods: surgeons, anesthesiologists, surgical nurses, and anesthesia nurses. Team members are simultaneously equally responsible for the patient during preoperative periods. Each member has an area of primary responsibility, but there is considerable overlap between them. Research on medical team performance reveals safety – critical constraints resulting from this team structure (Helmreich & Schaefer, 1994). Whereas physicians and nursing staff have a strong hierarchical separation, there is no clear division of authority between the senior surgeon and the senior anesthesiologist. Further, team composition is continually changing with consultants, for example, coming and going to discharge other duties. This might result in causes for errors, when a team loses cohesion and mutual support (Schöbel & Kleindienst, 2001).

In this chapter we want to focus on socio-psychological processes of coordinated team work. One crucial feature of operating teams is that there is no formal work coordination of team work between different subgroups (surgery, anaesthesia). Especially in critical work situations (when complications occur) the dynamic and adapted coordination of team performance is essential for a good outcome (Salas, Dickinson, Converse & Tannenbaum, 1992). We argue that interpersonal trust is one important prerequisite for coordination, communication and cooperation between team members in the operating theatre. Therefore, trust may contribute to successful team performance. We present some considerations and empirical data about trust decisions in collaborative and critical team situations which cover important factors and antecedents.

---

* *Correspondence: Cornelia Kleindienst, Cornelia.Kleindienst@tu-berlin.de*

Definition and determinants of interpersonal trust in the context of work and organization

When reading scientific literature on organizations, there seems to emerge an expanding interest in the phenomenon of trust in organizations in general (for example Kramer, 1999; Costa, Roe & Taillieu, 2001). Meanwhile, it is common sense that trust improves cooperation and communication (Dirks, 1999; Kegan & Rubinstein, 1973), especially in the light of the loss of importance of formal control and sanctions for the regulation of individual behavior in organizations and work processes.

Interpersonal trust is seen as a person's expectation that an interaction partner is able and willing to behave promotively toward that person, even when the interaction partner is free to choose among alternative behaviors that could lead to negative consequences for the person (Koller, 1988). Hardin (1992) emphasizes the connotation of trust as rational choice. Individuals can trust someone, if they have adequate reasons for believing, it will be in that person's interest to be trustworthy in a relevant way at a relevant time. In addition, he highlights the relational model of trust as well: Trust needs to be conceptualized not only as a calculative orientation toward risk, but also as a social orientation towards other people and towards society as a whole.

On the basis of these formulations, we define trust in the context of task-oriented work relations, as a deciding factor in a social process that results in a conscious decision which includes: risk or willingness to being vulnerable, and a positive expectation towards the behavior of the trustee. Hence, trust is seen as a property of interpersonal relationship in particular situations that is actualized in observable behavior like a trust decision. The decision to trust someone is based on the expectation that another party will meet the performance requirements. The degree of trust can be said to be higher the stronger the individual holds this expectation.

The determinants of trusting behavior within organizations can be understood as antecedent conditions that promote the emergence of trust. We assume that there are two classes of factors which coincide and therefore influence individuals' willingness to engage in trusting behavior. First, factors that influence the expectations about others' trustworthiness and second, task-relevant factors within the specific work context over which trust is conferred.

Good (1988) defines trustworthiness as the extent to which individuals expect others to behave according to their implicit and explicit claims. This judgement has cognitive and emotional grounds. Depending on situational demands the evaluation of the other party can be based on its competence or benevolence (McAllister, 1995). Furthermore, the trusting person has different sources of information about the trustee. Research on trust development has shown that individuals' perceptions of others' trustworthiness and their willingness to engage in trusting behavior are largely history-dependent processes (Kramer, 1999). Interactional history provides a basis for drawing inferences in order to judge others' trustworthiness and predict future behavior. History-based trust can be seen as an important form of knowledge-based or personalized trust in organizations (Kramer, 1999). While personalized knowledge about other organizational members represents one possible foundation of trust, this kind of knowledge is often not obtainable. Within most organizations, decision makers have difficulties in collecting sufficient knowledge about all persons with whom they interact or on whom they depend. The size and degree of social and structural differentiation found within most organizations precludes the sort of repeated interactions and dense social relations required for the development of personalized trust. As a consequence, 'proxies' or substitutes for a direct, personalized knowledge are often utilized. Third-parties serve as conduits of trust by giving 'second-handknowledge' about others.

Another form of presumptive trust found within organizations is role-based trust (Kramer, 1999). It constitutes a form of depersonalized trust based on knowledge that a person occupies a particular role in an organization. For example, Barber (1983) stated that strong expectations regarding technically competent role performance are typically aligned with roles in organizations, as well as expectations that role occupants will fulfill the fiduciary responsibilities and obligations associated with the roles they occupy. Thus, to the extent that people within an organization have confidence in the fact that role occupancy signals both an intent to fulfill such obligations and competence in carrying them out, individuals can adopt a sort of presumptive trust based upon knowledge of role relations, even in the absence of personalized knowledge or history of prior interaction. It is not the person in the role that is trusted so much as the system of expertise that produces and maintains role-appropriate behavior of role occupants. In this respect, the hierarchical position of a trustee could be seen as a kind of role-related information.

In addition, the readiness to trust can increase as a result of situational factors (Oswald & Fuchs, 1998). For example, Luhmann (1973) suggests a basic need for trust since trust may reduce the perceived complexity of a situation. Therefore it can be assumed that the degree of trust an individual forms toward an interaction partner can be a function of the degree of risk that is involved in the situation. However, it remains open how and what perceived risks affect trust decisions. Individuals may trust others, if they believe not being able to control the occurrence of negative consequences. They may not trust others, if they believe that their interaction partner may display an act of behavior that leads to negative consequences for the individual, based on the fact that the interaction partner has a higher degree of control over the situation than the individual.

These theoretical considerations support the view that trust plays an important role in regulating interpersonal behavior at work. Due to the fact that team performance in the operating theatre is characterized by only a few standardized or formal coordination mechanisms, we assume that trusting behavior between the actors with different professions and hierarchical ranking coordinates their performance, especially when they are confronted with dynamic changes of work task constraints where patient safety is at odds. Study 1 explores the importance of the determinants of trusting relationships outlined above. Study 2 was designed to analyse the impact of situational factors and the characteristics of the trustee on trust decisions of anaesthesiologists by means of a laboratory experiment.

Study 1: Exploration of 'trusting' teamwork in the operating team

Study 1 aims at exploring the importance of trusting behavior in the operating theatre. The main objective was to examine the attributes which constitute the trustworthiness of other team members as well as the situational factors that potentially influence trusting behavior.

Method

Seven semi-structured in-depth interviews with experts from the medical field (surgeons, anaesthesists and nurses) were carried out. The questions dealt with perceptions of team and work structures in the operating theatre, cooperation in the operating team in general and with trust within the team and with regard to co-workers in particular (for example: What characteristics of a coworker are important for a trustful decision in a critical situation during surgical operation? What is the adequate relation of control and trust in a critical situation?). Furthermore the experts were asked to describe examples of trust-relevant critical situations in the operating team. The interviews lasted in average 2 hours with a range from one to three and a half hours. The experts were asked for registration of the interview and nobody refused. Subsequently the interviews were transliterated and were analyzed by content analysis methods (Mayring, 1988).

Results and discussion

The result demonstrated that the experts distinguish between two functional sub-teams in the operating theatre. There is a division into the surgical and the anaesthesiological sub-team. Both are working together relatively autonomously during the surgical operation. If complications appear in the course of the operation, the senior surgeon and the senior anaesthesiologist have to collaborate directly. The coordination and matching of their actions is crucial for the successful coping with the complication.

In general, trust was seen as a prerequisite for efficient teamwork. There was no difference in this evaluation between the diverse professional groups. Trustworthiness of team-members was mainly attributed to their competence. Competence relates on the one hand to medical knowledge, on the other hand to abilities of stress-regulation and coordination in the team with respect to social competencies. The coordination of action within a subteam and between subteams is mainly attributed to leadership behavior. Especially surgeon's behavior was seen as a crucial component of the perceived 'general trust level' within teams. Furthermore, the interviews revealed that experience in teamwork with other co-workers was stated as the main basis for trust. In addition, the importance of affect (good feeling) is emphasized, evoked by the assessment of the trustee's cooperativeness.

The necessity and functionality of trust was found to be connected with situational features as well. Uncertainty and risk associated with the emergence of critical situations motivate team members to evaluate the trustworthiness of their colleagues.

Study 2: Interacting determinants of trust decisions in the operating team

The goal of study 2 was to determine how characteristics of the task and perceived trustworthiness of the interaction partner will contribute to a trust decision in a critical situation during the surgical operation of a patient. From the results of the first study we assume that higher levels of trust should correspond with an increasing complexity of the work situation. In addition, we predict higher levels of trust (1) when the trustee has a higher hierarchical ranking as the trusting person, (2) when trustee is known as a professional expert (competence) in comparison to his social abilities (cooperativeness), and (3) when information about the trustee stems from direct experience in relation to third party information.

Method

152 anaesthesiologists from different German university hospitals participated in an online-survey. There was a request for participation sent by email to different departments of anaesthesiology. In order to analyze trusting behavior in the operating theatre the participants were confronted with four

scenarios which were designed in co-operation with an experienced anaesthesiologist.

The basic situation building the basis of each of the four scenarios described a surgical operation. It was presented from the perspective of an anaesthesiologist, who works together with a surgeon. In the course of the operation there appears a loss of blood. There is no unit of crossed blood from stock transfusion in the operating room, which would be necessary for an immediate transplantation. The surgeon states that he has everything under control, which means, that he will stop the bleeding sufficiently directly. The dilemma of the anaesthesiologist in the described scenario is as follows: Trust the surgeon or order a unit of crossed-stocked blood.

The following factors were randomly varied in the four scenarios according to an analysis of variance design: the base of trust-decision and the source of information about the trustee were varied as within-factors. The complexity of the situation and the hierarchical position of the trustee were varied as between-factors.

The first between-factor was the complexity of the situation. On the one hand the patient was an old female patient with gall bladder resection and some more diseases (overweight, etc.); on the other hand the patient was a young female with appendectomy and no other diseases. The latter should represent a task with low to middle complexity and difficulty in contrast to the first situation where a non-routine operation was depicted.

The second between-factor was the hierarchical position of the surgeon. In one condition the surgeon was a senior consultant, in the other condition it was an intern surgeon on the same hierarchical level as the anaesthesiologist.

The base of the trust decisions was varied by providing information about the competence of the surgeon or about his cooperativeness. The source of this information was varied by simulating sound experience in working together with the surgeon or, in contrast, obtaining information about the surgeon given by the nurse as third party.

The first dependent variable was the trust decision. Participants should assess on an 11-point-scale the probability (0-100%) that the anaesthesiologist would not ask for a unit of crossed stocked blood. Two other dependent variables were also measured on 11-point-scales. First, the probability of complications (0-100%) in the described situation should be assessed in order to control the perceived severity of the situation. The third dependent variable was the assessment of the surgeon's ability to stop the bleeding (0-100%).

Results and discussion

In order to test our predictions, we conducted repeated analysis of variances with complexity of the situation and hierarchical ranking of the trustee as between-factors and source and base of information about the trustee as within-factors. The results reveal that the complexity of the situation is crucial for the trust-decision. Contrary to our prediction, the anaesthesiologists showed significantly more trust (no order of a unit of crossed stock blood) in the situation with the young patient with better health status ($M = 63.72$) compared to the situation of the old patient ($M = 22.66$), where participants significantly trusted less, $F(1.15) = 18.3$, $p = 0.00$. Considering participants assessment of surgeon's ability to stop the bleeding, we found no significant difference between both conditions, $p = .18$, whereas the probability of the occurrence of complication was significantly higher judged for the operation of the old patient ($M = 35.73$) compared to the operation of the young patient ($M = 13.94$), $F(1.14) = 19.03$, $p = .00$. It seems that in our stimulus situation the positive expectation of the behavior of the surgeon did only indirectly affect the trust decision. Instead of that it can be assumed that a critical factor of trusting is the risk involved in the situation per se, or in other words, is a property of the task.

With regard to the factors that are important for the assessment of the trust-worthiness of the interaction partner, we found a higher degree of trust if the surgeon had a higher hierarchical position as the anaesthesiologist ($M = 48.14$) in comparison to the scenario where both had the same hierarchical position ($M = 38.31$), $F(1.15) = 3.9$, $p = 0.05$. In addition, we found two significant interactions. The participants tended to trust more, if there is perceived competence based on experience of their own. Third-party information affected the trust decision when it emphasizes the cooperativeness of the surgeon, $F(1.15) = 5.51$, $p = 0.02$.

General discussion

From the results of both studies we may tentatively conclude that trusting behavior plays an important role as coordination mechanism in the operating theatre. We make this conclusion from the finding of study 1 that the experts highlight the impact of trusting behavior in critical teamwork situations. Moreover, the results of study 2 show that experts trust in an 'imagined' real-life teamwork situation. Regarding the determinants of trusting behavior, both studies reveal that not only the trustworthiness is an important aspect of trust decisions, also the risk done in the task situation is crucial for trusting. The meaning of risk is here twofold: On the one hand, the risk that the trustee does not show the expected behavior, on the other hand the risk that the behavior of both, trustor and trustee, leads to negative consequences, independently of their trusting behavior. Hence, the magnitude and the probability of potential negative consequences are crucial for trusting. It can be assumed that this feature is particularly important in the medical field because there is a strong influence of accountability. The anaesthesiologists prefer to control the situation on their own if a situation bears the possibility of strong negative consequences.

In addition, both studies demonstrate that *role-based trust*, building on the assumed competence of higher ranked trustees, plays an important role in the operating theatre. In our studies, role-based trust reaches higher importance than personalized trust. Especially when team composition is continually changing, it is essential for trust decisions what kind of information in what quality is connected to the role-information. One potential hazard in this regard could be, that hierarchical higher persons elicit trust decisions that are not balanced with the situational demands. The capability of the hierarchical higher ranked surgeon to control the situation could be overestimated in regard to the risk of complication.

Another interesting finding is that the importance of the base for the trust decision is changing with the source of this information. Information content about the competence of the trustee is relevant for trust decisions if this knowledge stems from one's own experience. Information content about the cooperativeness of the trustee is relevant if it stems from third-party information. It can be assumed that the information by the nurse is judged as not reliable in regard to competence but more to cooperativeness.

One important question still remains open. As indicated in study 1, emotions may play an important role as a determinant of situational trust-building. One should consider how the assessment of situational risk or complication is influenced by emotions as well as the assessment of the trustworthiness of interaction partners (for example Loewenstein, Weber, Hsee & Welch, 2001). Especially in work situations like in the operating team where there is a relatively unstructured and complex (sub-)team hierarchy, emotional processing of situational information seems relevant for trust decisions.

References

Barber, B. (1983). *The logic and limits of trust*. New Brunswick, N.J.: Rutgers Univ. Press.

Costa, A. C., Roe, R. A. & Taillieu, T. (2001). Trust within teams: The relation with performance effectiveness. *European journal of work and organizational psychology, 10*(3), 225-244.

Dirks, K. T. (1999). The effects of interpersonal trust on work group performance. *Journal of Applied Psychology, 84*(3), 445-455.

Good, D. (1988). Individuals, interpersonal relations and trust. In D. Gambetta (Ed.), *Trust making and breaking cooperative relations* (pp. 31-47). New York: Basil Blackwell.

Hardin, R. (1992). The Street-Level Epistemology of Trust. *Analyse und Kritik, 14*, 152-176.

Helmreich, R. L. & Schaefer, H.-G. (1994). Team performance in the operating room. In M. S. Bogner (Ed.), *Human error in medicine. Hillsdale.* N.J.: Lawrence Erlbaum Ass. Publ.

Kegan, D. & Rubenstein, A. (1973). Trust, effectiveness and organizational development: A field study in R&D. *Journal of Applied Behavioral Science, 9*, 498-513.

Koller, M. (1988). Risk as a determinant of trust. *Basic and Applied Social Psychology, 9*, 265-276.

Kramer, R. M. (1999). Trust and distrust in organizations: Emerging perspectives, enduring questions. *Annual Review of Psychology, 50*, 569-598.

Loewenstein, G. F., Weber, E. U., Hsee, C. K. & Welch, N. (2001). Risk as Feelings. *Psychological Bulletin, 127*(2), 267-286.

Luhmann, N. (1973). *Vertrauen. Ein Mechanismus der Reduktion sozialer Komplexität.* Stuttgart: Enke.

Mayring, P. (1988). *Qualitative Inhaltsanalyse. Grundlagen und Techniken.* Weinheim: Beltz.

McAllister, D. J. (1995). Affect- and cognition-based trust as foundations for interpersonal cooperation in organizations. *Acadademy of Management Journal, 38*, 25-59.

Oswald, M. E. & Fuchs, T. (1998). Readiness to trust in complex situations. *Swiss Journal of Psychology, 57*(4), 248-254.

Salas, E., Dickinson, T. L., Converse, S. A. & Tannenbaum, S. I. (1992). Toward an understanding of team performance and training. In R. W. Swezey & E. Salas (Eds.), *Teams: their training and performance* (pp. 3-29). Norwood, N.J.: Ablex.

Schöbel, M. & Kleindienst, C. (2001). The psychology of team interaction. *Acta Neurochirurgica, Supplement 78*, 33-38.

Experiences in the German model project 'Interprofessional communication in hospitals'

Silke Pawils[*1]*, Bernadette Klapper*[1]*, Doris Schaeffer*[2] *& Uwe Koch*[1]
[1] *Institut für Medizinische Psychologie, Zentrum für Psychosoziale Medizin, Universitätsklinikum Hamburg Eppendorf, Germany*
[2] *Institut für Pflegewissenschaften, Universität Bielefeld, Germany*

Background of our model project

The initial situation in the public health sector is requiring the participation of both the affected as well as the sensitisation of professional helpers as to how medical care quality can be improved in every realm. 2.263 German hospitals carry out 16 million stationary treatments per year (Reister, 1999). Every day half a million citizens require a hospital bed and stay 10.7 days on the average (Arnold, Litsch & Schellschmidt, 2000). In the face of the anticipated demographic development there are trenchant legal reforms (Health reforms in 1989 and 2000, SGB V – social legislation book V) and considerable endeavours in science and practice (i.e., the federal projects 'DemoProQM' or 'KTQ' (Aufderheide, 1998).

We started our project – described below – in view of the fact that there are new perspectives and patients' positions which have to be integrated and that there are social factors such as technicalization, public health restructuring and increasing cost pressure which have to be considered. They demand newly defined nursing and medical staff qualification (Sachverständigenrat für die Konzentrierte Aktion im Gesundheitswesen, 2001). Such alterations as i.e., the implementation of new diagnosis related groups (DRGs) have to be taken into account within professional cooperation and communication (Simon, 2000). In order to attain an amelioration of patient treatment together with a simultaneous price reduction internal quality management and external quality assessment were implemented and it was found out that the interprofessional cooperation was a potential weak point for the goal of an effective treatment (Schmerfeld & Schmerfeld, 2000). As to professional communication between nurses and physicians it is generally criticised that there is a lack of information flow (Büssing, 1997). Both professions have specific

---

[*] *Correspondence: Silke Pawils, s.pawils@uke.uni-hamburg.de*

This article is a summary of the InterKiK final report, which is available as pdf and can be purchased via http://www.bundesaerztekammer.de/30/Fachberufe/50Interkik/. The InterKiK-Toolbox can be obtained via Hans Huber Verlag, Göttingen.

expectations directed towards the other due to different access to patients and fields of duties. Facing the active integration of patients into the care it is necessary to combine cooperatively these differing perspectives in the work routine.

On the basis of former model projects about the amelioration potential of interactive competence (compare Köhle, Böck & Graumann, 1977; Uexküll, 1992) as well as on latest treatment research results (compare Höhmann, Müller-Mundt & Schulz, 1998) our model project comprises the development, implementation and evaluation of an intervention concept which will better meet the requirements of patients in admittance, ward rounds and discharges.

The project design (Interprofessional communication in hospitals)

Our project 'Inter-professional Communication in Hospitals' (InterKiK) had a duration of three years (1999-2002) and was financed by the Federal Ministry of Public Health aiming at the development of a manual helping to improve the communication and cooperation in federal acute care wards. Our department of Medical Psychology of the University Hospital Hamburg-Eppendorf and the Institute of Care Sciences of the University Bielefeld were asked by the Federal Medical Chamber (Bundesärztekammer) and by the Associations of the German Care Committee (Verbände des Deutschen Pflegerates) to carry this project into effect. Research object was the communication among patients, physicians and nurses in central interfaces within hospitals. As our field of investigation we chose medicinal and surgery wards in three different hospitals in order to obtain a broad and typical survey of hospital communication activities.

Scientific evaluations in the hospital realm comprising a perspective of external experts beside the description of results and aspects of staff members are quite rarely (Büssing, Barkhausen & Glaser, 1999). InterKiK integrates several perspectives similar to Büssings evaluation study (1999) but uses another evaluation design due its differing goal.

The evaluation design is quasi-experimental (Bortz & Döring, 1995). The pre-post-comparison of both quality assessments is carried out by comparable instruments. Furthermore we added a group design for comparison reasons according to which one out of three wards functions as control station receiving no intervention (Schwartz, 1993). The effects of quality groups and communication training in wards should be assessed equally.

Our aim was the scientific, multi-perspective evaluation of definite changes similar to the evaluation study of Büssing, Barkhausen and Glaser (1999). In addition we wanted to develop a transfer option enabling practitioners an access to a scientifically evaluated procedure. This transfer option has above all to offer the practicability of a scientifically evaluated procedure. As our main endeavour was to develop this transfer option we had to answer following questions via our model project:

- What kind of instrument is adequate for a comprehensive, detailed and scientifically valid description of the actual situation.

- How and in which way can this instrument be made available for practitioners if the procedure is guided internally.

The consideration of practical priorities as well as necessities such as staff resources, qualification of future users, availability of money and time will determine the success of organisational development procedures. In case of hospital application the execution will no longer be guided externally but internally.

The model project comprises a complete evaluation cycle:

Assessment of the actual situation

Result feedback to wards and hospital management

Intervention by quality groups and/or communication training

Assessment of the situation after intervention

Method of the project

InterKiK had to meet following important requirements:

To describe extensively, in detail and validly inter-professional communication and cooperation on wards during admittance, ward rounds and patient discharge

To infer intervention measures from the results

To describe and assess changes from the viewpoint of different perspectives

To offer a procedure which enables other hospitals to carry out each project step independently thus improving their inter-professional communication without external guidance.

The first step comprised the development and application of an instrument which describes the respective ward specific communication and cooperation during admission, ward rounds and patient discharge as a kind of 'ward diagnosis' in a comprehensive, detailed and valid way (see figure 1).

Figure 1: Design of the project

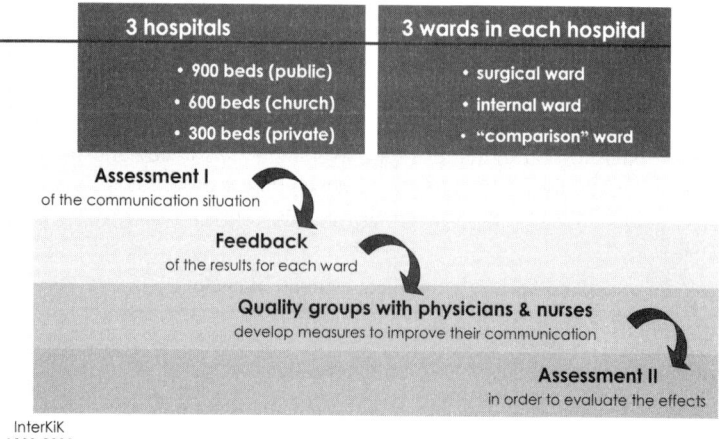

Georgopoulos (1986) suggests three main methods to evaluate the quality of patient care in hospitals:

Analysis of existing documents as i.e., patient files

Observation of actual patient care activities

Surveys basing on questionnaire data or on interviews with hospital staff and others

In order to describe the quality of communication and cooperation within the experimental wards we decided to use methods using all three accesses. The use of different methods describing an object of research is called triangulation procedure (Flick, 2000).

Our method set (see figure 2) is composed of:

Aim of the structure and concept assessment is to systematically register relevant structure and concept characteristics of model hospitals and experimental wards. The registered parameters will be used to document the actual situation of formal aspects and thus supplying a reference structure for the result analysis.

Interviews with nurses and physicians ($n = 47$ ward members) in experimental wards are supposed to show the subjective perspective of participating staff members. On the basis of this internal perspective strong and weak points of communication and coordination processes in their ward specific shape and in their details are to be brought out. In addition the interviews offer material for further methodological development of quantitative evaluation instruments.

Similarly to the interviews the observation of admittance, ward rounds and patient discharge are supposed to show details and ward specifics in communication and cooperation. This method enables us to include the external perspective of the researcher into the assessment.

The patient document analysis ($n = 900$) is supposed to register the information flow among physicians and nurses and to assess the facilitation of their inter-professional communication by the existing documentation system as well as of the support in the communication with patients if the care process is applied.

Questionnaires as to patient content ($n = 436$ patients) should be used as a standardized assessment of the ward from the patient's point of view (Lecher, 2002).

Analogously, questionnaires as to staff content ($n = 132$ ward members) should be used as a standardized assessment of the ward from the staff's point of view. With regard to the envisaged intervention the staff will also be assessed as to their change motivation and improvement recommendations will be gathered.

There are no qualitative interviews with patients as the choice of suitable patients being ready to participate would be highly selective and would only comprise a minor part of the overall patient group quite in contrast to the staff interviews. Considering these reservations the considerable effort to carry out qualitative interviews could not be justified economically. Psychometric indicators and information about reliability and validity of the instruments can be seen in the final report and in specified publications (Lecher, 2002).

Our quality assessment comprised the determination of resources and deficits of patient admittance, ward rounds and patient discharge based on multi-methodological instruments including a basis assessment with responsive observation, half-structured interviews with nurses, physicians and a core assessment of patient documentation and questionnaires as to patient and staff satisfaction (see figure 2).

Beside the assessment and the feedback of research results our project also comprised a six months intervention phase during which quality groups or communication training with ward members were carried in case of need. It was supposed to work on communication problems on wards and on a future successful communication culture (see figure 1). The intervention effects were evaluated by quality assessment on the wards and were reported as feedback in order to stimulate a further sensitisation for a further amelioration. Single results of participating hospitals will be comprehensively described in our final report and in specified publications.

Figure 2: Assessment of interprofessional communication

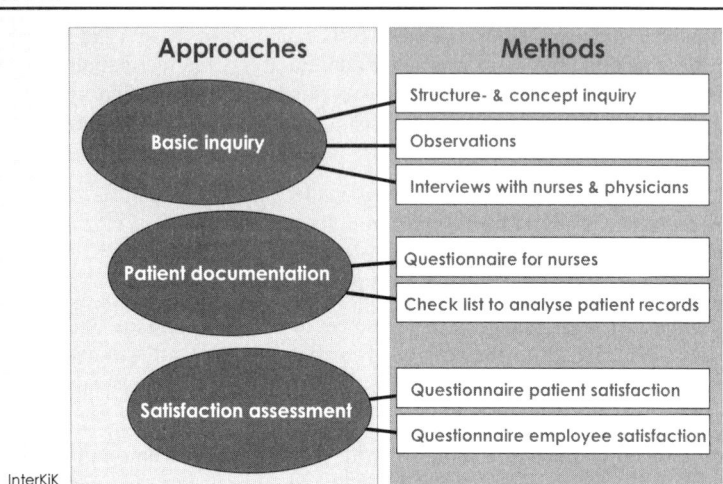

Predictors for successful quality groups and communication training

To sum up the quality groups presented a heterogeneous picture (see figure 3). In dependence of the respective internal preconditions and support of the group work it was possible to find and transfer solutions.

The communication training was supposed to be adjusted to the goals and forms of learning within the respective group as well as on the results of assessment phase I and on the actual requirements. The preparation of the communication training consisted of setting up supplier criteria for the selection of professional trainers. The communication training groups were organised by the respective hospitals and were thus offered quite differently.

Figure 3: Participation and results in quality groups

Participation in quality groups

KHS	Ward	Subjects	Participants	Solution founded	Solution realised
1	A	Regularly ward meetings	Nurses	No	No
	B	Better transfer of Informations	Nurses	No	No
2	A	Better organisation of the ward round	Nurses & doctors	Yes	Yes
	C	Improvement of patient documentation	Nurses & doctors	Yes	Yes
3	A	Interdisciplinary advanced training	Nurses & doctors	No	No
	B	New organisation of the ward round	Nurses & doctors	Half	Short-term

InterKiK
1999-2002

Our analysis of the reasons of such a heterogeneous intervention transfer in the included hospitals revealed some specific success factors for a recommendation for further projects:

Wards have to solve professionally overlapping problems themselves but it is also true that the solution cannot be found on the ward alone and cannot be directed by one professional group alone either. The success thus depends on preparatory discussions in the respective hospitals as to the question of participation or non-participation in the project.

The coordination of the communication project should be carried out be a person who a) is able to cooperate with different disciplines and who is neither subordinate to the nursing nor to the medical staff and b) he or she should have an exposed position so that it is possible to communicate with all profession groups and hierarchical levels and to take enough influence.

Experience in quality management has a positive influence in the envisaged success. This is due for the ward members who are responsible for the respective transfer but also this is due for all other colleagues including their individual experience in quality circles. For the quality management in general there are similar important success criteria as for quality group work (Antoni, 1988) as a) real preparedness to change and b) a hospital culture determined by ideas of participation and comprehensive quality.

In order to carry out organisational developments in a hospital it is a good precondition to engage a coordination group on management level being able to derive guiding decisions. For explicitly inter-professional projects such as InterKiK this approach appears to be a necessary prerequisite and optimal possibility to transfer improvement recommendations into long-term obligations.

As to the organisation of communication training groups it is an important precondition for the hospital to be prepared for the necessary financial investigation. The careful selection of the trainer is also of utmost importance. Furthermore it seems to be significant that a ward related implementation is carried out which focuses on the evaluated deficits.

Quality groups and communication training have to be thoroughly planned, organised and attended continuously (Walther & Walther, 1998). Their success is deeply depending on a) a continuous flow of information between project co-ordination and ward members as to planned and executed activities and b) on the careful organisation of intervention sequences as incentive for participation and free time compensation.

Results of the model project

In order to ameliorate the communicative routine among patients, physicians and nurses in acute care a systematic approach is necessary. It is favourable if there is a compatibility with the quality efforts in hospitals as well as a development of an internal quality management system. These endeavours require suitable assessment instruments in order to enable internal and external quality consultants to carry out an extensive organisational diagnostic.

The assessment developed in the course of our project focuses on resources and deficits during patient admission, ward rounds and discharge of patients with the help of multi-methodological instruments. We presented exemplary procedure backgrounds, contents and results of the pre-post-designed assessment instrument. Extensive data from different research accesses (structural and concept analyses, observation reports, interviews, patient documentation, questionnaires to patients and ward members) on nine wards in three hospitals of different carriers and different number of beds were assessed anonymously and were used for the evaluation of inter-professional co-operation.

The limits of data assimilation within the field of hospitals became quite evident. There are differing expectations of different participants such as patients, ward members and hospital management as to the executed analysis. Specific fears and negative experiences fence in the possibilities of field investigation. Practical considerations as time deficits demand simple strategies. Furthermore there is a lack of knowledge particularly on ward level about present and expected requirements as to an integrated, cooperative and patient orientated care practice. This is proved by numerous investigation results in ward reports and by feedback meetings. Individual results as to discharge procedures reveal that the main consideration of the professional helpers is focused on the ward and not on the overall care system of the patient beyond the hospital care. Due to these deficits there is a restriction in direct communication with patients.

Right from the start of our project while we developed our instruments we had to take careful consideration of the individual conditions, of the role expectations and of the envisaged probable interventions. The necessity to adopt the interviews and the interventions to the specific hospital settings was impressively confirmed by the heterogeneity of our research results. It was quite noticeable that the participation of physicians in the quality groups was poor. This finding is confirmed by further studies (Güntert & Horisberger, 1991; Höhmann, Müller-Mundt & Schulz., 1998; Mühlbauer & Strack, 1997). There also was a high fluctuation ratio from the side of the nurses. This circumstance caused a steady change in the group composition and impeded the lasting integration of achieved results. Thus the improvement of communication and co-operation between physicians and nurses presupposes the participation of the management level and in particular of the head physician and nurse managers. In addition the individual hospital conditions with respect to the transfer ratio of extensive quality management interventions as well as formal positions, competence and engagement of the respective quality management official are decisive for the success of alteration projects.

With regard to the necessity of improvement of the co-operation on wards we also have to consider the fact that the number of research and /or quality management projects reaches inflationary dimensions and thus already have caused understandable resistance in engaged hospitals. Future project should take these effects into consideration.

Despite these different research and content related problems we were able to fulfil our project order to develop an assessment instrument which can describe the multi-dimensional object of 'communication & co-operation' in hospital wards according to reality and which possesses the necessary sensibility to evaluate changes in respective communication situations (Lecher, Klapper, Schaefer & Koch, 2003. Its preciseness however can only favour the envisaged changes in the ward routine with the assistance of other project processes. One decisive step is the organisation of the feedback. We also could offer a procedure for this purpose

producing a comprehensibility of scientific results for practitioners

integrating due to its specific conception probable hierarchically related conflicts and favours the repeated engagement of all project members offering concrete hints of intervention needs on the basis of the respective ward resources

These procedures with the CD-manual InterKiK-Toolbox set up in the course of our project are now available to all hospitals.

Our project results reveal that lasting successes in organisational development can be achieved even in difficult areas being shaped and moulded by traditional work division. The combination of a precise instrument with a feedback carried out in empathy as well as a carefully drafted and a continuously executed intervention are the necessary prerequisites.

So far the final results of our model project 'Inter-professional Communication in Hospitals' can be called a success just in face of the numerous practical problems. It should be an encouragement to continue with the increasingly important topic of inter-professional cooperation for a future efficient a patient orientated care.

References

Antoni, C. (1988). Probleme bei der Implementierung von Qualitätszirkeln. *Zeitschrift für Arbeits- und Organisationspsychologie, 32*, 80-91.

Arnold, M., Litsch, M. & Schellschmidt, H. (Eds.) (2000). *Krankenhausreport 1999*. Stuttgart: Schattauer.

Aufderheide, A. (1998). Qualitätsmanagement im Krankenhaus. Projekte des BMG als Beitrag zur Verbesserung der Kommunikation und Kooperation. In G. Stadt München (Ed.), *Vertrauen durch Qualität!: Wege und Erfahrungen (7. Münchner Qualitätsforum 1997)* (S. 73-75). München: Gesundheitsreferat, Abt. 1-QM.

Bortz, J. & Döring, N. (1995). *Forschungsmethoden und Evaluation für Sozialwissenschaftler*. Heidelberg: Springer.

Büssing, A. (Ed.) (1997). *Reorganisation von Dienstleistungsprozessen im Krankenhaus*. Göttingen: Verlag für Angewandte Psychologie.

Büssing, A., Barkhausen, M. & Glaser, J. (1999). Evaluation von Organisationsentwicklung im Krankenhaus – Methodologische und methodische Anforderungen und deren Realisierung. *Zeitschrift für Gesundheitswissenschaften, 7*(2), 131-148.

Flick, U. (2000). Triangulation in der qualitativen Forschung. In U. Flick, E. v. Kardoff & I. Steinke (Eds.), *Qualitative Forschung. Ein Handbuch* (S. 309-318). Hamburg: Rohwolt Taschenbuch Verlag GmbH.

Georgopoulos, B. S. (1986). *Organizational Structure, Problem Solving, and Effectiveness*. San Francisco London: Jossey- Bass Publishers.

Güntert, B. & Horisberger, B. (1991). Qualitätssicherung im Krankenhaus. Können Qualitätszirkel (QZ) helfen? *f & w - führen & wirtschaften im Krankenhaus, 3*, 179-183.

Höhmann, U., Müller-Mundt, G. & Schulz, B. (1998). *Qualität durch Kooperation.* Frankfurt am Main: Mabuse-Verlag.

Köhle, K., Böck, D. & Grauhan, A. (Eds.) (1977). *Die internistisch-psychosomatische Krankenstation. Ein Werkstattbericht.* Basel: Rocom.

Lecher, S. (2002). *Patientenbefragung im Krankenhaus. Der Hamburger Fragebogen zum Krankenhausaufenthalt (HFK) als Instrument zur Defizitanalyse aus Patientensicht.* Regensburg: Roderer Verlag.

Lecher, S., Klapper, B., Schaeffer, D. & Koch, U. (2003). *InterKiK-Toolbox. Bewertung und Verbesserung der interprofessionellen Kooperation im Krankenhaus. Reihe Management im Gesundheitswesen.* Bern: Verlag Hans Huber.

Mühlbauer, B. H. & Strack, D. (1997). Qualitätszirkel als Teil der Krankenhausnormalität? *f&w - führen & wirtschaften im Krankenhaus, 14*(2), 103-109.

Reister, M. (1999). Die Entwicklung der Versorgungsanforderungen im Gesundheitswesen - die statistische Basis. In Asklepios Kliniken GmbH (Ed.), *Strukturen im Gesundheitswesen und Zukunftsorientiertes Qualitätsmanagement – Wege in die Zukunft, Rüstung für den Wandel. Königstein-Frankfurt: Asklepios Kliniken Eigenverlag.*

Sachverständigenrat für die Konzentrierte Aktion im Gesundheitswesen (2001). *Gutachten 2000/2001: Bedarfsgerechtigkeit und Wirtschaftlichkeit.* Available: www.svr-gesundheit.de.

Schmerfeld, K. & Schmerfeld, K. (2000). Interprofessionelle Kooperation im Krankenhaus. In T. Gerlinger, M. Herrmann, L. Hinricher, G. Hungeling, U. Lenhardt, M. Simon, K. Stegmüller & N. Wolf (Eds.), *Jahrbuch für Kritische Medizin 33: Kostendruck im Krankenhaus* (Vol. 94-109). Hamburg: Argument-Verlag.

Schwartz, F. W. (1993). Evaluation und Qualitätssicherung im Gesundheitswesen. In K. Hurrelmann & U. Laaser (Eds.), *Gesundheitswissenschaften. Handbuch für Lehre, Forschung und Praxis* (pp. 399-420). Weinheim und Basel: Beltz-Verlag.

Simon, M. (2000). Kein Ende des Experimentierens: Zur geplanten Einführung eines DRG-basierten Fallpauschalensystems. In T. Gerlinger, M. Herrmann, L. Hinricher, U. Hungeling, U. Lenhardt, M. Simon, K. Stegmüller & N. Wolf (Eds.), *Jahrbuch für Kritische Medizin 33: Kostendruck im Krankenhaus* (Vol. 10-36). Hamburg: Argument-Verlag.

Uexküll, T. v. (1992). *Integrierte Psychosomatische Medizin in Praxis und Klinik.* Lenzheide: Schattauer.

Walther, M. & Walther, A. (1998). *Qualitätszirkel im Krankenhaus: Gestalten – organisieren – moderieren.* Ulm: Fischer.

Stress and recovery of social care professionals: Development of a screening version of the Recovery-Stress-Questionnaire for work

Paulino Jiménez & K. Wolfgang Kallus[*]
Department of Work, Organizational and Environmental Psychology, University of Graz, Austria

A look at the publication statistics shows that topics related to breaks and recovery at work received increasing interest in the past twenty years, while they hardly showed up in the key concepts together with job, work or occupation in the eighties. This development is in contrast to the publication rates of stress and strain with relation to work, job and occupation. These show a high level but no further increases since a couple of years. As recovery within and between work periods is a basic topic in work psychology from the beginning on (Kraepelin, 1902) the assessment of the quality of recovery seems overdue. A lack of recovery is a crucial factor for decreases in motivation, job-satisfaction and performance, increases of errors, health problems, burnout and absenteeism, especially in stressful working conditions. A couple of interesting recovery related concepts and ideas have been promoted in the past years. New results on the problem of unwinding after work show striking differences between female and male managers as reflected in daytime and evening catecholamine levels (Frankenhaeuser, 1991; Lundberg & Frankenhaeuser, 1999). Unwinding is dependent on work related individual differences like the ability to change perspective and distance oneself or a Type A Behavior Pattern. For high levels of job strain a carry-over effect of high blood pressure into the spare time and night could be demonstrated (e.g., Rau, 2001) and spill over effects to leisure time activities have been reported (Bamberg, Rueckert & Udris, 1986; Sonnentag, 2003), just to mention a few empirical results (see also Frankenhaeuser, 1979, 1986; Meijman & Mulder, 1998; Kirkcaldy & Shephard, 2001; Richter & Hacker, 1998; Wieland-Eckelmann, Allmer, Kallus & Otto, 1994). Questionnaires to assess aspects of recovery have been provided by Kirkcaldy (e.g., Kirkcaldy & Shephard, 2001) and by Weyer, Hodapp and Neuhäuser (1980). These developments together with some promising preliminary results on the simultaneous assessment of stress and recovery in a stress recovery balance at the work place (Blanka, 2000; Gombocz, 2003; Platzer, 2000; Wagner, 1994) call for a psychometric instrument to assess stress and recovery in the work place. The stress recovery questionnaire (RESTQ, Kallus, 1995) might provide a basis of

---

[*] *Correspondence: Wolfgang Kallus, wolfgang.kallus@uni-graz.at*

high value for this purpose. The RESTQ is the only psychometric instrument which allows to assess a detailed recovery stress profile (Kentä & Hassmén, 1998), and it allow to include additional modules for specific area of application.

The RESTQ assess the state of an individual with respect to the most important facets of stress and recovery (cf. Janke, 1976) based on the frequency of stress and recovery related events and states in the past days. The scores from the RESTQ reflect important aspects of the state of the individual. It turned out, that e.g., for top athletes the recovery stress state is related to a broad spectrum of criteria, which range from mood state, physical symptoms and psychophysiological parameters to performance in competitions (Kallus, 2002).

An area specific module for sports has already been developed (RESTQ-SPORT, Kellmann & Kallus, 2001, cf. Kallus & Kellmann, 2000) and preliminary work for work specific modules to include burnout and off-work activities has already been conducted. The sports specific version received broad interest in research and application. The sports specific version is used as a monitoring instrument in training camps during the preparation for championships, as it can be used to predict performance outcomes (Kellmann, 2002).

An interesting result with high relevance for the working world concerns the performance decrements in athletes with a weak stress-recovery balance. While classical stress concepts explained stress related performance changes with deviation from an optimal level of activation, recovery seems to be more closely related to motivational states and resources (Beckmann, 2002).

The RESTQ-Work has been designed for an area specific assessment of the stress-recovery-profile for the occupational area as does the RESTQ-SPORT for the area of high performance sports. An important aspect has to be considered for a modern instrument assessing stress (and recovery) in the workplace: The principles and requirements concerning methods for measuring and assessing mental workload which are stated in the future international Norm ISO 10075-3:2004 (2004) require high levels for reliability and validity of instruments. For accurate measurement processes (precision level 1, ISO 10075-3:2004, table 1, p. 10) reliability must be $\geq$ .9 and validity must be $\geq$ .5. To reach this, we decided to combine existing instruments like the RESTQ and an instrument assessing work strain and burnout (AWSB, Jiménez, 2003a). The requirements in this norm are lower for screening purposes (level 2) and for orienting purposes (level 3). The planned work specific module for the RESTQ to provide a RESTQ-Work also should be usable for these levels. In this paper a first short version with few items and scales for the purpose of screenings is presented.

There are some theoretical aspects which should be addressed and included in an analysis of stress-recovery interactions. Recovery from stress has to be distinguished from coping with stress (Kallus, 2002), and the relationship between recovery and classical stress moderators like action latitude, participation and social support has to be analysed. Items for social support and for recovery in social situations are confounded in some social support questionnaires. Stress moderators contribute to the resources, which allow to cope with highly demanding situations. Recovery re-establishes resources after they have been taxed. An analysis of stress-recovery processes, which take place after termination of a stressor or in phases between intermittent occurrences of stress, might help to increase the impact of our occupational stress models.

The RESTQ-Work includes five dimensions of work strain and burnout from a preliminary questionnaire (Analysis of Work Strain and Burnout, AWSB, Jiménez, 2003a, in press) and some subtests to include theoretically interesting dimensions from the area of 'stress buffers'. The AWSB has been developed to measure aspects of burnout that are beyond those especially related to human services. Both the original version and the German version of the MBI, the MBI-D (Büssing & Perrar, 1992), include items which are very strongly related to human services. In contrast to this approach the items of the Analysis of Work Strain and Burnout are formulated without typical directions to 'patients' or 'clients'. The second aim was to have a very short list of items so the scale can be used in typical employee surveys where it is critical to use a longer questionnaire.

For the RESTQ-Work an additional set of work specific subtests was composed to include the possible links between recovery in social situations and social support, the problem of obligations in off-work time, the area of burnout, and the spill over from work to private life. These subtests assess specific aspects, which are relevant for the interpretation of the stress recovery profile in the work place. Of course, the work specific subtests will overlap with the general dimensions of RESTQ.

A short form of the work specific version of the RESTQ (RESTQ-WORK, cf. Jimenez & Kallus, 2003) will be introduced in the following passages. This version has the aim to fulfil the requirements of ISO 10075-3:2004 to have an instrument for screening purposes (level 2) and for orienting purposes (level 3). The data were obtained in a master thesis at the University of Graz (Hecht, 2003).

Method

Sample and procedure

The participants of the study worked in a professional community care setting for children and young adults. The organization consists of 17 different departments. 148 completed questionnaires were returned (response rate 54.6%). The sample consisted of 68.3% women and 31.7% men. The mean age was about 36 years (age was measured in categories: 0.7% up to 20 years, 29.3% 21 to 30 years, 39.5% 31 to 40 years, 22.4% 41 to 50 years, 8.2% above 51 years). 31.4% worked up to 5 years in the organization, 34.3% worked between 5 and 10 years and 34.3% worked more than 10 years in the organization.

Material

Recovery-Stress Questionnaire. (RESTQ, Kallus, 1995; Kellmann & Kallus, 2001). The RESTQ addresses different aspects of stress and recovery activities and states (physical indicators, emotional symptoms, behavioral and performance-related symptoms and social activities) during the preceding seven days/nights. The instrument has twelve scales with four items per subtest, seven subtests for stress and five for recovery. The answer scale assesses frequency in the past seven days/nights and ranges from 'never' (0) to 'always' (6). A short version of the RESTQ (Version RESTQ/24, cf. RESTQ-Sport-58, Kellmann & Kallus, 2001) was used with only two items per subtest. For this short version three scores can be computed assessing social emotional stress, performance related stress and recovery. These global scores correspond to the three factor solution for the basic version of the RESTQ.

Work related subtests of the Recovery-Stress Questionnaire assessing work strain and burnout. These items consist of a special scale for the analysis for work strain and burnout (Jiménez, 2003a; Platzer & Jiménez, 2001) as mentioned before. The internal consistency and retest reliability of the five scales (three items per scale) are good to acceptable (Jiménez & Kallus, 2003; Platzer & Jiménez, 2001).

The dimensions, internal consistency and retest reliability coefficient for 1 week for these scales are as follows (Jiménez, in press): Loss of control (α = .83, r = .64), meaningfulness of job (α = .86, r = .68), emotional exhaustion (α = .84, r = .57), social withdrawal (as analogues to depersonalisation) (α = .77, r = .84), reduced power (α = .64, r = .31). The rating scale ranges from 0 (never) to 6 (always) and corresponds to the RESTQ.

Work related subtests of the Recovery-Stress Questionnaire assessing stress and recovery at work. These items were developed to cover special aspects of stress and recovery at work, and to highlight the relationship between work stress, work related stress buffers and recovery. Most of the items are based on preliminary studies (cf. Gombocz, 2003; Platzer, 2000; Wagner, 1994) and have been selected for this study according to the results of the reliability analyses in the previous studies mentioned before. The scales used in this study were a subset of the preliminary version of the scales.

The RESTQ-Work in this version had in total 63 items. The questionnaire package included some additional questionnaires which are not presented here.

Results

Reliability analysis

The aim of the construction of the short version (screening version in the sense of ISO 10075-3:2004) of the RESTQ-Work is to have an economic but sufficiently reliable instrument. To fulfil the first aim the number of items per scale was reduced in this study (the Spearman-Brown formula was used to obtain the reliability estimates for scales with two items) and also some scales were removed of a longer version of the RESTQ-Work.

RESTQ-General

The internal consistency values for the scales of the global subtests of the Recovery-Stress Questionnaire for Work are presented in table 1. As this instrument is already widely used and published (e.g., RESTQ, Kallus, 1995; Kellmann & Kallus, 2001) further analyses focus on the work related modules of the RESTQ-Work.

Table 1: Cronbach's α for scales of RESTQ-General, analysis of work related strain/burnout, stress and recovery at work and the corresponding values

RESTQ-General	Cronbach's α
Social emotional stress	.78
Performance related stress	.80
Recovery	.79
Subscales from AWSB for work strain and burnout	
Loss of meaning	.69
Social withdrawal	.60

Reduced power	.58	
Loss of control	.67	
Emotional exhaustion	.77	
Subscales for stress and recovery at work		
Conflicts with colleagues	.72	a
Spill over	.83	
Disturbed breaks	.71	a
Spare time stress	.65	a
Obligations	.62	a
Leisure	.75	
Efficient breaks	.88	a
Meeting friends	.79	
Social support family	.85	a
Flow/success	.82	

[a] Spearman-Brown formula was used to obtain the reliability estimates for scales with two items.

The short version of the RESTQ with 24 items was used (Kallus, 1995). The internal consistency for the RESTQ-General is acceptable for the three global scores. This implies that the global scores of strain and recovery can be used for individual diagnoses. The profile information of the 24 Item version of the RESTQ has to be handled with some care as a two item per subtest version does not meet the level 2 requirements of ISO 10075-3:2004 for all subtests.

RESTQ-Work related parts

Cronbach's α for the Analysis of *work related strain/burnout* shows values from .58 for reduced power to .77 for emotional exhaustion. The scales of the next part, *stress and recovery at work*, also show acceptable to good values for Cronbach's α (from .62 to .88).

In general the values for Cronbach's α are acceptable or good for most scales for both parts, RESTQ-General and the RESTQ-Work related part. Scales for screening and orientation do not need to use the profile information for deeper interpretation. As a requirement of the ISO 10075-3:2004 is to have $\alpha > .7$ the scales of the module of the work related part were analysed with factor analyses to allow a combination of work specific subtests.

Factor analysis of the work specific subtests

The scales for the work related part of the RESTQ-Work were factor analysed using a principal component analysis (PCA). The resulting factors (according to the Scree test) were rotated according to VARIMAX-criteria.

The factorial loadings of the work specific subtests and the communalities are shown in table 2.

Table 2: Factor loadings (a > 0.3) for work related part of RESTQ from social care professionals and a reference group of blue collar workers (n = 98)

	Social care workers				Blue collar workers			
	Factor 1	Factor 2	Factor 3	Commu- nality	Factor 1	Factor 2	Factor 3	Commu- nality
Loss of meaning	.77		.40	.76	.82			.67
Social withdrawal	.75			.61	.69		.37	.67
Reduced power	.71			.55	.71		.34	.69
Loss of control	.70			.58	.84			.76
Conflicts with col- leagues	.65			.47	.68			.48
Emotional exhaustion	.71	.37		.64	.55	.47		.59
Spill over	.71			.57	.42	.47	.37	.53
Disturbed breaks	.51	.38	-.44	.59		.83		.74
Spare time stress		.79		.66		.79		.70
Obligations		.72		.58		.62		.48
Leisure		-.81		.75		-.54	-.66	.77
Efficient breaks		-.64		.48		-.56	-.47	.58
Meeting friends		-.43	-.43	.38			-.70	.58
Social support family			-.55	.30			-.74	.57
Flow/success			-.79	.70	-.40	.34	-.48	.50
Explained variance	.27	.19	.11		.24	.21	.17	

Factor loadings < .3 are not shown in this table

The factorial solution with four factors with eigenvalues larger 1 did not result in a satisfactory solution so three factors were extracted. The first three factors explain 57% of the variance. The communalities for 'meeting friends' and 'social support family' are low; all other values are acceptable or good.

The first factor (27% of the variance) displays mainly the scales for *work strain/burnout*. Scales like 'loss of meaning', 'social withdrawal', 'conflicts with colleagues' determine this factor. The 'spill over' of work to spare time is also important for this factor in the sample of social care professionals. The first factor summarizes the feeling of strain at work which is directly induced by the aspects of work. Note that the role of spill over and disturbed breaks seem to be different in a sample of blue collar workers (cf. table 2).

The second factor (19% of the variance) can be identified primarily as displaying a bipolar factor with the poles *recovery* and *obligations*. One pole is characterized by 'stress in spare time' ("In my spare time I was not able to do what I wanted.") and 'obligations' on the other side there are 'leisure' ("I had the opportunity for recuperation and relaxation") and 'efficient breaks'. The aspect of leisure is different in the reference sample of blue collar workers (cf. table 2).

The remaining scales 'meeting friends', 'social support family' and 'flow/success' form factor 3 (12% of the variance). As the scales can be seen in a function of moderating stress effects, the factor can be labelled as *strain moderators*.

Discussion

The work specific supplement to the general subtests of the RESTQ again support the view, that strain and recovery are far from being different sides of the same coin – at least as far as frequency of occurrence is concerned. Even more interesting seems the fact, that classical stress moderators like social support ('stress buffers') show a relative independence to recovery. In the work specific context of community care recovery has an opposite pole, which is formed by obligations and disturbed recovery (and not stress!). Note that 'meeting friends' shows high loadings on recovery and on strain moderators. This is an interesting result as different forms of social support might play different roles in the stress-health relationship, as Elfering, Semmer, Schade, Grund and Boos (2002) showed for back pain symptoms in employees.

All in all the work specific part of the RESTQ-Work allows to assess burnout and two classes of moderators: classical moderators and recovery. The results of the reliability analysis show, that some scales don't fulfil the requirement of $\alpha > .7$ in the screening version. As presented, the internal consistencies for the scales of the analysis of work strain/burnout have been found better in other samples (Jiménez, 2003a; Platzer & Jiménez, 2001). Therefore global scores for the three factors, which were found in this study, should be used for screening. The requirements for level 2 and 3 must be analysed in a future independent study, and a longer version with reliable profile information will be provided as it has been done for the RESTQ-Sport.

Limitations

The short version of the RESTQ-Work was constructed with a smaller subset of the initial scales from previous studies (e.g., Gombocz, 2003). The main reason was to get an instrument that is economically suitable for practical applications and doesn't overlap with other instruments (e.g., social support scales) and suits the requirements of ISO 10075-3:2004 for level 2 and 3. Especially scales with close relation to the construct of job satisfaction were removed. The modifications did not change the basic factorial structure of the work specific part as described by Gombocz (2003) for a sample of blue collar workers (cf. table 3). The factor *recovery and obligations* is essentially the same but not as clear as before. The differences in the structures can be led back to the different working settings: Social care workers are more likely in situations where they think about their work still at home so spill over and efficient breaks play a different role for them. Results indicate that recovery and stress buffers might be two separate approaches to reduce stress related health and performance risks in the work place.

The advantage of the RESTQ-Work is that it consists of two modules for assessing the stress recovery process: A general part and the work related part where the results support each other. As shown with the RESTQ-SPORT (Kellmann & Kallus, 2001; cf. Kallus & Kellmann, 2000) the instrument has a higher acceptance with area specific items (here work related) than used only with general aspects. The scores of the general part can be compared with other populations also e.g., with athletes. The work specific part helps experts in practice to identify facets for interventions.

RESTQ-WORK and job satisfaction. The previous mentioned aim of the work related part of the RESTQ-Work is the usage in practice together with typical parts of employee surveys like job satisfaction. So a future question is the differentiation between constructs: Do we measure job satisfaction again or a separate construct? Büssing and Perrar (1992) pointed out that job satisfaction can be seen as linked with work strain or burnout depending of the conceptual point of view. If job satisfaction is seen as an attitude to different aspects of work then the constructs are more distant. If looking to a dynamical view of job satisfaction as in the way of Bruggemann (1976) or Büssing and Bissels (1998; see also Büssing, Bissels, Fuchs & Perrar, 1999; Büssing, Bissels, Herbig & Krüsken, 2000) then the constructs are close to each other as both, satisfaction and strain, are the result of an appraisal process. Especially the cybernetic model of job satisfaction of Jiménez (2000, 2002, in press) describes the dynamic aspects which leads to non linear feedback loops. This aspect is important for the practical usage of the instrument and will be addressed in future validity studies.

From a practitioners point of view it is crucial to get insights to approaches of interventions. This aim was also very important for the construction of the RESTQ-WORK: It is not enough to have many different figures which don't allow making the next necessary step in an organization. This is necessary for interventions for the individual and the organization in modern job design. Kompier (2003) and many others (cf. Cox, Griffith & Rial-Gonzalez, 2000; Schabracq, 2003; Schaufeli & Buunk, 2003) demand that interventions should be based on theoretical frameworks which are – on the other hand – very often far from useful for practitioners as there is a big gap between theory and practice. Very often stress management programmes are 'off the shelf' regardless of the underlying problems.

The RESTQ-WORK provides a profile which supports practitioners to get insight into the very important risk assessment of stress and strain at work extending the view to the forgotten aspect of recovery. The work is in progress and the described instrument is very promising, current research will bring more insight into validity and applicability.

References

Bamberg, E., Rueckert, D. & Udris, I. (1986). Interactive effects of social support from wife, non-work activities and blue-collar occupational stress. *International Review of Applied Psychology, 35*(3), 397-413.

Beckmann, J. (2002). Interaction of volition and recovery. In M. Kellmann (Ed.), *Enhancing recovery: Preventing underperformance in athletes* (pp. 269-282). Champaign, Ill: Human Kinetics.

Blanka, E. (2000). *Arbeitszufriedenheit, Burnout, Ressourcen und Fehlzeitenanalyse in einem Unternehmen mit Teamarbeit [Job satisfaction, burnout, resources and analysis of absence in a company with teamwork]*. Unpublished master's thesis, University of Graz, Graz, Austria.

Bruggemann, A. (1976). Zur empirischen Untersuchung verschiedener Formen von Arbeitszufriedenheit [The empirical study of different forms of job satisfaction]. *Zeitschrift für Arbeitswissenschaft, 30*, 71-74.

Büssing, A. & Bissels, Th. (1998). Different Forms of Work Satisfaction: Concept and Qualitative Research. *European Psychologist, 3*(3), 209-218.

Büssing, A. & Perrar, K. M. (1992). Die Messung von Burnout. Untersuchung einer deutschen Fassung des Maslach Burnout Inventory (MBI-D) [The Measurement of Burnout. Studies of a German Version of the Maslach Burnout Inventory (MBI-D)]. *Diagnostica, 38*(4), 328-353.

Büssing, A., Bissels, T., Fuchs, V. & Perrar, K. M. (1999). A Dynamic Model of Work Satisfaction: Qualitative Approaches. *Human Relations, 52*(8), 999-1028.

Büssing, A., Bissels, Th., Herbig, B. & Krüsken, J. (2000). Formen von Arbeitszufriedenheit im Experiment: Differentielle Auswirkungen auf die Beziehung von Wissen und Handeln [Forms of work satisfaction in an experiment: differential effects on the relationship of knowledge and action]. *Zeitschrift für Arbeits- und Organisationspsychologie, 44*(1), 27-37.

Cox, T., Griffiths, A. & Rial-Gonzalez, R. (2000). *Research on Work-Related Stress*. Bilbao: European Agency for Safety and Health at Work.

Elfering, A., Semmer, N., Schade, V., Grund, S. & Boos, N. (2002). Supportive colleague, unsupportive supervisor: The role of provider-specific constellations of social support at work in the development of low back pain. *Journal of Occupational Health Psychology, 7*(2), 130-140.

Frankenhaeuser, M. (1979). Psychoneuroendocrine approaches to the study of emotion as related to stress and coping. In H. E. Howe, Jr. & R. A. Dienstbier (Eds.), *Nebraska Symposium on Motivation, 1978: Human Emotion* (pp. 123-161). Lincoln: University of Nebraska.

Frankenhaeuser, M. (1986). A psychobiological framework for research on human stress and coping. In M. H. Appley & R. Trumbll (Eds.), *Dynamics of stress: Physiological, psychological, and social perspectives*. New York: Plenum.

Frankenhaeuser, M. (1991). The psychophysiology of workload, stress, and health: Comparison between the sexes. *Annals of Behavioral Medicine, 13*(4), 197-204.

Gombocz, T. (2003). *Fortentwicklung einer arbeitsspezifischen Version des Erholungs-Belastungs-Fragebogens [Revision and update of a work specific version of the Recovery-Stress Questionnaire]*. Unpublished master's thesis, University of Graz, Graz, Austria.

Hecht, K. (2003). *Formen der Arbeitszufriedenheit im zeitlichen Verlauf [Forms of job satisfaction in the course of time]*. Unpublished master's thesis, University of Graz, Graz, Austria.

Janke, W. (1976). Psychophysiologische Grundlagen des Verhaltens. [Psychophysiological basis of behaviour]. In M. von Kerekjarto (Ed.), *Medizinische Psychologie* (pp. 1-101). Berlin: Springer.

ISO 10075-3:2004 (2004). *Ergonomic principles related to mental workload - Part 3: Principles and requirements concerning methods for measuring*. Brussels: European committee for standardization.

Jiménez, P. (2000). Job Satisfaction And Burnout From A Cybernetic View - An Integrative Model, First Project-Results. *International Journal of Psychology, 3/4*(35), 309.

Jiménez, P. (2002). Specific influences of job satisfaction and work characteristics on the intention to quit: Results of different studies. *Psychologische Beiträge, 44*(4), 596-603.

Jiménez, P. (2003a). *Belastungserleben als Prädiktor für die Absicht zu wechseln – der moderierende Einfluss des Selbstwirksamkeitserlebens [Work strain as predictor for the intention to quit – the moderating effect of perceived self-efficacy]*. Paper presented at the 9. Dresdner Symposium für Psychologie der Arbeit, February, Dresden, Germany.

Jiménez, P. (in press). Call Center in Österreich: Arbeitsbezogenes Beanspruchungserleben und Arbeitszufriedenheit als Prädiktoren für die Wechselbereitschaft [Call centers in

Austria: Work related strain and job satisfaction as predictors for intention to quit]. In R. Wieland, P. Richter & A. M. Metz (Hrsg.), *Call Center. Effiziente Arbeitsgestaltung – optimales Human Resource Management.*

Jiménez, P. & Kallus, W. (2003). *RESTQ-Work, Recovery-Stress-Questionnaire for Work.* Poster presented at the 8. European Conference on Organizational Psychology and Health Care, October, Vienna, Austria.

Kallus, K. W. (1995). *Der Erholungs-Belastungs-Fragebogen (EBF) [The Recovery-Stress Questionnaire].* Frankfurt, Germany: Swets & Zeitlinger.

Kallus, K. W. (2002). Impact of recovery in different areas of application. In M. Kellmann (Ed.), *Enhancing recovery: Preventing underperformance in athletes,* (pp. 281-298). Champaign, Ill: Human Kinetics.

Kallus, K. W. & Kellmann, M. (2000). Burnout in athletes and coaches. In Y. L. Hanin (Ed.), *Emotions in Sports* (pp. 209-230). Champaign, Ill.: Human Kinetics.

Kellmann, M. (Hrsg.) (2002). *Enhancing recovery: Preventing underperformance in athletes.* Champaign, IL: Human Kinetics.

Kellmann, M. & Kallus, K. W. (2001). *Recovery-Stress Questionnaire for Athletes: User manual.* Champaign, IL: Human Kinetics.

Kenttä, G. & Hassmén, P. (1998). Overtraining and recovery. *Sports Medicine, 26,* 1-16.

Kirkcaldy, B. & Shephard, R. J. (2001). Occupational stress, work satisfaction and health among the helping professions. *European Review of Applied Psychology, 51,* 243-253.

Kompier, M. (2003). Job design and Well-Being. In. M. Schabracq, J. Winnubst & C. Cooper (Eds.), *The Handbook of Work and Health Psychology* (pp. 429-454). Chichester: John Wiley.

Kraepelin, E. (1902). Die Arbeitskurve. In W. Wundt (Hrsg.), Philos. Studien, 19, 450.Lundberg, U. & Frankenhaeuser, M. (1999). Stress and workload of men and women in high-ranking positions. *Journal of Occupational Health Psychology. 4*(2), 142-151.

Meijman, T. F. & Mulder, G. (1998). Psychological Aspects of Workload. In P. J. D. Drenth, H. Thierry & C. J. de Wolff (Eds.), *Handbook of Work and Organizational Psychology* (Vol. 2, 2nd ed., pp. 5-33). Hove: Psychology Press.

Platzer, A. (2000). *Soziale Unterstützung, Burnout, Belastung und Erholung. Eine empirische Studie an Betreuerinnen und Betreuern in der Behindertenhilfe [Social support, burnout, stress and recovery. An empirical study at care workers of handicapped persons].* Unpublished master's thesis, University of Graz, Graz, Austria.

Platzer, A. & Jiménez, P. (2001). *Profile Analysis of Work Satisfaction - Validation of a new instrument for queries on work satisfaction.* Paper presented at the 10th European Congress on Work and Organizational Psychology, May, Prag, Czech Republic.

Rau, R. (2001). Objective characteristics of jobs affect blood pressure at work, after work and at night. In J. Fahrenberg & M. Myrtek (Eds.), *Progress in Ambulatory Assessment* (pp. 361-386). Seattle, Toronto, Bern, Göttingen: Hogrefe & Huber.

Richter, P. & Hacker, W. (1998). *Belastung und Beanspruchung [Stress and strain].* Heidelberg: Asanger.

Schabracq, M. (2003). What an Organisation Can Do about its Employees' Well-Being and Health: An Overview. In. M. Schabracq, J. Winnubst & C. Cooper (Eds.), *The Handbook of Work and Health Psychology* (pp. 429-454). Chichester: John Wiley.

Schaufeli, W. & Buunk, B. (2003). Burnout: An Overview of 25 Years of Research and Theorizing. In. M. Schabracq, J. Winnubst & C. Cooper (Eds.), *The Handbook of Work and Health Psychology* (pp. 429-454). Chichester: John Wiley.

Sonnentag, S. (2003). Recovery, work engagement, and proactive behavior: a new look at the interface between non work and work. *Journal of Applied Psychology, 88*(3), 518-528.

Wagner, S. H. (1994). *Empirische Untersuchung zu Belastungsfaktoren bei Krankenpflegekräften im Mehrebenenmodell unter Einbeziehung arbeits- und umweltpsychologischer Ansätze [Empirical study on stress in nurses using a multilevel approach based on methods from work psychology and from environmental psychology].* Unpublished master's thesis, University of Würzburg, Würzburg, Germany.

Weyer, G., Hodapp, V. & Neuhäuser, S. (1980). Weiterentwicklung von Fragebogenskalen zur Erfassung der subjektiven Belastung und Unzufriedenheit im beruflichen Bereich (SBUS-B). [Further developement of a questionnaire to assess subjective strain and dissatisfaction in occupational settings]. *Psychologische Beiträge, 22,* 335- 355.

Wieland-Eckelmann, R., Allmer, H. J., Kallus, K. W. & Otto, J. H. (Hrsg.). (1994). Erholungsforschung. Beiträge der Emotionspsychologie, Sportpsychologie und Arbeitspsychologie [Recovery research. Contributions from the psychology of emotions, sports psychology and work psychology]. Weinheim: Psychologie Verlagsunion.

A questionnaire for assessing ethical aspects and organisational quality of on-line counselling websites (WEBCQUAL)

Michael Trimmel* & Gerlinde Rohrauer
Center for Public Health, Medical University of Vienna, Austria

Introduction

There is still a growing number of services offering on-line counselling (E-counselling) or even on-line psychotherapy (E-therapy) via the Internet (c.f., Childress & Asamen, 1998). For these types of on-line mental health services diverse authorities describe a number of design recommendations (see below). In this paper an empirically proved questionnaire is suggested in order to assess ethical aspects and the organisational quality of such websites, based on diverse recommendations.

Various benefits of on-line counselling, like the possibility of E-counselling serving as a potential entry to the mental health system, which is important concerning people who may not see a therapist or counsellor otherwise (Childress, 2000), are currently being discussed. Furthermore, E-counselling is considered to be convenient (Manhal-Baugus, 2001) and also more affordable than face-to-face counselling or therapy (Lazlo, Esterman & Zabko, 1999). Due to the asynchronous and text-based characteristics of communication, Suler (2001) suggested that E-therapy offers enhanced possibilities for reflection and might have positive effects similar to journal writing or bibliotherapy, or might reduce clients' inhibitions due to the absence of face-to-face contact.

Nevertheless, several risks and deficits have been reported concerning the provision of this type of mental health services. Many of the concerns deal with implications of a lack of face-to-face contact: For example, there is an increased potential for misunderstandings (Childress, 2000; Manhal-Baugus, 2001), it is more difficult to handle emergency situations (Manhal-Baugus, 2001), and the ability of therapists to provide full assessment and diagnosis is severely diminished (Childress, 2000; Shapiro & Schulman, 1996). According to Barthelmeus (1999) online mental health services differ greatly in the

---

* Correspondence: Michael Trimmel, michael.trimmel@univie.ac.at

The authors wish to thank Karin Trimmel for help in preparing the manuscript.

extent to which they inform clients about the benefits, risks and limitations of E-Therapy services ('informed consent information'). Lang (2001) reported the existence of a misleading discrepancy between the naming of the services and the actual professional education of the counsellors. DiBlassio et al. (1999) conducted an examination about on-line behavioural health care resources and pointed out that the quality of this type of sites is not regulated and varies extensively. Barak (1999) concluded that practically all providers of psychological services (e.g., information resources, therapy, testing) use unsecured websites.

Meanwhile, a number of organisations, which aim at protecting clients by developing ethical guidelines, quality suggestions or quality initiatives, have emerged. Nevertheless, no systematic tool is offered to evaluate ethical aspects and the organisational quality of on-line mental help sites efficiently has been offered so far (DiBlassio et al., 1999). The purpose of this study was to develop a rating scale in order to assess the quality of on-line counselling websites. Suggestions or rules related to the quality of health websites and specifically to the quality of E-counselling and E-therapy services launched by pertinent initiatives, professional organisations or regulatory authorities have been explored. All suggested aspects were collected and served as items for the composition of the questionnaire. Subsequently the rating scale's suitability to assess significant differences between some exemplary websites in respect to the quality categories was investigated in order to demonstrate the sensitivity of the questionnaire. Furthermore, 5 subscales which can be combined to an overall score will be described and finally, the inter-rater reliability demonstrates a high reliability of all items.

Method

Existing recommendations

In order to identify criteria for ethical aspects and organisational quality for E-counselling and E-therapy applications, the following ethical guidelines have been reviewed (cited in Manhal-Baugus, 2001): The "Ethical Standards for Internet On-line Counselling" (American Counselling Association, 1999), the "Suggested Principles for the Online Provision of Mental Health Services Version 3.11" (International Society for Mental Health Online, 2000), the "Standards for the Ethical Practice of WebCounselling" (Center for Credentialing and Education, 2003; National Board for Certified Counsellors, 2001), the "APA Statement on Services by Telephone, Teleconferencing, and Internet" (American Psychological Association, 1997), and the "Guidelines for the Clinical Use of Electronic Mail with Patients" (Kane & Sands, 1998).

In addition, the following publications offering quality suggestions or rules were reviewed: The 'Certificate for Psychological Online Counselling" released by the Association of German Professional Psychologists (BDP) (Lang, 2001), the 'Star Ratings', judging the E-Therapy websites listed at the 'Metanioa' directory (Ainsworth, 1995–2001b), the 'Health Web Site Standards Version 1.0' (URAC, 2001), which was selected for review as it is based on a number of relevant quality initiatives and ethical codes, and the "Position Paper on Internet Text-based Therapy" (Clinical Social Work Federation, 2001). According to a press release at the web page of the German Psychological Association (BDP Verband, 2002), the German 'Teledienstgesetz' (law governing the use of electronic information and communication services) applies to psychotherapists too, and was therefore reviewed as well. Ethical guidelines and suggestions related to the quality of health websites or on-line mental health services launched by professional organisations or regulatory authorities served as basis for the construction of the rating form (e.g., Ainsworth, 1995-2001; American Psychological Association, 1997; American Counselling Association, 1999; BDP Verband, 2002; International Society for Mental Health Online, 2000; Kane & Sands, 1998; Lang, 2001; National Board for Certified Counsellors, 2001). There was a great overlap of relevant topics in the suggested standards and the related publications. It was mentioned that a website should provide information about: organisation/person/owner offering the service (name, address), financial interests, qualifications of the person offering the service (how to confirm the qualifications), the specific services that are offered, the conditions of using the service, response times, ethical aspects of use (e.g., appropriate use of service, limitations of service, emergency situations), ethical standards of the profession in question, users' rights and privacy (collection and deletion or removal of person related information, triage of E-mails, secure communication). Thirty-five items were generated and twenty-three items remained after factor analysis (Kaiser criterion; see table 2). For most items a 6-point-rating scale ranging from 0 (very poor/not at all) to 5 (excellent) was used (see table 1 for the exact response format for each item).

Table 1: Answering formats of response scales (from items in table 2).

Response-scale A	0 = not at all, 1 = poor, 2 = moderate, 3 = fair, 4 = good, 5 = excellent
Response-scale B	0 = no, 3 = some of the counsellors, 5 = yes
Response-scale C	0 = very poor, 1 = poor, 2 = moderate, 3 = fair, 4 = good, 5 = excellent
Response-scale D	0 = no, 5 = yes

Selection of the websites

Similar to a potential client searching for an E-counselling service on the Internet, a search engine was used to identify five websites. The search items '+psychologische' '+online' '+beratung' (psychological online counselling) entered into the search engine 'Altavista.de' revealed more than 9,000 websites. The first 5 websites matching to E-counselling have been opted out. Sorted by the order given by the search engine, the following websites were selected: (1) 'Drewes Psychologie online' (Volker Drewes, Anke Fischbach) in the following referred as the 'Drewes website', URL: http://www. beratung-therapie.de/. (2) 'Psychologie Online, Informationen zu Psychologie und Psychotherapie' (Eugen Sondermann) in the following referred as the 'Sondermann website', URL: http://www.psy-online.de/psychotherapie /psy.htm. (3) 'Psychologische Beratung Online' (Andrea Schütze) in the following referred as the 'Schütze website', URL: http://www. psychologische-beratung-online.de/. (4) 'Online-Praxis. Beratung Supervision Coaching Weiterbildung' (Willi Bauer) in the following referred as the 'Bauer website', URL: http://home.t-online.de/home/proWiAnd/Homepage .htm. (5) 'psybera – Psychologische Beratung im Internet' (Marcus Rautenberg, Felix Weiss, Carola Ort) following referred as the 'Rautenberg website", URL: http://www.psychologische-beratung.net/.

Procedure and participants

The rating scale and the links to the 5 websites to be examined were presented at a website on the Internet. The web based presentation of the examination was chosen as it is asynchronous and therefore time independent, subjects could participate independently from any location, and there was no direct interaction with the researcher, data are therefore independent from the researcher (Batinic & Bosnjak, 2000).

Of course there are also disadvantages inherent to web based examinations. For example, the presentation of the documents at the subjects' screens could not be controlled, which is especially problematic when images are part of the experiments (Janetzko, 1999). In the present study, layout issues were not addressed in detail. At least, most of the subjects (87.5 %) used the same Internet browser (MS Internet Explorer). Furthermore, environmental conditions such as noise and interferences cannot be controlled when conducting Internet surveys (Janetzko, 1999), which is a clear disadvantage for a comparison after an experimental design. Therefore, subjects were instructed to take care not to be disturbed. Another problem is that the collection of the participants' personal data over the Internet can impact their right to privacy (Batinic & Bosnjak, 2000). This problem was resolved in the way that participants obtained a specific password. Data were therefore transferred and stored anonymously. The problem that no direct contact to the subjects could be established whilst filling in the on-line questionnaire (Batinic & Bosnjak, 2000) was not specifically addressed. However, participants could initiate contact via E-mail.

The participants logged in an on-line survey tool on the Internet. They were instructed to evaluate all 5 websites consecutively, but to take a break of 10 minutes after each website. The entire examination lasted from 1 to 2 hours, which was another reason for not investigating more than 5 websites, as motivation and/or exactness in assessing more websites would presumably be rather shortened. The sequence of websites was presented in a balanced order in order to avoid position effects and effects of sequence in evaluating it. Forty persons participated in this study. The sample consisted of 21 women and 19 men, age ranged from 19 to 40 years (mean age = 28.38 y). Concerning the educational background, 1 participant reported to have attended secondary school (2.5%), 21 participants were high school graduates (52.3 %), 15 reported being university graduates and 3 participants reported other educational backgrounds (7.5 %). In respect of the occupational position, 14 participants (35 %) reported that they have not been employed yet, 3 (7.5%) are self-employed, 21 (52.5 %) are white collar workers, 1 participant (2.5 %) works in the public service, and 1 participant (2.5 %) is a blue collar worker.

Results

Dimensions

A factor analysis (see table 1 for corresponding items and loadings) suggested 5 interpretable factors, explaining 67 % of the total variance. Factor 1 represents '(information about) privacy and confidentiality" (total variance explained: 34 %, Cronbach α = .90). Factor 2 can be interpreted as '(information about the) capabilities of counsellors/services" (total variance explained: 12.4 %, Cronbach α = .86). Factor 3 represents '(information about the) risks and limitations of E-therapy services" (total variance explained: 7.4 %, Cronbach α = .87). Factor 4 represents 'contact information" (total variance explained = 6.5 %, Cronbach α = .65). Factor 5 represents '(information about) website/service conditions", which includes the website conditions (design and clarity of the website) and information about the service conditions (total variance explained 5.7 %, Cronbach α = .63). For the five dimensions as well as for a 'total score' – which is the average of the 5 dimensions – scores were summed up and transformed to a range from 0 to 100.

Inter-rater reliability

Inter-rater reliability was assessed by computing Cronbach's α for each item (see table 2). Cronbach's α was in the range from .74 to .99 with a mean value of Cronbach's $\alpha = .95$.

Table 2: Item number (item #) of items, format of response scale, number of factor (factor #), factor loadings (loading) at the respective factor (factor #) and Cronbach α (α) of inter-rater reliability.

Item #	Item	Response scale	Factor #	Loading	α
1	The website informs about the nature of the service(s) offered	A	5	.57	.74
2	The website informs when clients can expect a response (e.g., 24 h, 72 h, 3 weeks)	A	5	.60	.94
3	Real name	B	2	-.58	.95
4	Address	B	4	.80	.93
5	Telephone number	B	4	.86	.93
6	Professional title/license (e.g., psychologist)	A	2	-.85	.98
7	Professional education/further education	A	2	-.90	.98
8	Professional experience	A	2	-.89	.98
9	The website provides enough details about the E-therapist's certification, license or other credentials, so that a client can independently verify this information (name, website URL or telephone number of the relevant institutions).	A	2	-.54	.93
10	The website informs that E-counselling cannot replace face-to-face consultation.	A	1	.65	.98
11	The website informs about the potential risks and limitations of receiving mental health services online (e.g., respecting communication, assessment and diagnosis, emergencies, etc.)	A	1	.78	.98

12	The website informs for which issues (circumstances) E-counselling may be (not) appropriate	A	3	-.65	.97
13	The website informs about potential benefits of text-based E-counselling services	A	2	-.74	.99
14	The website informs about fees and calculation modes (e.g., if counsellors charge per hour, per E-mail, per test, etc.)	A	5	.53	.79
15	The design and clarity of the website is ...	A	5	.75	.92
16	The website informs about the client's right to his/her confidentiality	A	1	.81	.98
17	The website informs if and to whom confidential information may be disclosed (e.g., to supervisors)	A	1	.78	.97
18	The website informs if, how, and how long confidential information may be preserved	A	1	.79	.98
19	The website informs about security measures that have been taken to protect the confidential information	A	1	.79	.97
20	Does the website provide the opportunity to encrypt the information transmitted (e.g., PGP encryption software, a secure form, a secure website)?	D	1	.80	.98
21	In my opinion the measures that are taken for secure information transmission are ...	C	1	.85	.98
22	The website informs about legal/ethical guidelines that cover the services offered	A	3	-.70	.95
23	The website informs about legal/ethical guidelines that cover the services offered	A	5	.58	.95

Examination of websites

Mean values of the five dimensions as well as of the total score are presented in figure 1. Most of the websites did not achieve a mean score higher than 70 points in any category, except for the website of Rautenberg which attained a mean score of 79 points in the category 'contact information'.

Figure 1: Normalised mean values of the 5 scales and of the total score of the quality of on-line counselling websites (WEBCQUAL) assessment for the five investigated websites

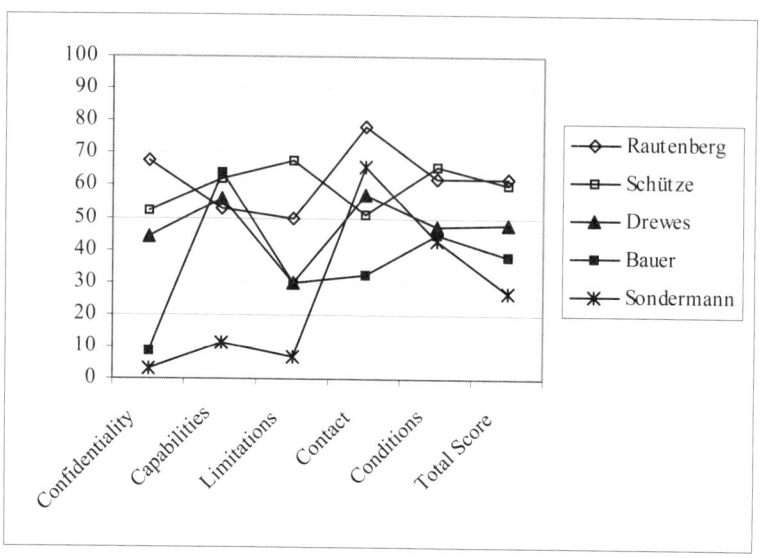

Due to violations of normality distribution, homogeneity of variance and sphericity assumptions in some cells, a non-parametric Friedman test was used to prove statistical significance. The non-parametric Friedman test revealed that the websites were significantly different in respect to 'confidentiality' (χ^2 = 129.20, p < .000), 'capabilities' (χ^2 = 78.68, p < .000), 'limitations' (χ^2 = 93.62, p < .000), 'contact' (χ^2 = 30.24, p < .000), 'conditions' (χ^2 = 45.22, p < .000), and the 'total score' (χ^2 = 99.74, p < .000) with df = 4 for all scales. The Rautenberg (mean rank = 1.74) and Schütze (mean rank = 1.80) websites achieved the highest overall rating ('total score'). The websites of Rautenberg and Schütze did not show a significant difference but were rated significantly better (p < .05) than those of Drewes (mean rank = 3.09), Bauer (mean rank = 3.85) and Sondermann (mean rank = 4.53) – which also differed significantly from each other by means of Scheffé test (p < .05).

Discussion

The purpose of this study was to develop a questionnaire to assess ethical aspects and organisational quality of websites offering E-counselling and/or E-therapy to clients. Based on suggestions of diverse health related organisations about ethical guidelines and the quality of on-line mental health services, items were generated and empirically tested by letting 40 participants rate 5 exemplary E-counselling websites, which are available on the Internet. A Factor Analysis suggested 5 factors which will be characterised in the following.

Factor one, '(information about) *privacy and confidentiality*' summarises the items 'information about the confidentiality right', 'information about data preservation', 'information about risks of unencrypted information transmission', 'information about potential disclosure of information to 3rd parties', 'information about security measures for information transmission' and 'availability of encryption opportunities'. For example, two of the rated websites (Bauer and Sondermann) did hardly inform about privacy and confidentiality or did not offer pertinent conditions (mean scores less than 10).

Factor two, '(information about the) *capabilities* of counsellors/services' summarises the items 'information about the counsellor's(s') professional education', 'information about the counsellor's(s') professional experience', 'information about the counsellor's(s') professional title and license', 'information about the benefits of E-counselling services', 'disclosure of the counsellor's(s') name(s)', and 'information to verify the professional title and license'. Four of the five rated websites (except for the Sondermann website) achieved mean scores of over 50. However, 'capabilities of counsellor's(s')/services" presented at the Sondermann website was rated 'very poor/absent" (mean score = 11).

Factor three '(information about the) *risks and limitations* of E-counselling services', summarises the items 'information about the risks and limitations of E-counselling services', 'information about the appropriateness of E-counselling services', and 'information that E-counselling cannot replace face-to-face consultation'. Three of the rated websites did not sufficiently inform about risks and limitations of E-counselling services (Sondermann, Bauer, and Drewes achieved mean scores ranging from 6 to 30).

Factor four, '*contact* information", summarises the items 'disclosure of counsellor's telephone number(s)' and 'disclosure of counsellor's address(es)'. Four of the 5 websites (except for the Bauer website) achieved scores of over 50 in category 'contact information' (mean scores ranging from 51 to 79). The Bauer website offered poor contact information with a mean score of 34.

Factor five, '(information about the) website/service *conditions*' summarises the items 'design and clarity of the website', 'information about response time', 'information which legal/ethical guidelines cover the services', 'information about the nature of the service(s)' and 'information about fees and calculation modes'. Three websites achieved moderate ratings (mean scores from 45 to 49) in this category (Bauer, Drewes, and Sondermann). Again, the websites of Rautenberg and Schütze achieved the best results (Rautenberg mean score = 62, Schütze mean score = 66).

The 'total score" reflects an overall judgement of the websites and summarises the scales 'confidentiality', 'capabilities', 'limitations', 'contact' and 'conditions'. The Rautenberg (M = 62) and Schütze (M = 60) websites achieved the highest 'total scores' and can therefore be considered as best out of 5 examined E-counselling websites. The Drewes website achieved a moderate 'total score' with a M of 47. The Bauer website was rated lower with a M of 38. The Sondermann website achieved the lowest ratings, and a very poor 'total score' with only 26 out of 100 obtainable points.

Moreover, the assessment of the 5 exemplary websites demonstrated the high sensitivity of the presented questionnaire on the 'quality of on-line counselling websites' (WEBCQUAL). The item analysis of the 5 subscales displayed a Cronbach α in the range from .65 to .90, suggesting a satisfying homogeneity of subscales and the mean inter-rater reliability of Cronbach α = .95 demonstrates a pretty high reliability of this instrument.

Limitations of this study could be seen in the moderate number of investigated subjects as well as in the investigation of a very limited number of websites. Nevertheless, results suggest that the presented assessment can be seen as a tool for quick and inexpensive rating of ethical and organisational characteristics of websites offering E-counselling or other on-line mental health services and can give quick and informative 'quality scores' of this kind of websites. This could be helpful for current attempts to establish and/or improve quality standards for governmental and non governmental use.

References

Ainsworth, M. (1995-2001b). *ABC's of 'Internet Therapy. Star Ratings.* Retrieved September 29, 2003, from http://www.metanoia.org/imhs/stars.htm.

American Counselling Association (1999). *Ethical Standards for Internet Online Counselling.* Retrieved September 29, 2003, from http://aca.convio.net/site/ PageServer?pagename=resources_internet.

American Psychological Association. (1997). *APA Statement on Services by Telephone, Teleconferencing, and Internet.* Retrieved September 29, 2003, from http://www.apa.org/ethics/stmnt01.html.

Barak, A. (1999). Psychological Applications on the Internet: A Discipline on the Threshold of a New Millennium. *Applied and Preventive Psychology, 8,* 231-246. Retrieved September 29, 2003, from http://construct.haifa.ac.il/~azy/app-r.htm.

Barthelmeus, S. H. (1999). *Disclosure of limitations, risks, and benefits by online counselling services: an investigation of the effects of differing amounts of information on perceived desirability.* Doctoral dissertation, University of Sarasota.

Batinic, B. & Bosnjak, M. (2000). Fragebogenuntersuchungen im Internet. In B. Batinic (Ed.), *Internet für Psychologen* (pp. 287-317). Göttingen: Hogrefe.

BDP Verband (2002). Eigene Homepage nicht ohne Tücken. Retrieved September 29, 2003, from http://www.bdp-verband.org/bdp/politik/011_homepagetuecken.shtml.

Childress, C.A. (2000). Ethical Issues in Providing Online Psychotherapeutic Interventions. *Journal of Medical Internet Research, 2*(1): e5. Retrieved September 29, 2003, from http://www.jmir.org/2000/1/e5.

Childress, C. A. & Asamen, J. K. (1998). The emerging relationship of psychology and the Internet: Proposed guidelines for conducting Internet intervention research. *Ethics & Behaviour, 8,* 19-35.

Clinical Social Work Federation (2001). *CSWF Position Paper on Internet Text-based Therapy.* Retrieved April 29, 2003, from http://www.cswf.org/therapy.html.

DiBlassio, J., Simonin, D., DeCarolis, A., Morse, L., Jean, J., Vassalotti, L., Franks, K. & Chambliss, C. (1999). Assessing the quality of psychological Healthcare sites available on the Internet. *Perspectives, 4*(1). Retrieved September 29, 2003, from http://mentalhelp.net/poc/ view_doc.php/type/doc/id/372 (p. 1) and http://mentalhelp.net/poc/view_doc.php/type /doc/id/373 (p. 2).

International Society for Mental Health Online (2000). *Suggested Principles for the Online Provision of Mental Health Services.* Retrieved September 29, 2003, from http://www.ismho.org/suggestions.html.

Janetzko, D. (1999). *Statistische Anwendungen im Internet. Daten in Netzumgebungen erheben, auswerten und präsentieren.* München: Addison-Wesley-Longman.

Kane, B. & Sands, D. Z. (1998). Guidelines for the Clinical Use of Electronic Mail with Patients. *Journal of the American Medical Informatics Association, 5,* 104-111.

Lang, F. (2001). Siegel zur psychologischen Beratung im Internet (Certificate for Psychological Online Counselling). *Report Psychologie, 26,* 510-511.

Laszlo, J.V., Esterman, G. & Zabko, S. (1999). Therapy over the Internet? Theory, Research & Finances. *CyberPsychology & Behavior, 2,* 293-307.

Manhal-Baugus, M. (2001). E-therapy: practical, ethical, and legal issues. *Cyberpsychology & Behavior, 4,* 551-563.

National Board for Certified Counselors. (2001). *The Practice of Internet Counselling.* Retrieved September 29, 2003, from http://www.nbcc.org/ethics/webethics.htm.

Shapiro, D. E. & Schulman, C. E. (1996). Ethical and legal issues in E-mail therapy. *Ethics and Behavior, 6,* 107-124.

Suler, J. R. (2001). Assessing a person's suitability for online therapy: the ISMHO clinical case study group. International Society for Mental Health Online. *Cyberpsychology & Behaviour, 4,* 675-679.

URAC (2001). *Health Website Standards Version 1.0.* Retrieved September 29, 2003, from http://webapps.urac.org/websiteaccreditation/portal/Consumer/Standards.asp.

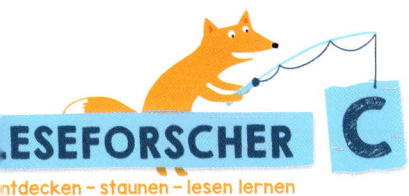

LESEFORSCHER C

entdecken – staunen – lesen lernen

Kathrin Köller

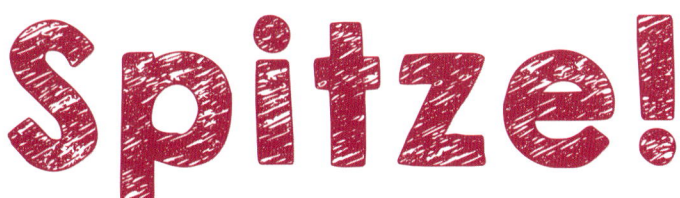

Spitze!

Von Ballett bis Hip-Hop

Mit Illustrationen von Julia Dürr

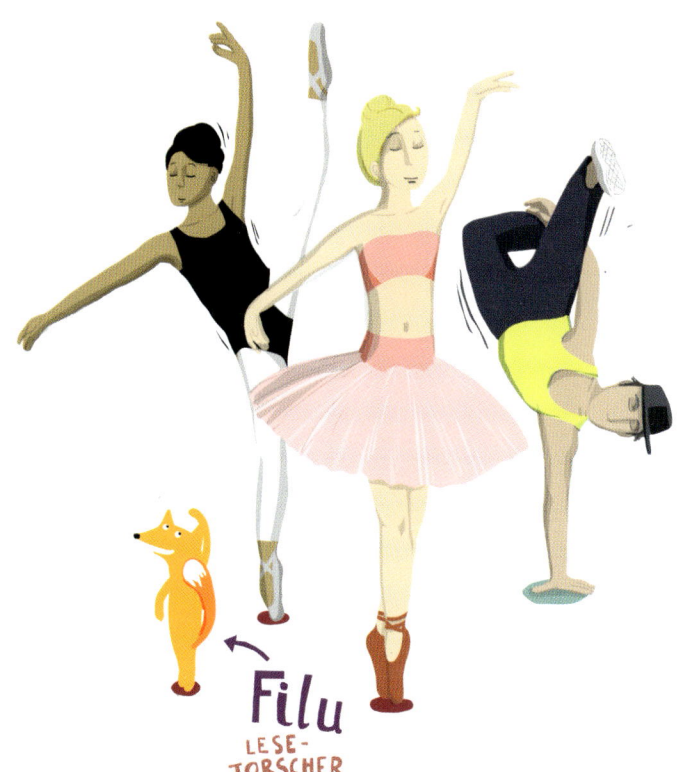

Filu
LESE-
FORSCHER

ueberreuter

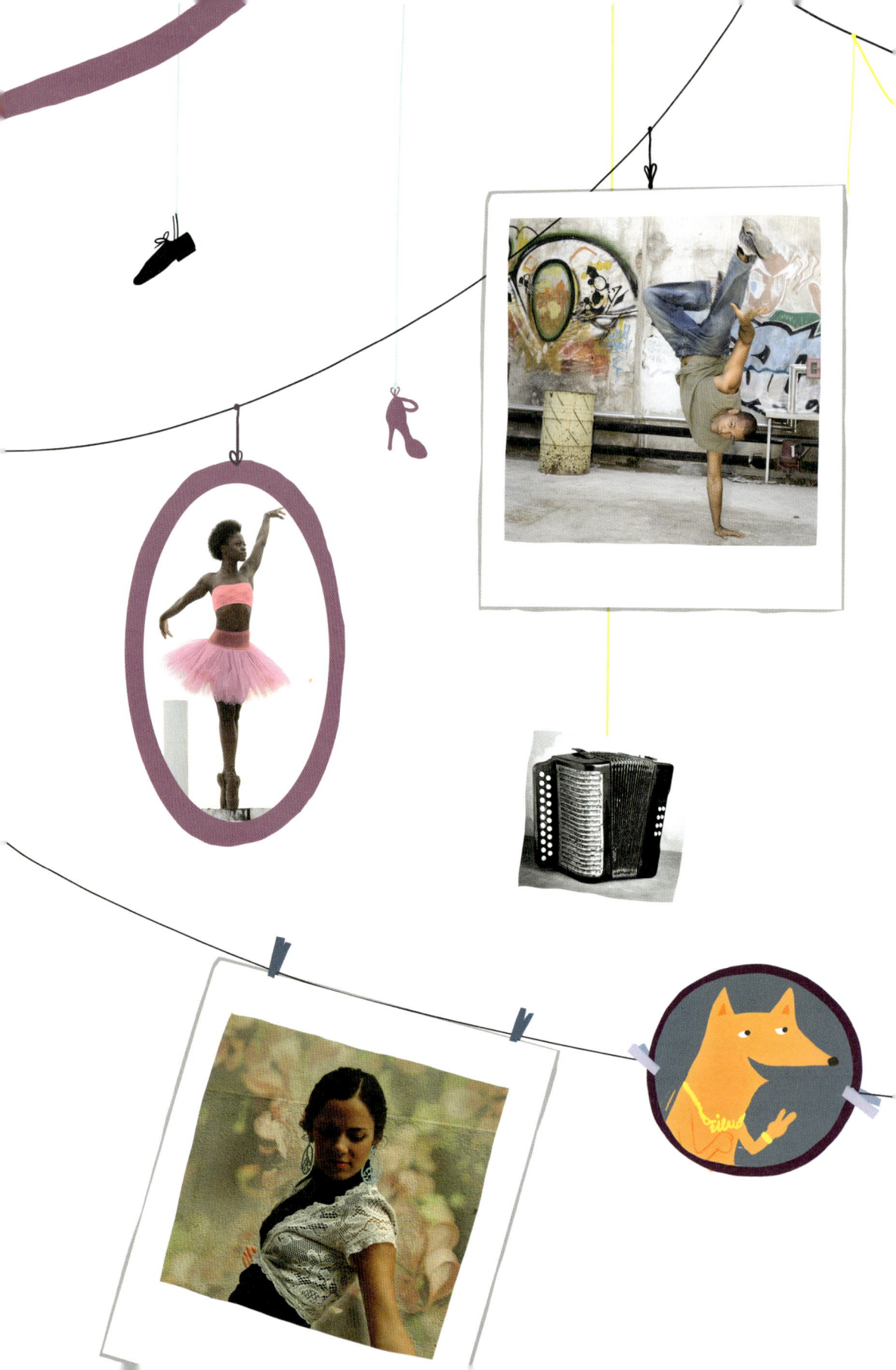

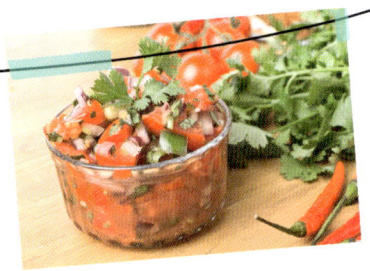

Inhalt

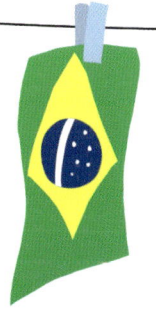

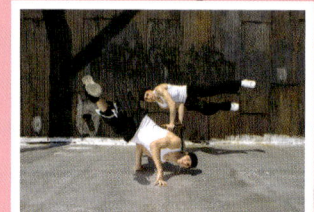

Hip-Hop

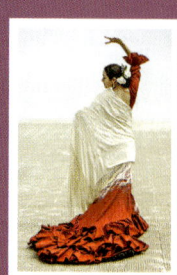

Flamenco

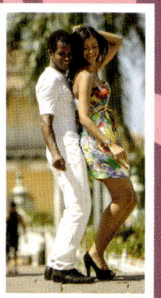

Salsa

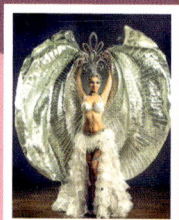

Samba

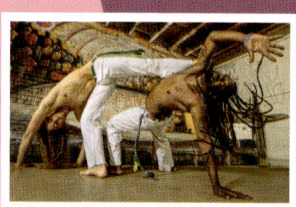

Capoeira

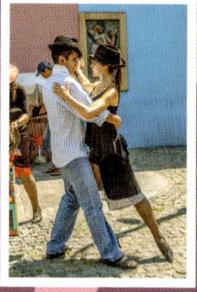

Tango

DIE WELT TANZT

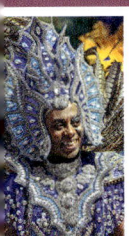

Karneval der Kulturen

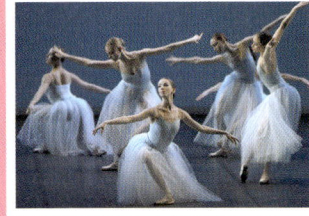

Ballett

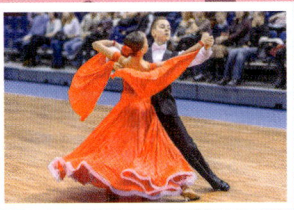

Wiener Walzer

Überall auf der Welt tanzen die Menschen. Mal auf der Straße, mal im Ballsaal. Mal wild, mal schön und elegant. Das schaue ich mir an. Und dann machen wir mit, okay?

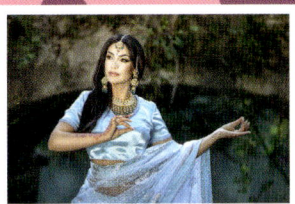

Bollywood

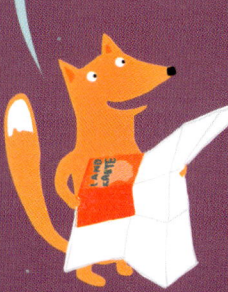

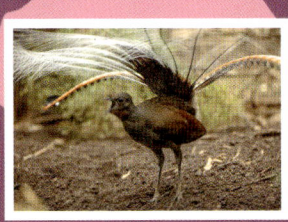

Meistertänzer

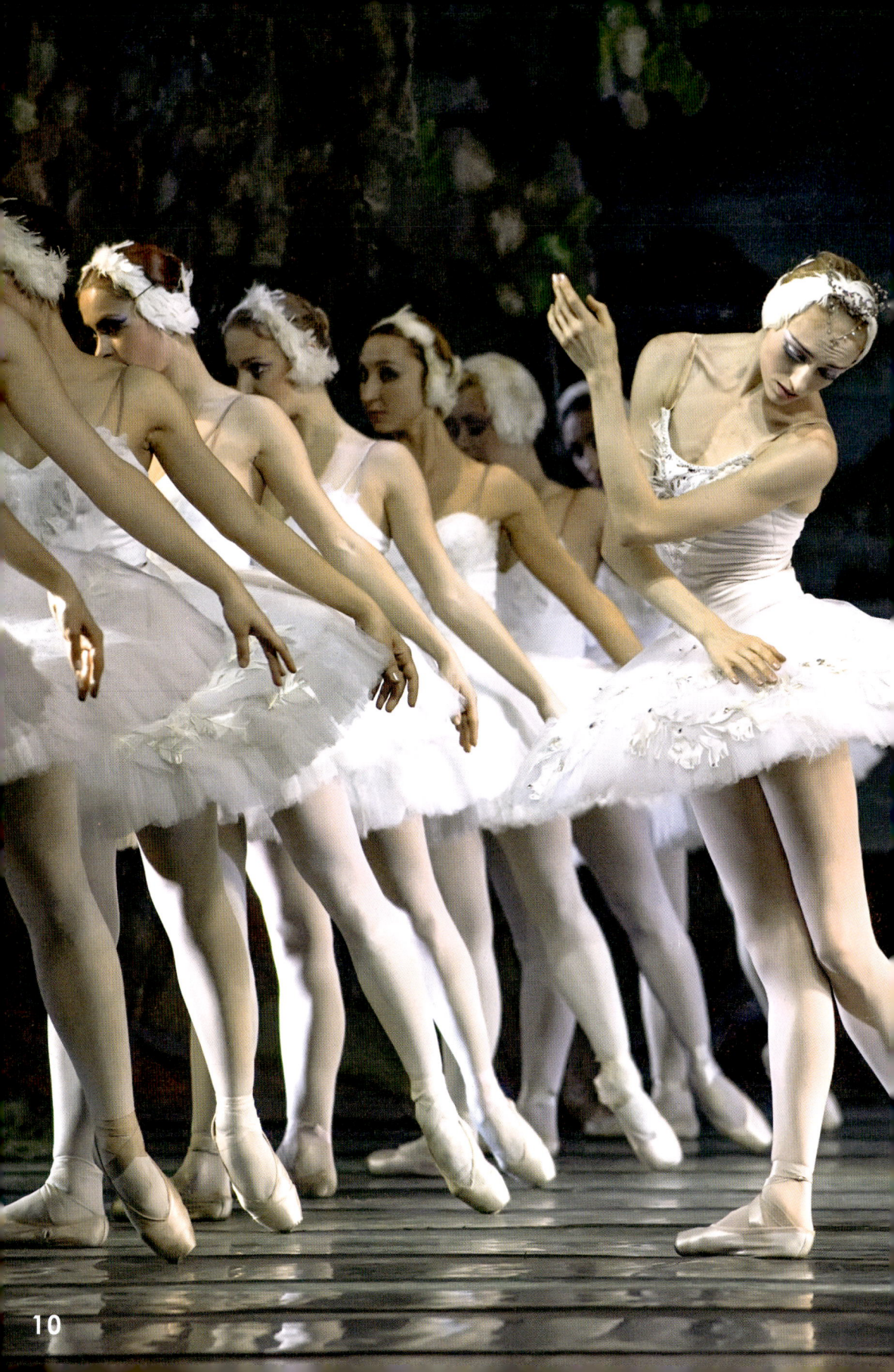

TECHNIK, TRAINING UND TUTUS

Gibt es etwas Schöneres als Ballett?

Für viele Menschen heißt tanzen ganz klar: Ballett tanzen.

Aber wie kam es eigentlich dazu?

Tanzen wie ein Gott

Angefangen hat alles an den Höfen der Fürsten in Italien. Die allerersten Tänzer waren übrigens Männer: Könige, Fürsten und Höflinge.

Der französische Sonnenkönig, Ludwig, der 14., war begeistert. Und so gründete er 1661 die erste Ballettschule der Welt. Deswegen haben die meisten Schritte und Positionen im Ballett französische Namen.

Russisches Ballett

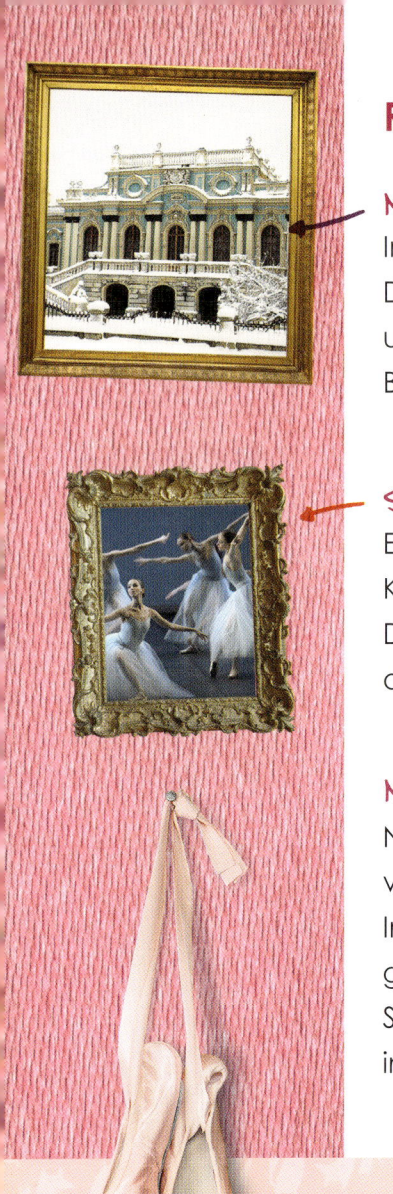

Mariinski

Im 19. Jahrhundert kam das Ballett nach Russland.
Die berühmtesten Theater waren das **Bolschoi** in Moskau
und das **Mariinski-Theater** in Sankt Petersburg.
Bis heute wird dort Ballett getanzt.

Schwanensee

Ende des 19. Jahrhunderts schrieb der
Komponist **Tschaikowsky** Schwanensee,
Dornröschen und Der Nussknacker,
die berühmtesten Ballettstücke aller Zeiten.

Modernes Ballett

Nach dem 2. Weltkrieg flohen
viele Balletttänzer aus Russland.
In den USA und in Frankreich
gründeten sie neue Schulen.
Sie sorgten dafür, dass das Ballett
immer wieder neue Ideen bekam.

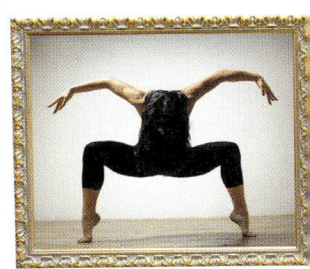

FRANZÖSISCH FÜR BALLERINEN

Arabesque,
sprich: Arabesk,
heißt „auf arabische Art"
und ist vielleicht die
berühmteste Position im
Ballett. Die Tänzerin steht
auf einem Bein, beziehungsweise auf der Fußspitze.
Das andere Bein ist weit
nach hinten gestreckt.

Barre, sprich: Bar,
die Stange, an der man
das Gleichgewicht übt

Corps de ballet,
sprich: Koadeballä,
Gruppe der Tänzerinnen,
die zusammen tanzen und
keine Einzeltänze machen

Ensemble,
sprich: Onsomble,
heißt „zusammen". Alle
Gruppentänzerinnen und
Einzeltänzerinnen, die
zusammen Aufführungen
machen, bilden ein
Ensemble.

Pirouette, sprich: Piruet,
Drehung auf einem Bein.
Das andere Bein wird am
Knie angelegt.

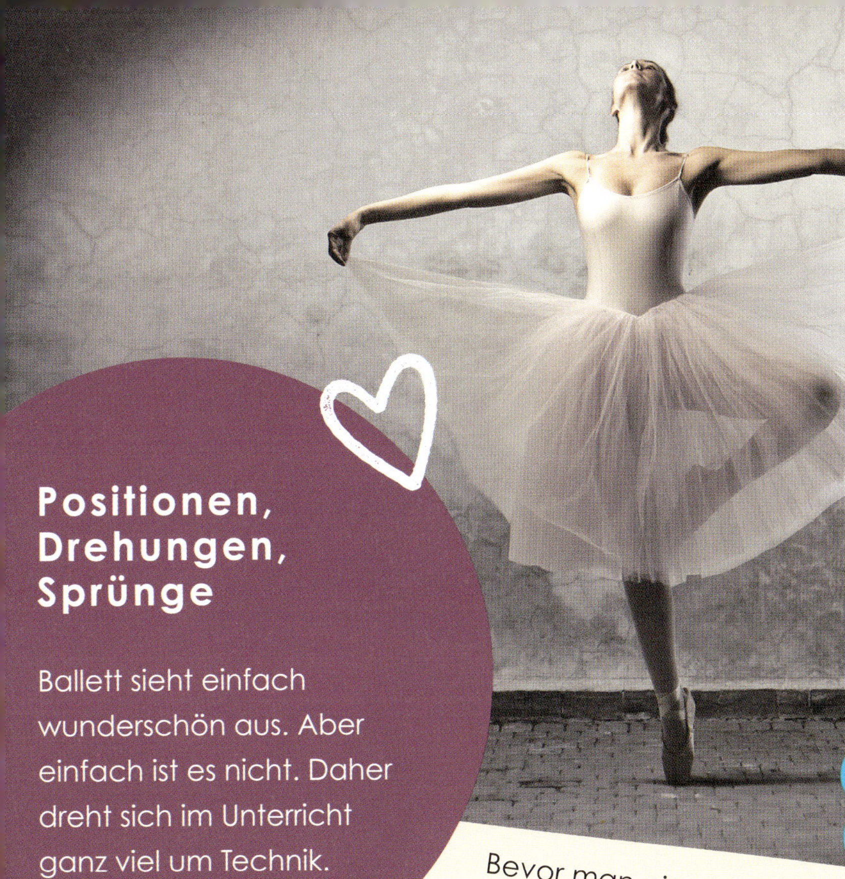

Positionen, Drehungen, Sprünge

Ballett sieht einfach wunderschön aus. Aber einfach ist es nicht. Daher dreht sich im Unterricht ganz viel um Technik.

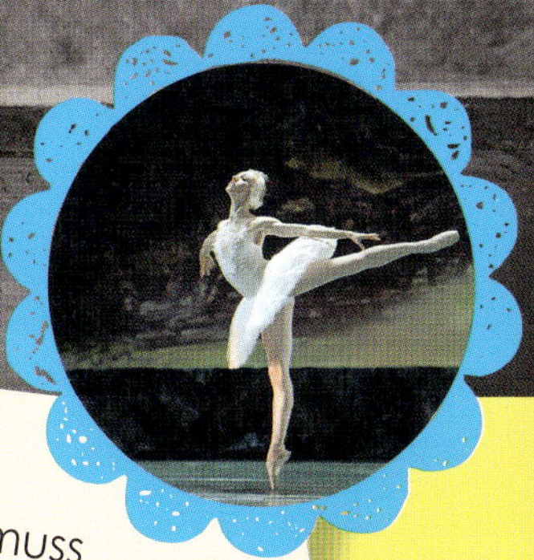

Bevor man eine schöne **Arabesque** hinbekommt, muss man lange an die **Barre** und Körperspannung üben.

Spitzentanz sieht toll aus. Als ob man schwebt. Dafür braucht es allerdings starke Füße, gute Spitzenschuhe und viel Geduld. Wer zu früh damit anfängt, schwebt nicht lange.

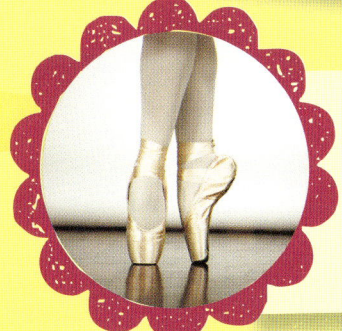

Toll ist auch die **Pirouette**. Das ist eine Drehung um sich selbst mit angezogenem Bein. Die Profis schaffen mehrere **Pirouetten** nacheinander.

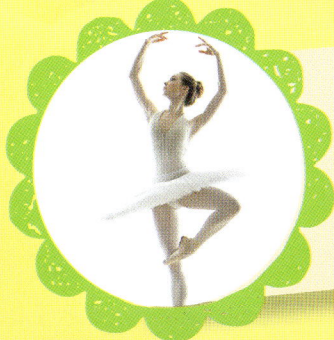

VOM WAISENKIND ZUM STAR

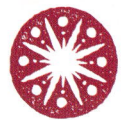

**Ballett ist viel Technik und noch mehr Training.
Und es ist für viele Menschen ein Traum.
Auch bei Michaela DePrince war das so.**

Im Waisenhaus

Michaela kam in Sierra Leone
zur Welt. Dort gab es einen
Bürgerkrieg. Michaela verlor
ihre Eltern und wurde von ihrem
Onkel ins Waisenhaus verkauft.

Der Traum vom Tanzen

Als sie drei Jahre alt war, fand sie
ein Bild mit einer Ballett-Tänzerin.
Seit diesem Tag wusste sie,
dass sie Ballett tanzen wollte.

Unglaublich, aber wahr

Eine amerikanische Familie
adoptierte sie. Michaela durfte
Ballett lernen. Als dunkelhäutige
Tänzerin hat sie es nicht leicht.
Aber Michaela hält an ihrem Traum
fest. Heute ist sie eine der besten
jungen Ballerinen der Welt.

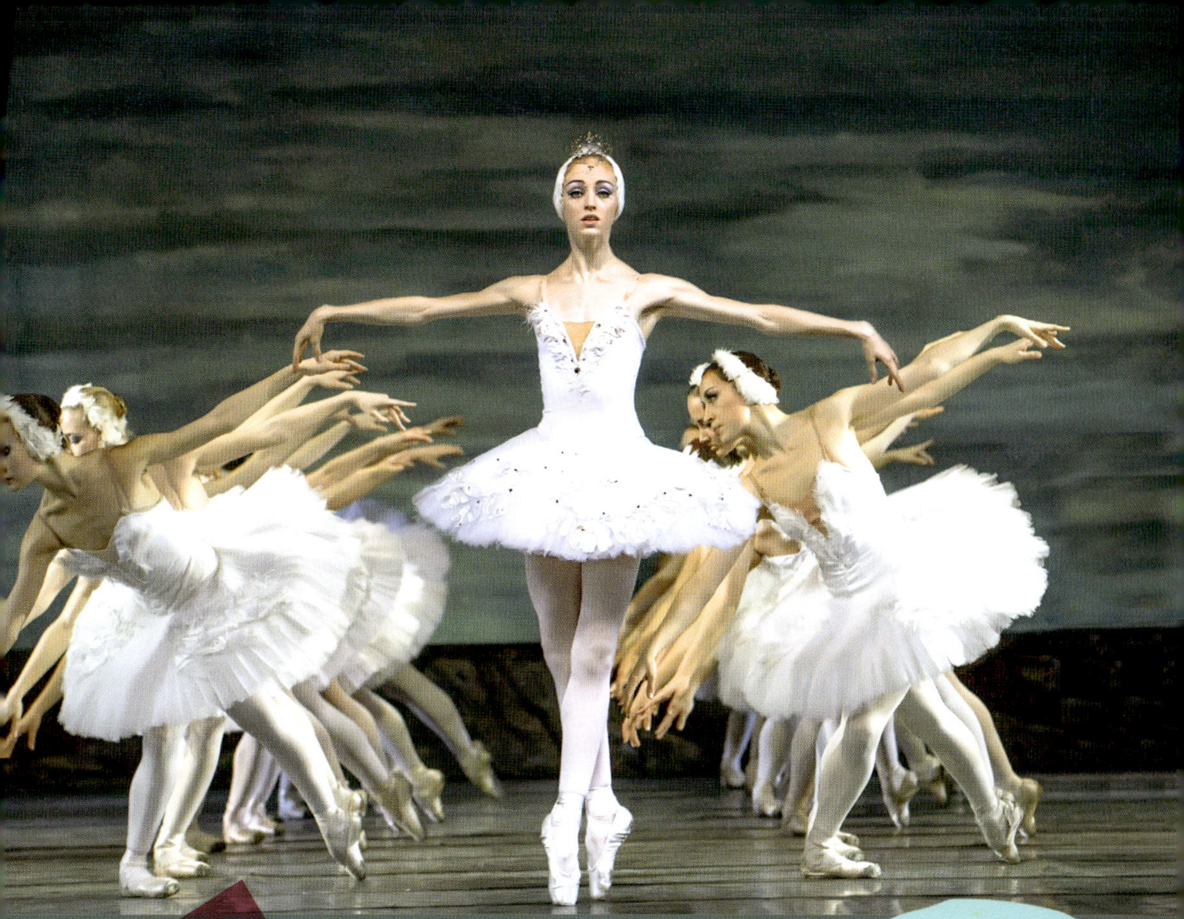

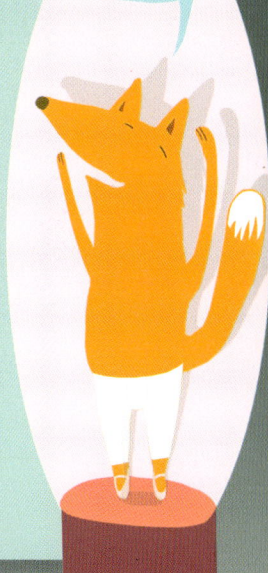

Ist doch prima!
Ich werde später
Ballerino.

„Jetzt sei doch nicht so eine Primaballerina."

Ein Spruch, wenn Eltern ihr Kind zu anstrengend finden. Dabei ist das ganz schön unlogisch. Nur besonders begabte Tänzerinnen werden zu **Primaballerinen**. Sie dürfen die schwierigen Solos tanzen und alleine im Rampenlicht stehen. Die meisten waren vorher jahrelang **Gruppentänzerinnen** im Corps de ballet. Sie mussten hart trainieren, bevor sie zu Primaballerinen wurden. Das sollten Eltern erst mal nachmachen!

DIE STOLZEN TÄNZE

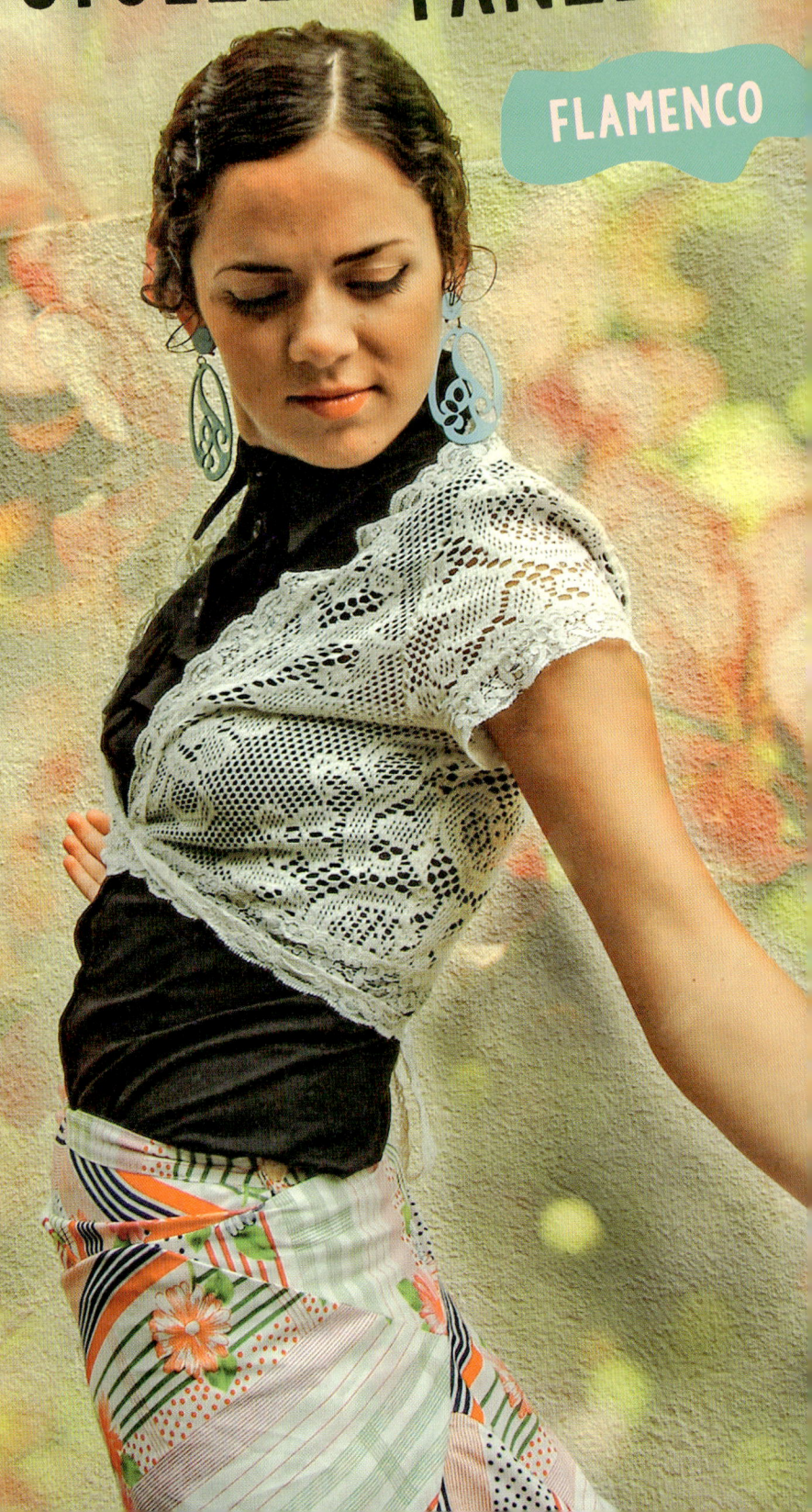

FLAMENCO

Heute wird Flamenco in Südspanien in der Schule unterrichtet. Das war nicht immer so. Erfunden haben den Tanz die unterdrückten Roma. Mit Flamenco konnten sie ihr Leid ausdrücken, sich wieder Mut machen und feiern.

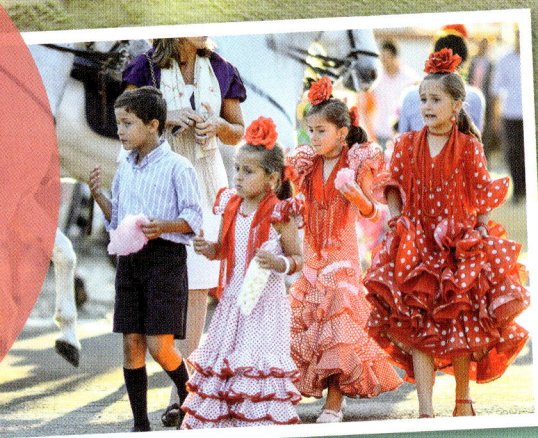

Fransentuch

weiter Rock, mit dem man beim Tanz spielen kann

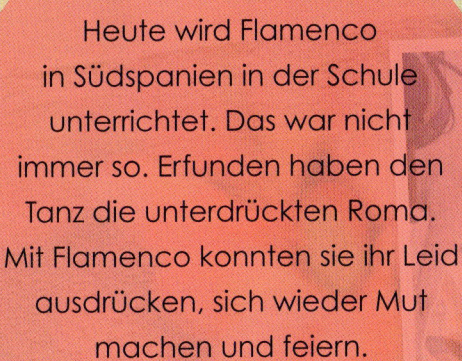

Heimat: Andalusien, Südspanien

Fangemeinde: weltweit

Erfinder: Roma, Mauren, jüdische Spanier

Zutaten:
1. tolle Tänzer
2. Gesang (spanisch: Cante)
3. Gitarre
4. Händeklatschen

Immer dabei:
Schuhe, die mit Nägeln beschlagen sind. Denn man muss Flamenco nicht nur sehen, sondern auch hören.

Typisch Flamenco:
– sehr rhythmischer Tanz
– schnelle Beinarbeit
– elegante Bewegungen mit dem Oberkörper
– Kastagnetten

17

TANGO

Vom verbotenen Tanz zum Kassenschlager

Der erste Tango

1880: In Buenos Aires treffen täglich neue Einwanderer aus Europa ein. Sie ziehen in die Armenviertel, in den Hafen der argentinischen Hauptstadt. Alle bringen ihre eigenen Tanzstile mit. Niemand weiß, wie genau und woher, aber es entwickelt sich ein neuer Tanz: Tango. Ein Tanz der Armen, von dem man in Argentinien eigentlich nichts wissen will.

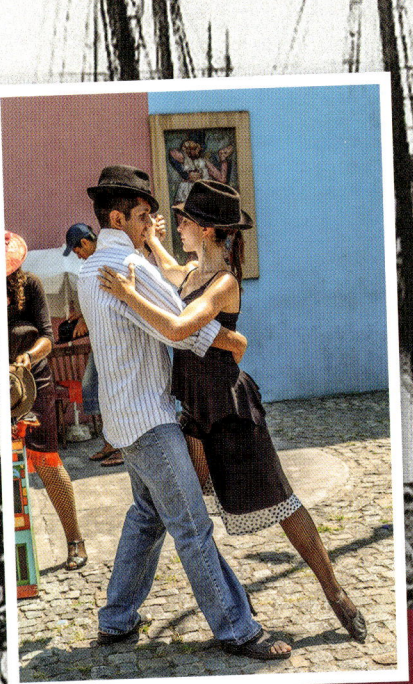

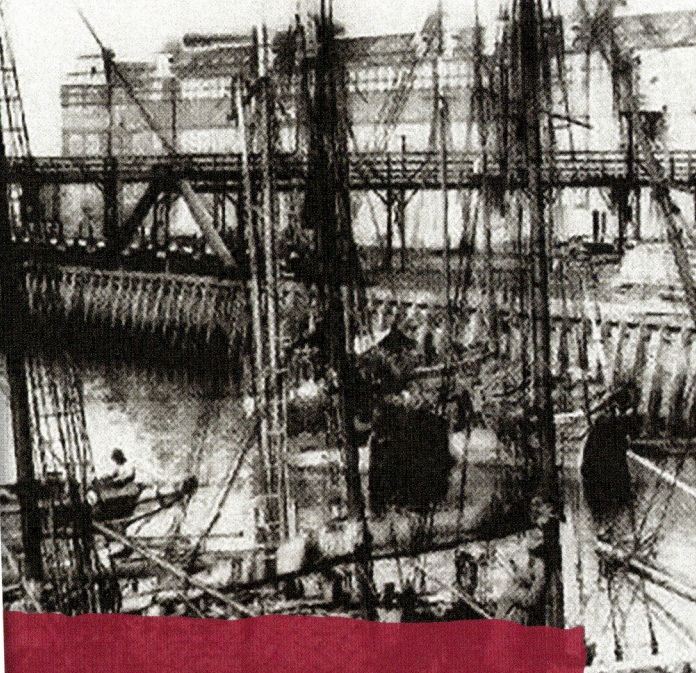

Tanzform: Paartanz, keine Frage

Wichtig: Der Mann!

Mann: Ja! Von mir geht alle Aktion aus.
Hältst du dem Blick in meine Augen stand?
Dann lass dich zum Tanz auffordern.
Und ich verspreche dir, es wird wild!

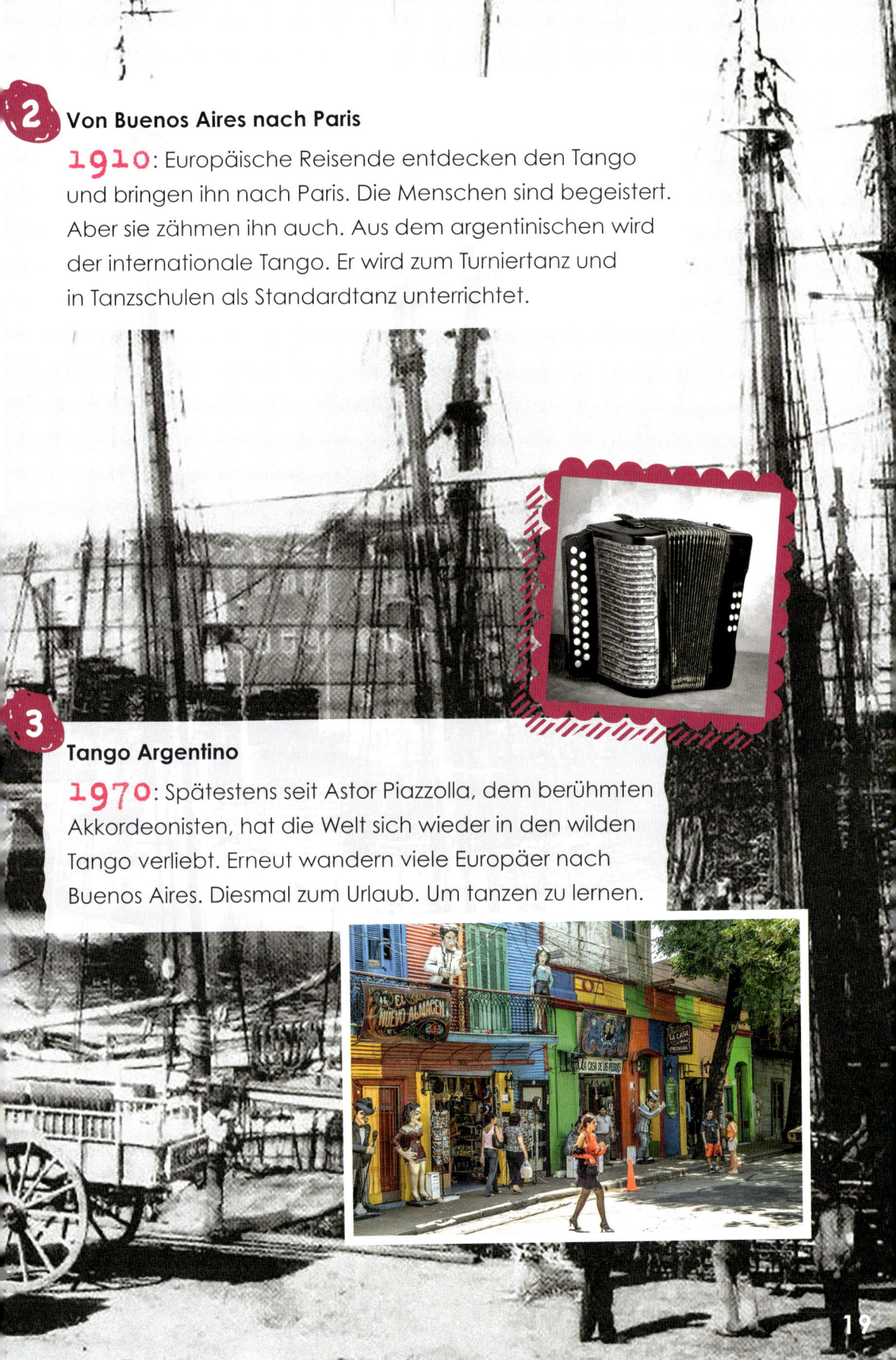

2 Von Buenos Aires nach Paris

1910: Europäische Reisende entdecken den Tango und bringen ihn nach Paris. Die Menschen sind begeistert. Aber sie zähmen ihn auch. Aus dem argentinischen wird der internationale Tango. Er wird zum Turniertanz und in Tanzschulen als Standardtanz unterrichtet.

3 Tango Argentino

1970: Spätestens seit Astor Piazzolla, dem berühmten Akkordeonisten, hat die Welt sich wieder in den wilden Tango verliebt. Erneut wandern viele Europäer nach Buenos Aires. Diesmal zum Urlaub. Um tanzen zu lernen.

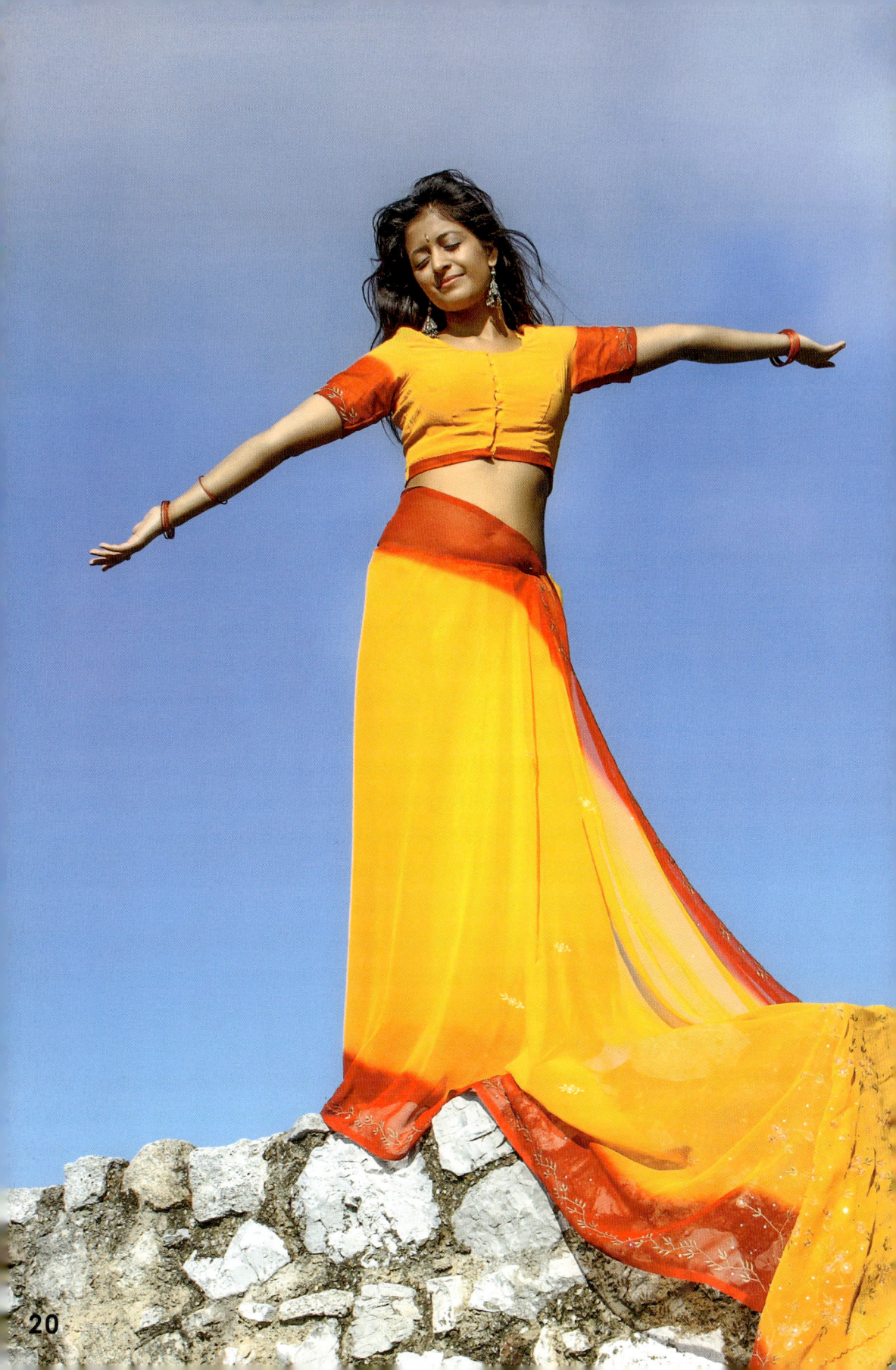

BOLLYWOOD

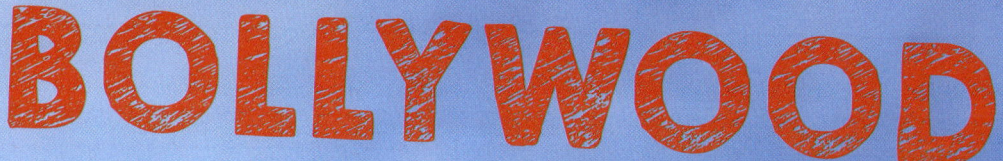

Will jemand Liebe tanzen?
Freude, Spannung, Tempo?
Andere mit Glück anstecken?
Kostüme in den tollsten Farben tragen?

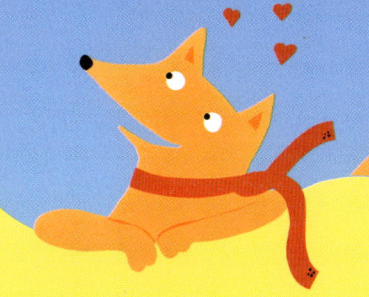

Willkommen in Bollywood!

Bollywood-Tänze haben ihren Namen von den
Bollywood-Filmen. Indische Tänze gibt es zwar schon
viel länger als die Filme. Aber erst durch die Filme
wurden die Tänze weltweit berühmt. Pro Jahr entstehen
in Indien rund 900 neue Bollywood-Filme. In diesen
Filmen geht es um Liebe und Gerechtigkeit und am
Ende um den Sieg des Guten über das Böse.

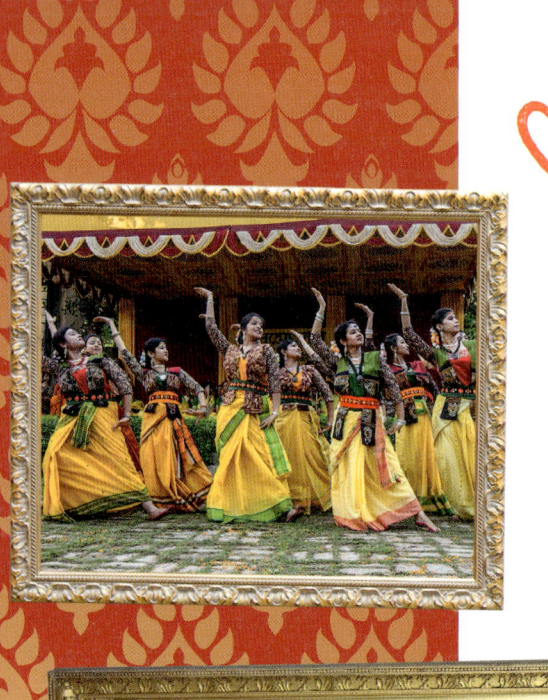

Es geht um Tanz

Richtig viel Tanz.
Ob auf einem Zug oder in den
Schweizer Bergen: Wer in einem
Bollywood-Film mitspielen will,
muss sehr gut tanzen können.

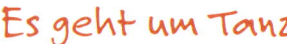

Übrigens auch die Jungs

In vielen Filmen treten die Jungs
in Teams gegen die Mädels an.
Die Bewegungen müssen extrem
gut sitzen. Zum Helden taugen
nur die allerbesten Tänzer.

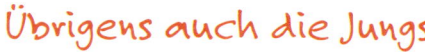

Traumtänze

Von den Bergen in die Großstadt ans
Meer? Das alles in weniger als einer
Minute und in wechselnden Outfits?
Bei den Traumtänzen geht es um
Sehnsucht und Liebe. Dafür braucht
man dramatische Orte und viele
verschiedene Kostüme!

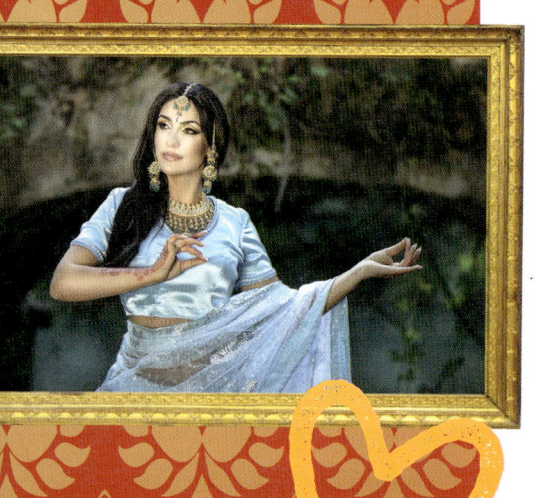

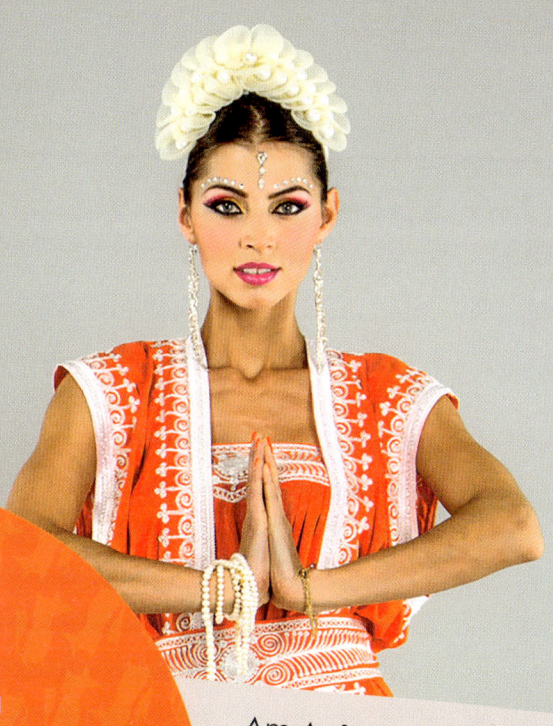

Echte Handarbeit

Eine Handbewegung sagt mehr als 1.000 Worte. Beim Bollywood-Tanz spielen die Hände immer eine Hauptrolle. **Mudras** heißen die Handbewegungen. Mit ihnen kann man Gefühle ausdrücken und Geschichten erzählen.

Am Anfang die **Begrüßung**: Hände fest zusammenpressen. Lächeln. Kopf nach rechts drehen. Kopf nach links drehen. Sei gegrüßt!

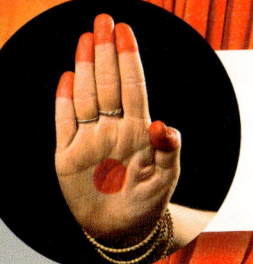

Wer sich freut, macht die **Pataka**, die Fahne. Die Finger sind ausgestreckt, der Daumen liegt an.

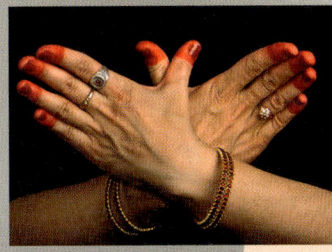

Ich bin frei wie ein Vogel. Oder: Ich fliege zu dir. Das kann man beides mit der **Garuda**, dem Vogel, ausdrücken. Die Daumen sind verschränkt, die Handinnenflächen zeigen zum Gesicht. Die Hände flattern.

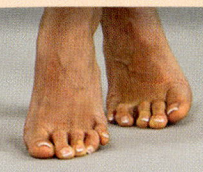

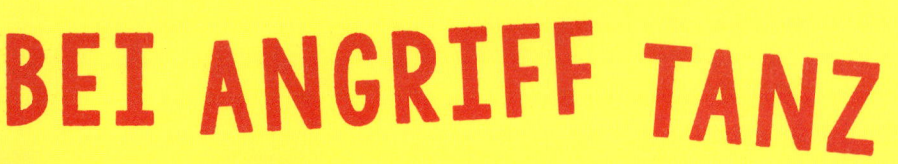

BEI ANGRIFF TANZ

CAPOEIRA

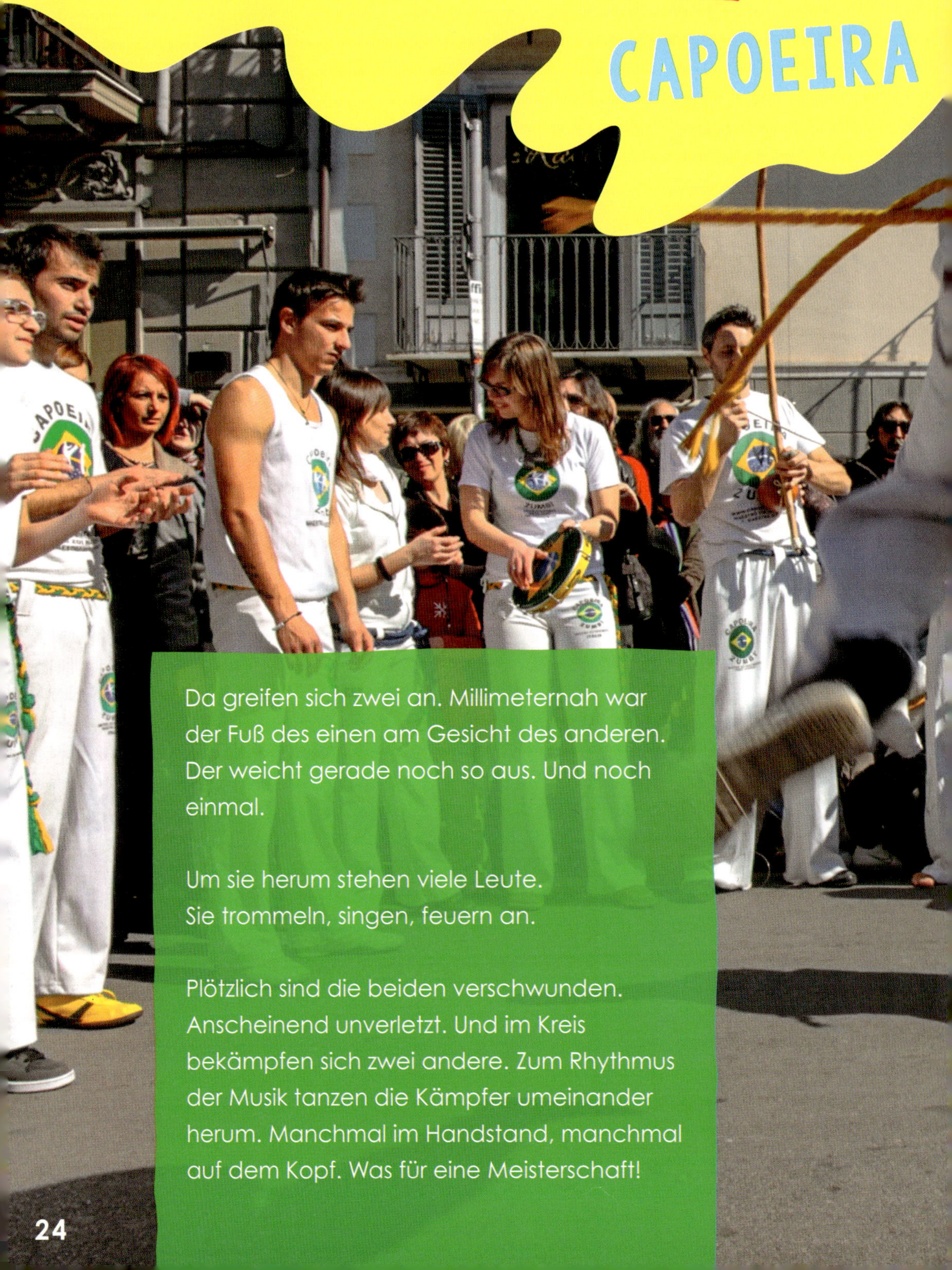

Da greifen sich zwei an. Millimeternah war der Fuß des einen am Gesicht des anderen. Der weicht gerade noch so aus. Und noch einmal.

Um sie herum stehen viele Leute. Sie trommeln, singen, feuern an.

Plötzlich sind die beiden verschwunden. Anscheinend unverletzt. Und im Kreis bekämpfen sich zwei andere. Zum Rhythmus der Musik tanzen die Kämpfer umeinander herum. Manchmal im Handstand, manchmal auf dem Kopf. Was für eine Meisterschaft!

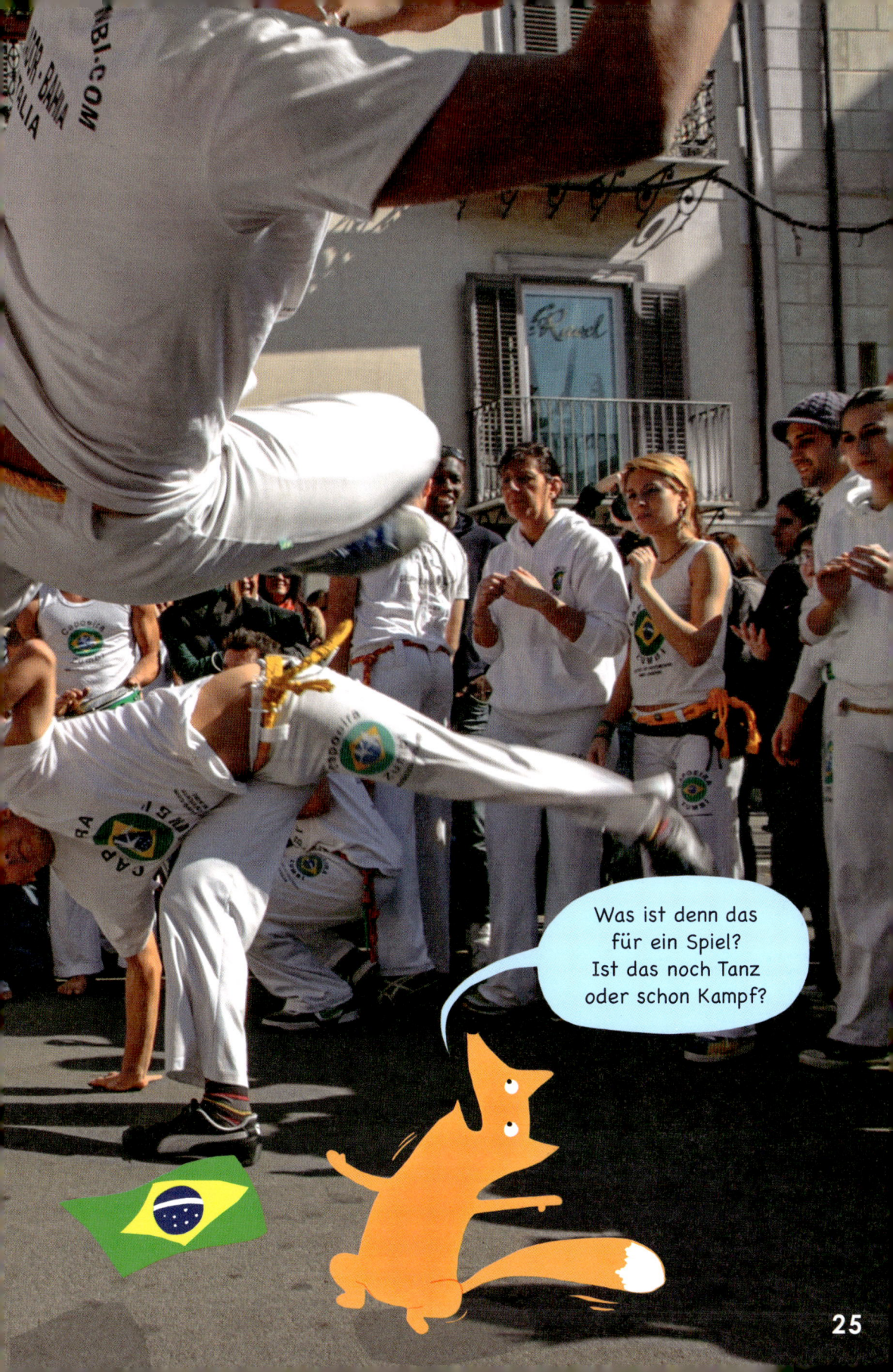

Was ist denn das für ein Spiel? Ist das noch Tanz oder schon Kampf?

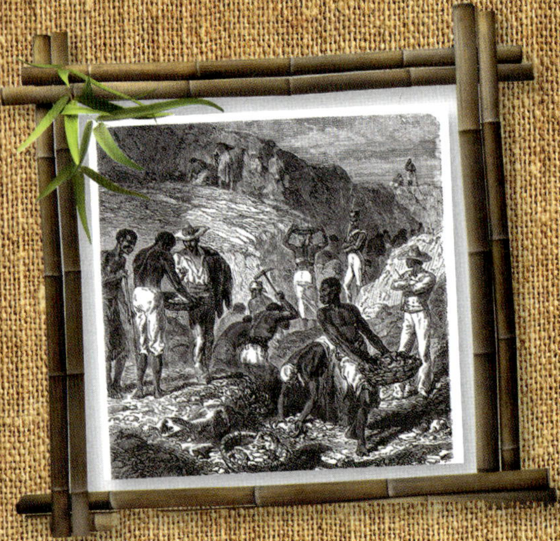

Brasilien im Jahr 1548

Die Portugiesen haben Brasilien erobert und brauchen Arbeiter für ihre **Zuckerrohrplantagen**. Sie verschleppen Tausende von Menschen aus Afrika nach Brasilien.

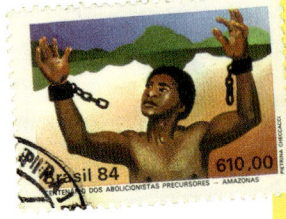

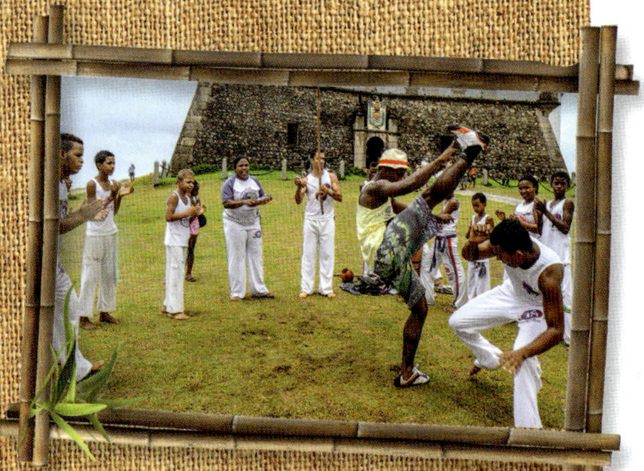

Schutz der Seele

Um sich zu wehren und nicht verrückt zu werden, entwickeln die afrikanischen Sklaven die **Capoeira**. Capoeira ist eine Mischung aus Kampf, Tanz und Akrobatik zu rhythmischer Musik. Mit Gesang.

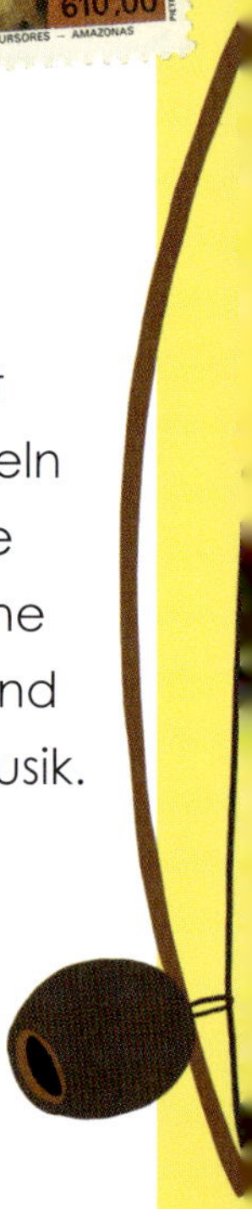

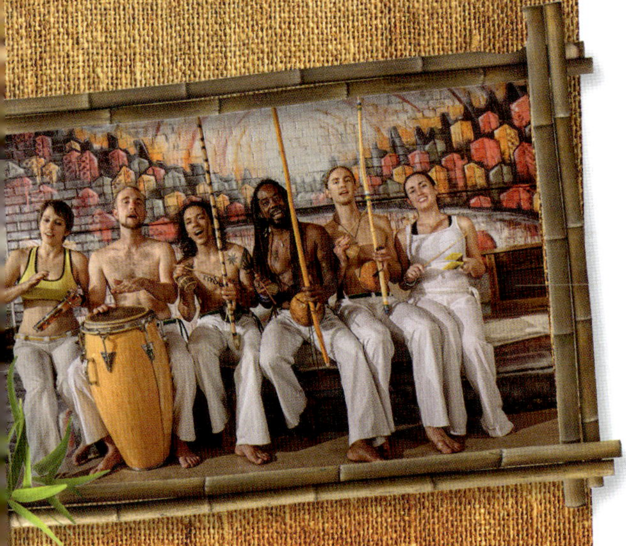

Das Orchester

Echtes Capoeira braucht Live-Musik. Nichts geht ohne die drei **Berimbaus**: Bogeninstrumente, die mit Stock und Stein gespielt werden. Dazu kommen noch Tamburin, Trommel und Gesang. Zusammen sorgen sie für die nötige Spannung.

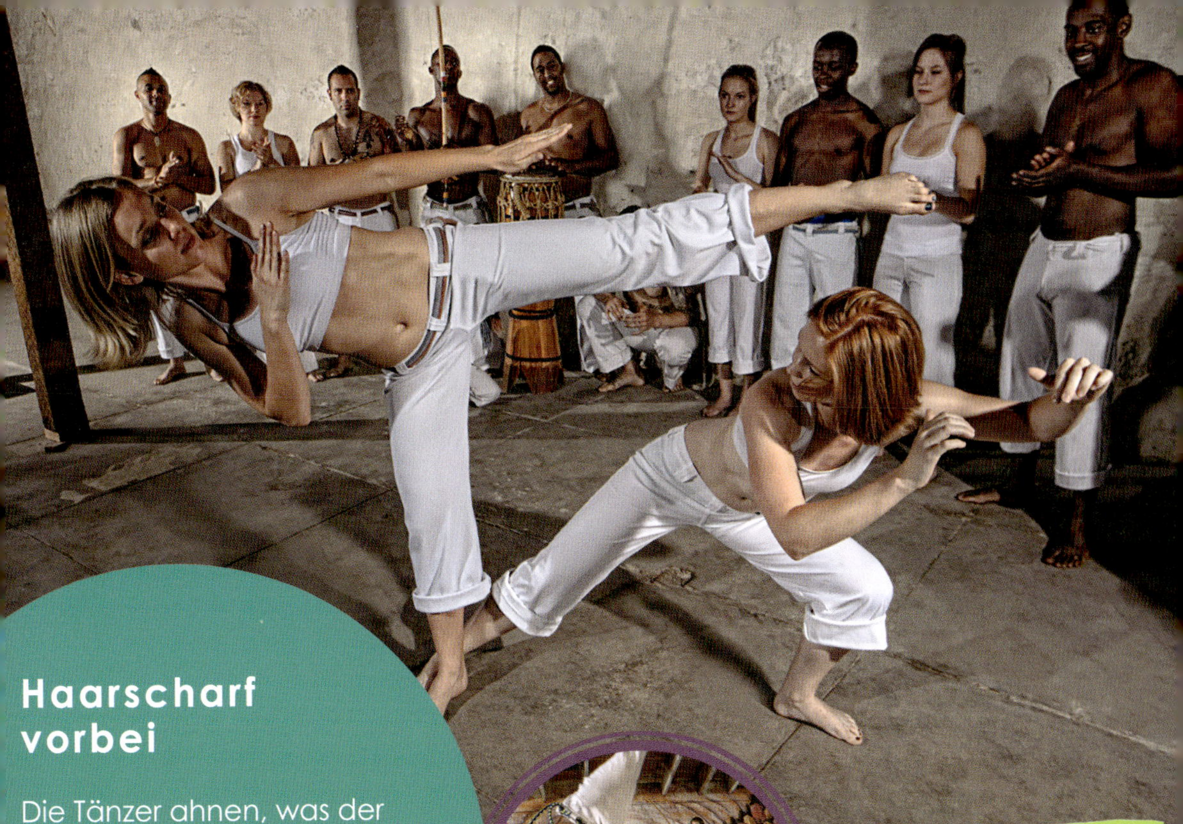

Haarscharf vorbei

Die Tänzer ahnen, was der andere als Nächstes tun wird. Blitzschnell reagieren sie und verwandeln mit ihrer Gegenbewegung den Kampf in Tanz.

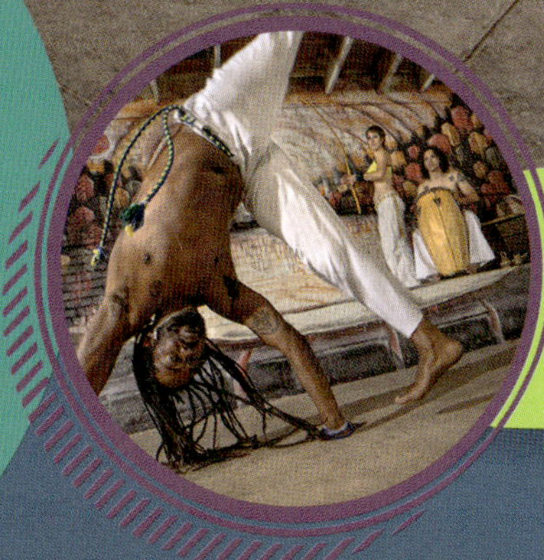

Mit einem **Radschlag** kann man angreifen und ausweichen.

Wenn man weiß, woher der Fuß kommt, kann man drunter **durchtauchen**.

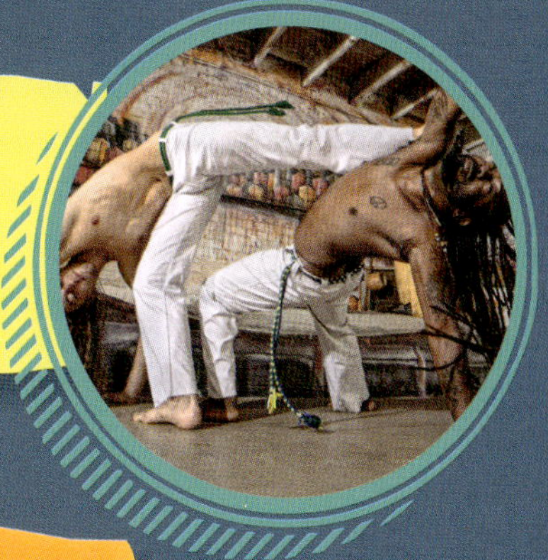

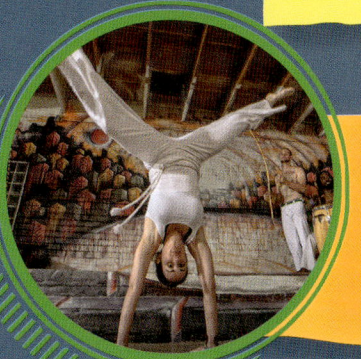

Auch mit einem **Handstand** nach hinten lässt sich gut einem Angriff entgehen.

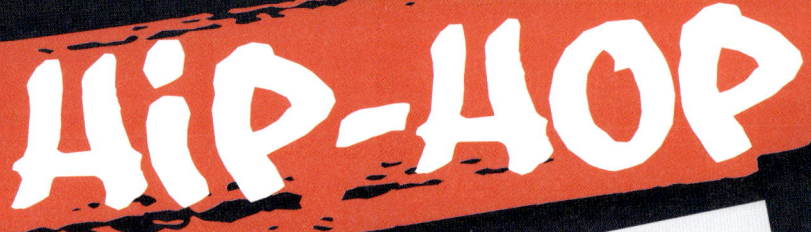

HiP-HOP

Hip-Hop ist nicht nur eine Musikrichtung.

Hip-Hop ist so viel mehr: Graffiti, Tanz, Rap, Basketball.

Hip-Hop ist eine Lebenseinstellung.

Los geht's auf die Straße

Ja, man kann heute in Tanzschulen Hip-Hop-Kurse machen. Das macht auch Sinn, denn die **Moves** sind nicht einfach. Damit es richtig cool aussieht, muss man viel trainieren. Trotzdem: Eigentlich lernt man das Tanzen auf der Straße von anderen Jugendlichen.

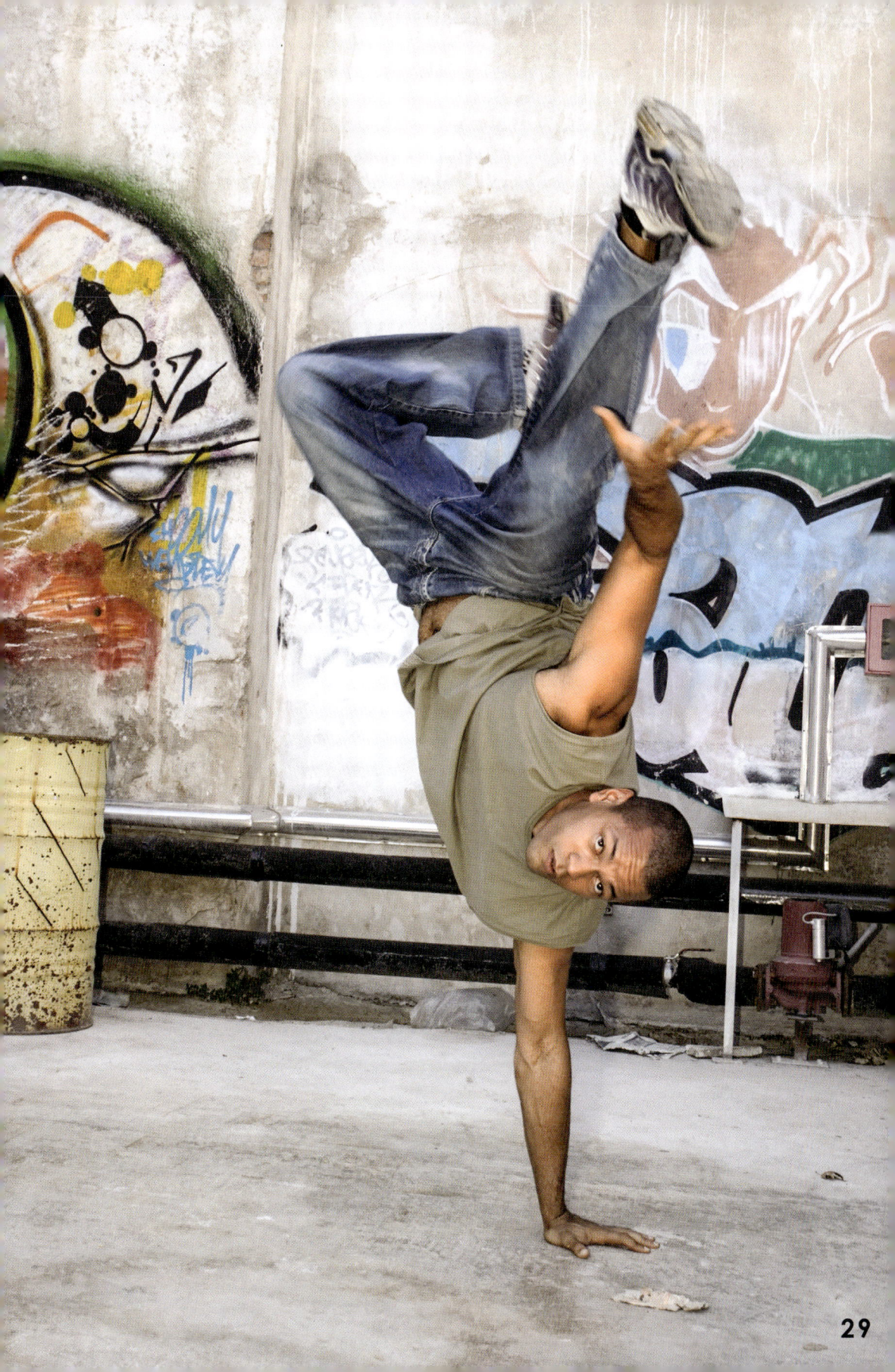

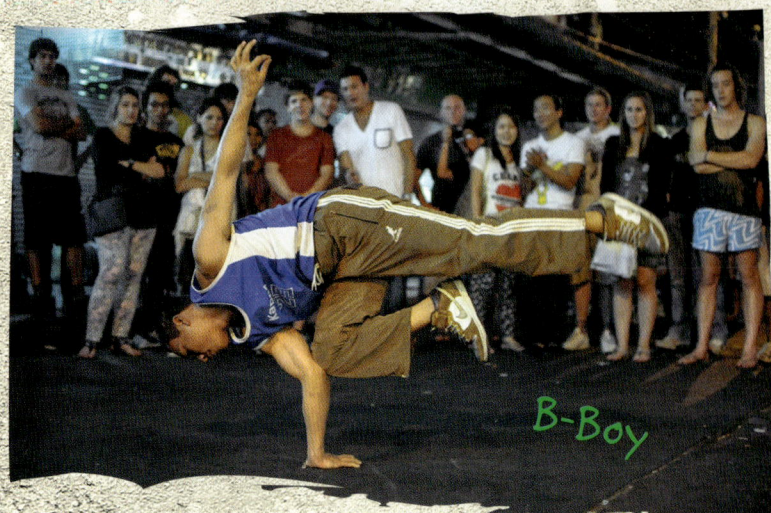

B-Boy

Zeig mir, was du kannst!

B-Boying entstand vor ungefähr 50 Jahren in den Armenvierteln von New York. Armut, keine Chance auf gute Schulen, Straßenbanden: Das Leben war gefährlich für viele Jugendliche.

Tanz-Battles

Sie kämpfen darum, wer der Beste ist. Aber sie benutzen keine Waffen. Sie treten mit Tänzen gegeneinander an. Drehungen auf dem Kopf, Tanz auf den Händen? Wer seinen Gegner beeindrucken will, muss viel draufhaben.

ENGLISCH FÜR B-BOYS UND B-GIRLS

Battle, sprich: Bättel, heißt wörtlich Kampf. Hier fliegen aber nur Arme und Beine, keine Fäuste.

B-Boys, sprich: Bibois
So nennen sie sich: die Jungs, die **breaken** (sprich: bräiken).
Hip-Hop war am Anfang Jungssache, heute gibt es auch geniale **B-Girls**.

Locking
Explosive Bewegung, für eine Sekunde einfrieren, dann die nächste Bewegung, eine Sekunde einfrieren und so weiter ...

Popping
Einzelne Muskeln werden bewegt, während der Rest des Körperteils ruhig bleibt.

Locking und Popping

Los Angeles, 50 Jahre vor unserer Zeit:
Die ersten Roboter kommen auf die Tanzfläche.
Nein, natürlich sind Locker und Popper echte
Menschen. Aber ihr Tanzstil ist von Robotern inspiriert.
Sie bewegen sich ruckartig und schaffen es,
ihre Muskeln einzeln zu bewegen. Dadurch sehen
die Tänzer fast wie ferngesteuert aus.

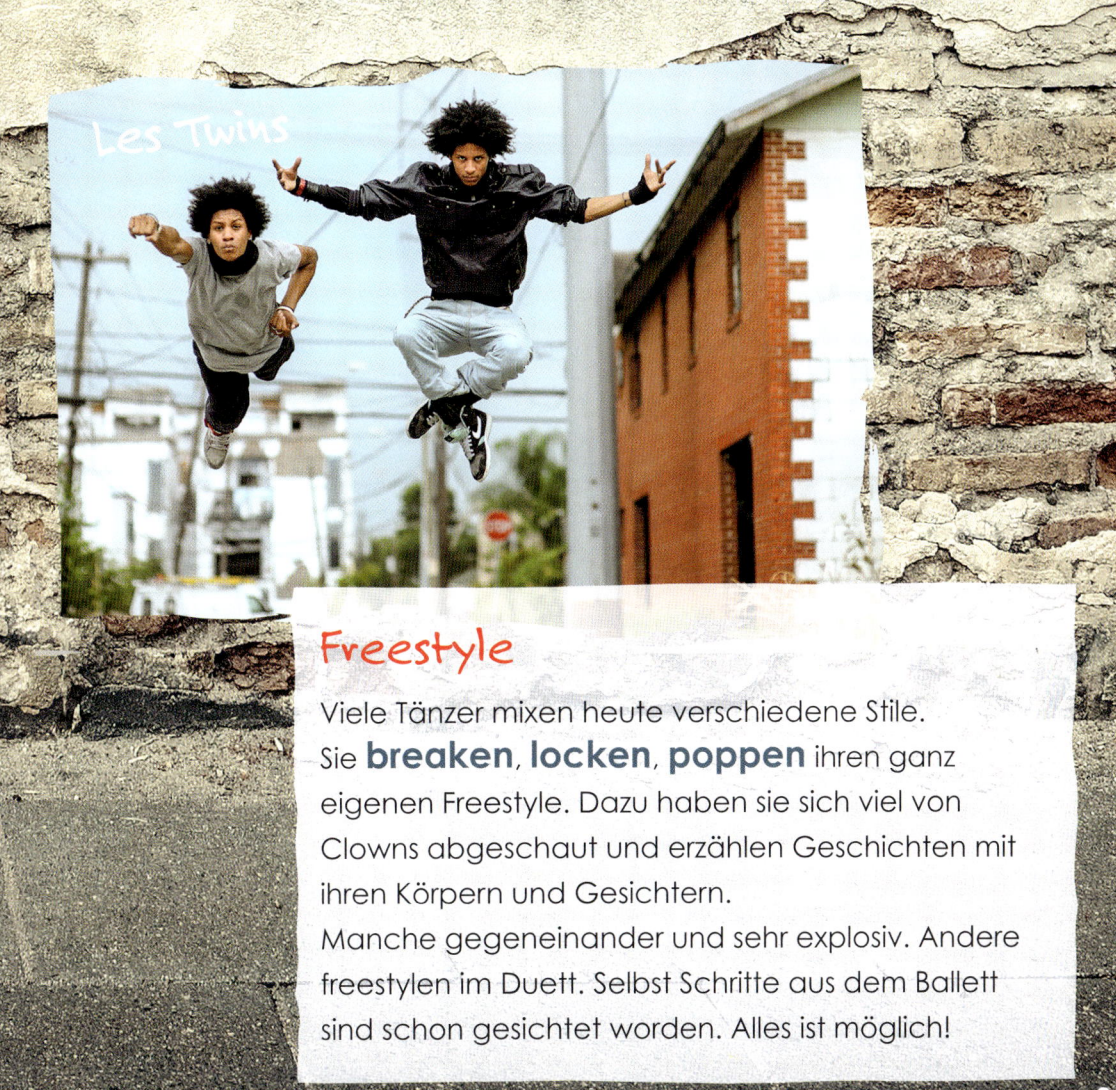

Les Twins

Freestyle

Viele Tänzer mixen heute verschiedene Stile.
Sie **breaken**, **locken**, **poppen** ihren ganz
eigenen Freestyle. Dazu haben sie sich viel von
Clowns abgeschaut und erzählen Geschichten mit
ihren Körpern und Gesichtern.
Manche gegeneinander und sehr explosiv. Andere
freestylen im Duett. Selbst Schritte aus dem Ballett
sind schon gesichtet worden. Alles ist möglich!

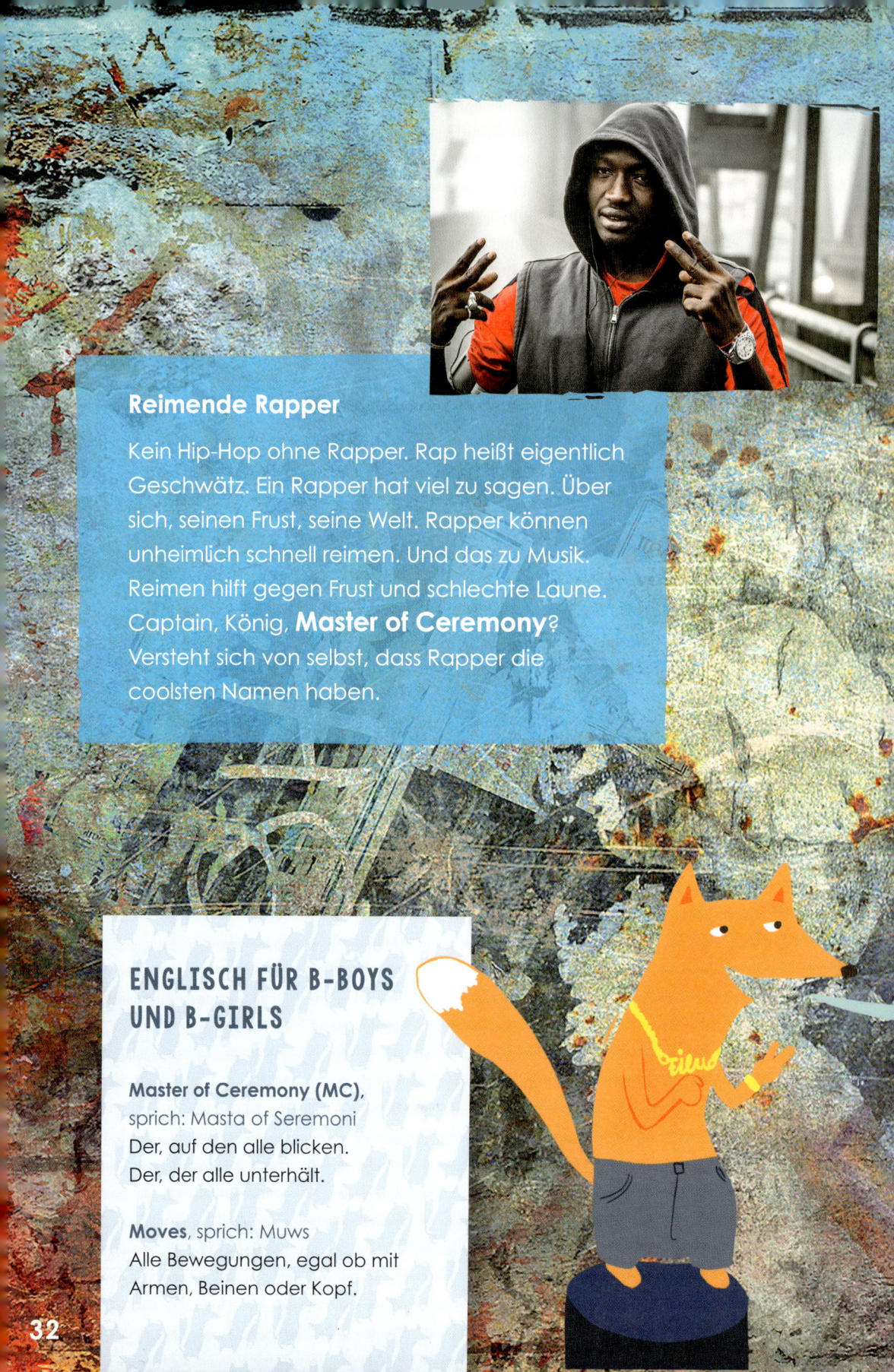

Reimende Rapper

Kein Hip-Hop ohne Rapper. Rap heißt eigentlich Geschwätz. Ein Rapper hat viel zu sagen. Über sich, seinen Frust, seine Welt. Rapper können unheimlich schnell reimen. Und das zu Musik. Reimen hilft gegen Frust und schlechte Laune. Captain, König, **Master of Ceremony**? Versteht sich von selbst, dass Rapper die coolsten Namen haben.

ENGLISCH FÜR B-BOYS UND B-GIRLS

Master of Ceremony (MC),
sprich: Masta of Seremoni
Der, auf den alle blicken.
Der, der alle unterhält.

Moves, sprich: Muws
Alle Bewegungen, egal ob mit
Armen, Beinen oder Kopf.

MACH DIR DEINEN EIGENEN REIM!

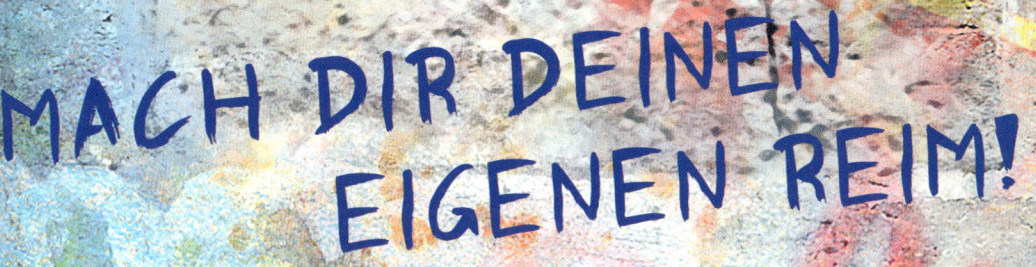

Bin kein Luchs, bin Fuchs.
Heiße nicht Balu. Hier spricht MC Filu!
Bin so schlau, hab immer eine Frage,
forsche, suche, messe, zähle, sage.

Will es wissen, ziehe durch die Welt,
bleibe nur dort, wo es mir gefällt.
Hab schon Pferde und Drachen besucht,
Könige, Ritter und Flieger gesucht.

Beschwere mich mit keinem Mucks,
bin der krasse Abenteuerfuchs.
Nenn mich einfach MC Filu.
Das bin ich und wer bist du?

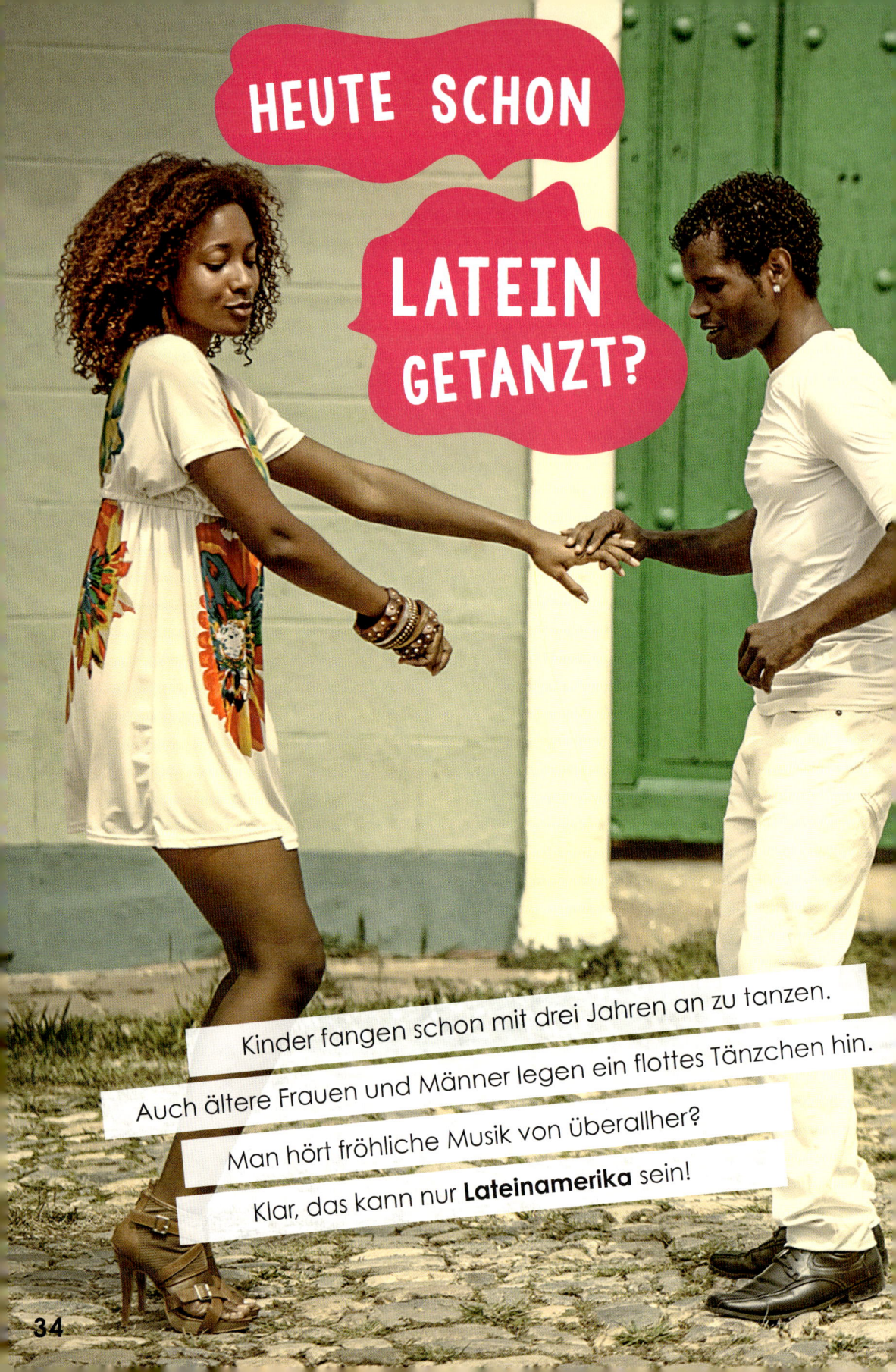

HEUTE SCHON

LATEIN GETANZT?

Kinder fangen schon mit drei Jahren an zu tanzen.

Auch ältere Frauen und Männer legen ein flottes Tänzchen hin.

Man hört fröhliche Musik von überallher?

Klar, das kann nur **Lateinamerika** sein!

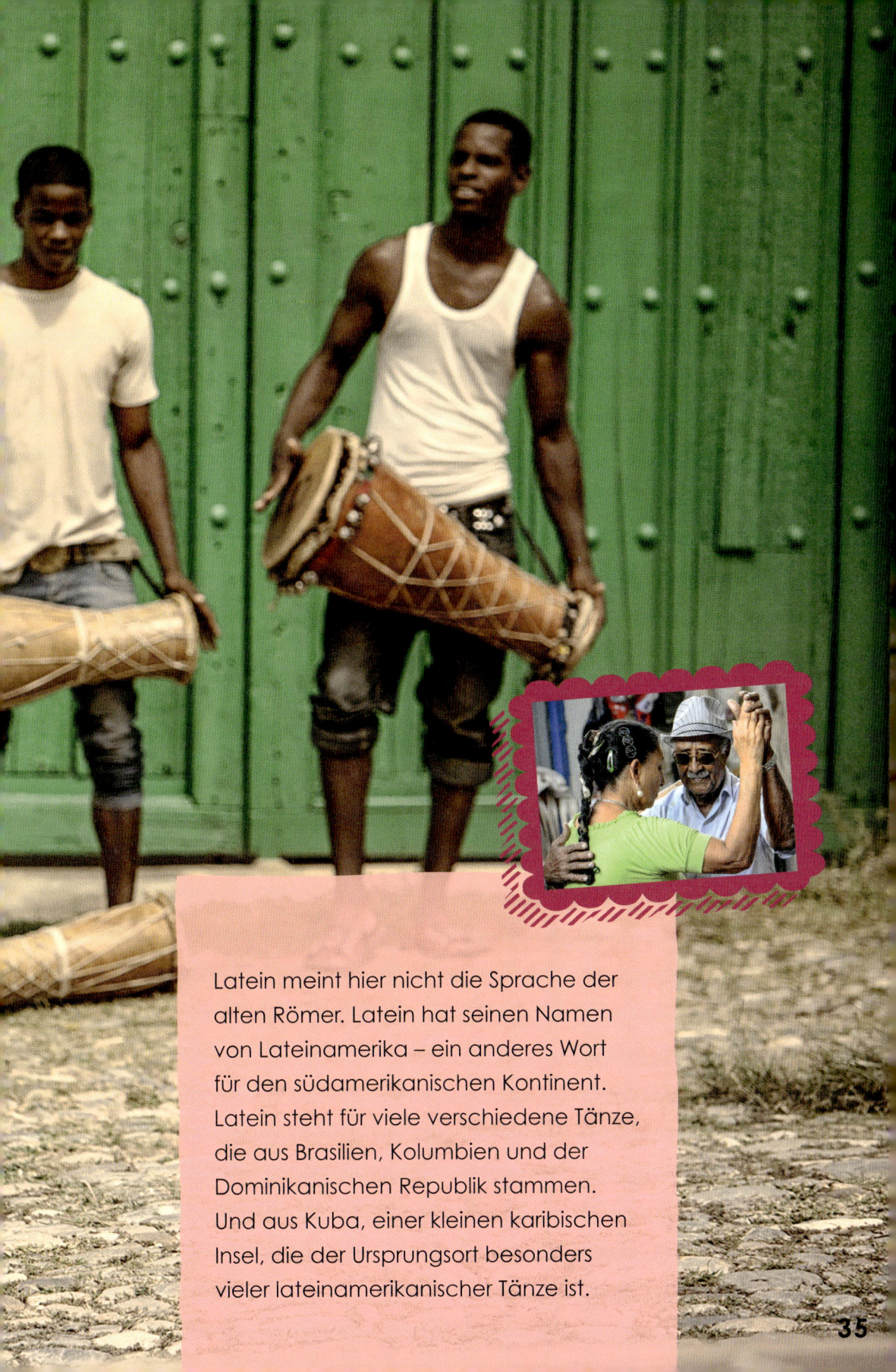

Latein meint hier nicht die Sprache der alten Römer. Latein hat seinen Namen von Lateinamerika – ein anderes Wort für den südamerikanischen Kontinent. Latein steht für viele verschiedene Tänze, die aus Brasilien, Kolumbien und der Dominikanischen Republik stammen. Und aus Kuba, einer kleinen karibischen Insel, die der Ursprungsort besonders vieler lateinamerikanischer Tänze ist.

Das lateinische **ABC**

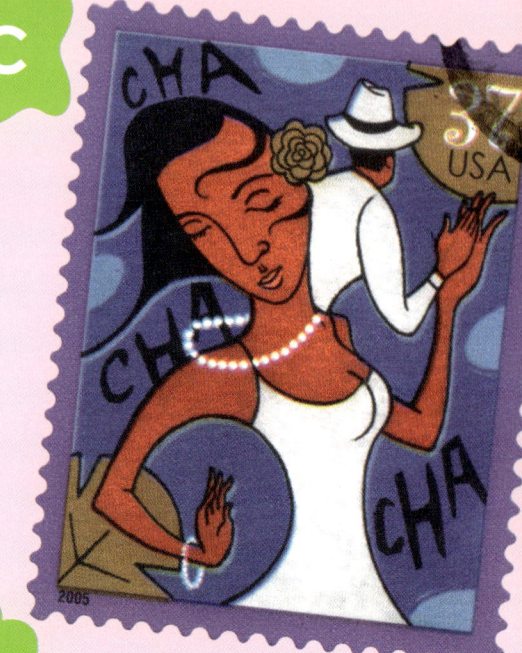

hat viele Buchstaben. Für viele Tänze. Und es entstehen immer wieder neue. Klassische Tänze werden von anderen Tanzstilen und Musikrichtungen beeinflusst.

LATEIN FÜR SCHNELLE TÄNZER

C umbia: kam mit den afrikanischen Sklaven nach Kolumbien. Mischte sich mit indianischen und spanischen Elementen. Heute beliebter Paartanz.

M ambo: Vorläufer des Cha-Cha-Cha. Oberkörper und Hüfte haben viel zu tun.

M erengue: sehr fröhlicher Tanz aus der Dominikanischen Republik, guter Einsteigertanz.

Z umba: die Fitnessvariante der lateinamerikanischen Tänze. Aerobic trifft Salsa, trifft Mambo, trifft Merengue.

C wie

Cha-Cha-Cha
sprich: Tscha-tscha-tscha

Cha-Cha-Cha hat seinen Namen vom Wechselschritt. Man zählt die Schritte: Schritt-Schritt-Cha-Cha-Cha.
Cha-Cha-Cha ist ein verspielter Paartanz. Man tanzt aufeinander zu, lächelt und dreht sich genauso schnell wieder weg.

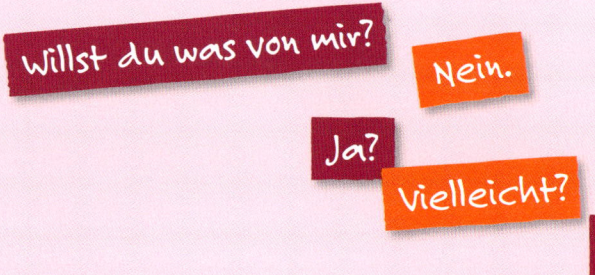

Willst du was von mir?

Nein.

Ja?

Vielleicht?

Ja?

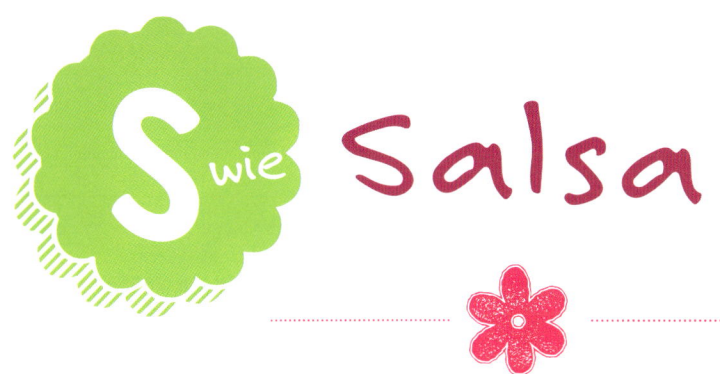

S wie Salsa

Salsa ist in Kuba und in Puerto Rico zu Hause und auf der ganzen Welt sehr beliebt.

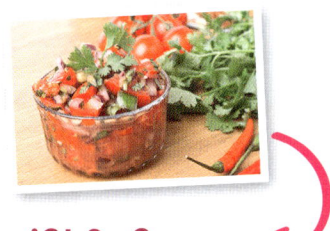

Salsa heißt Soße

In diese Soße sind verschiedene Traditionen eingerührt. Und es gibt diese Soße in ganz verschiedenen Geschmacksrichtungen.

Salsa ist weit gereist

Als erste Zutat kam der europäische Kontratanz des 17. Jahrhunderts. Dann ging es in die Karibik und nach Kuba. Spanische Gitarrenklänge mischten sich mit afrikanischen Trommelrhythmen.

Salsa ist schnell

Salsa ist ein schneller Paartanz voller Drehungen. Die Jungs halten die Mädels an einer Hand. Und die Mädels wirbeln um sie herum. Mal ganz nah und dann schnell wieder weg.

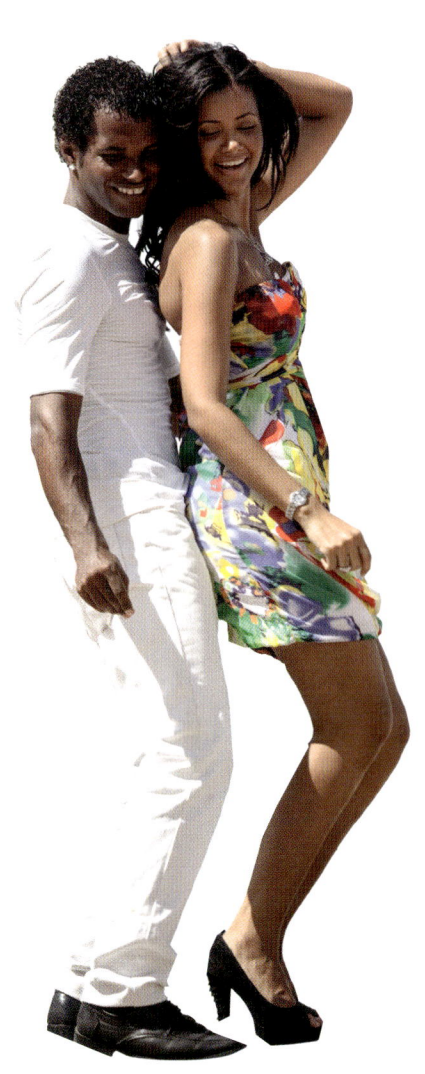

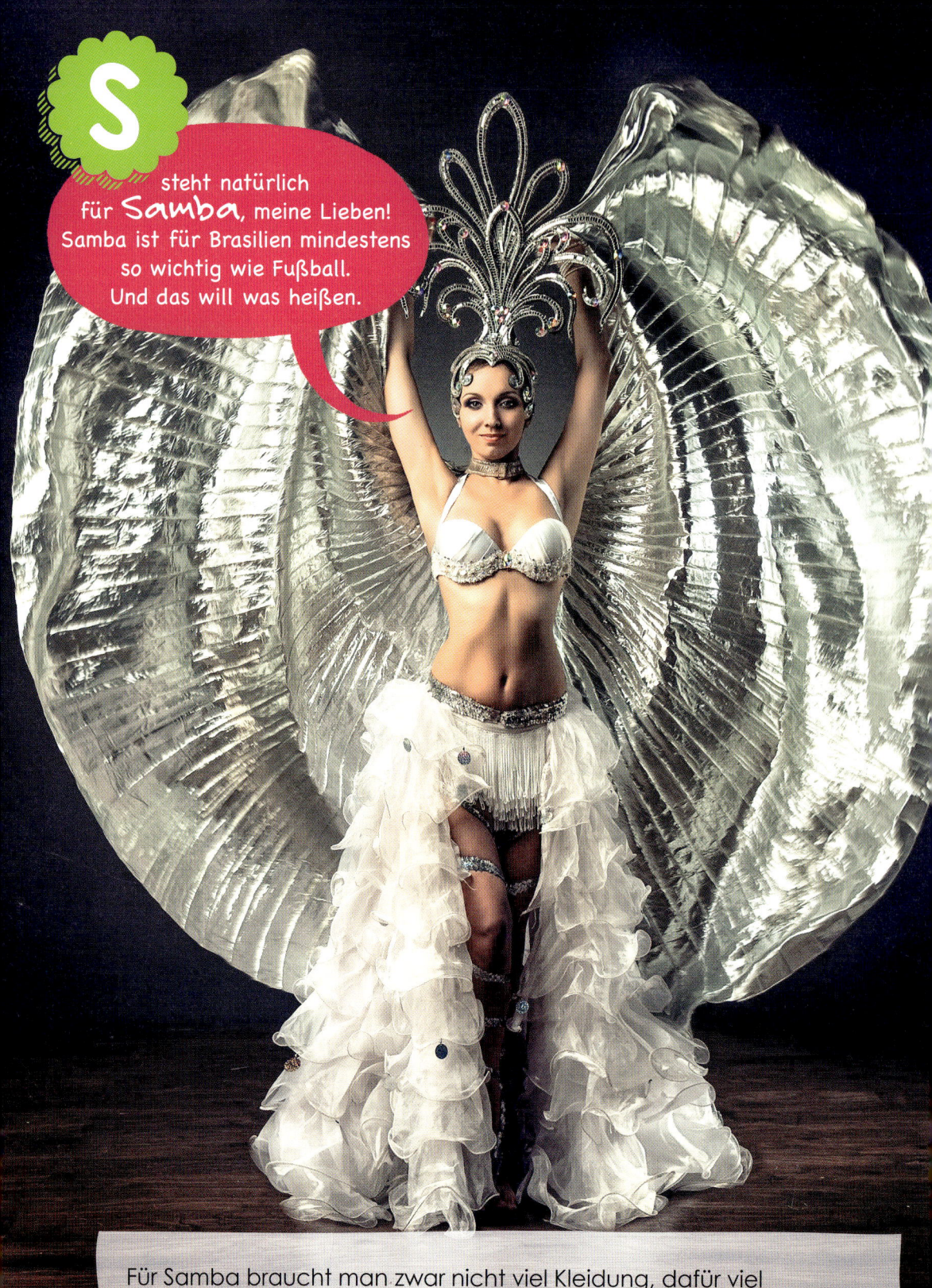

S steht natürlich für **Samba**, meine Lieben! Samba ist für Brasilien mindestens so wichtig wie Fußball. Und das will was heißen.

Für Samba braucht man zwar nicht viel Kleidung, dafür viel **Verkleidung**. Beim Karneval, wenn die verschiedenen Samba-schulen um die Wette tanzen, muss man schließlich gut aussehen.

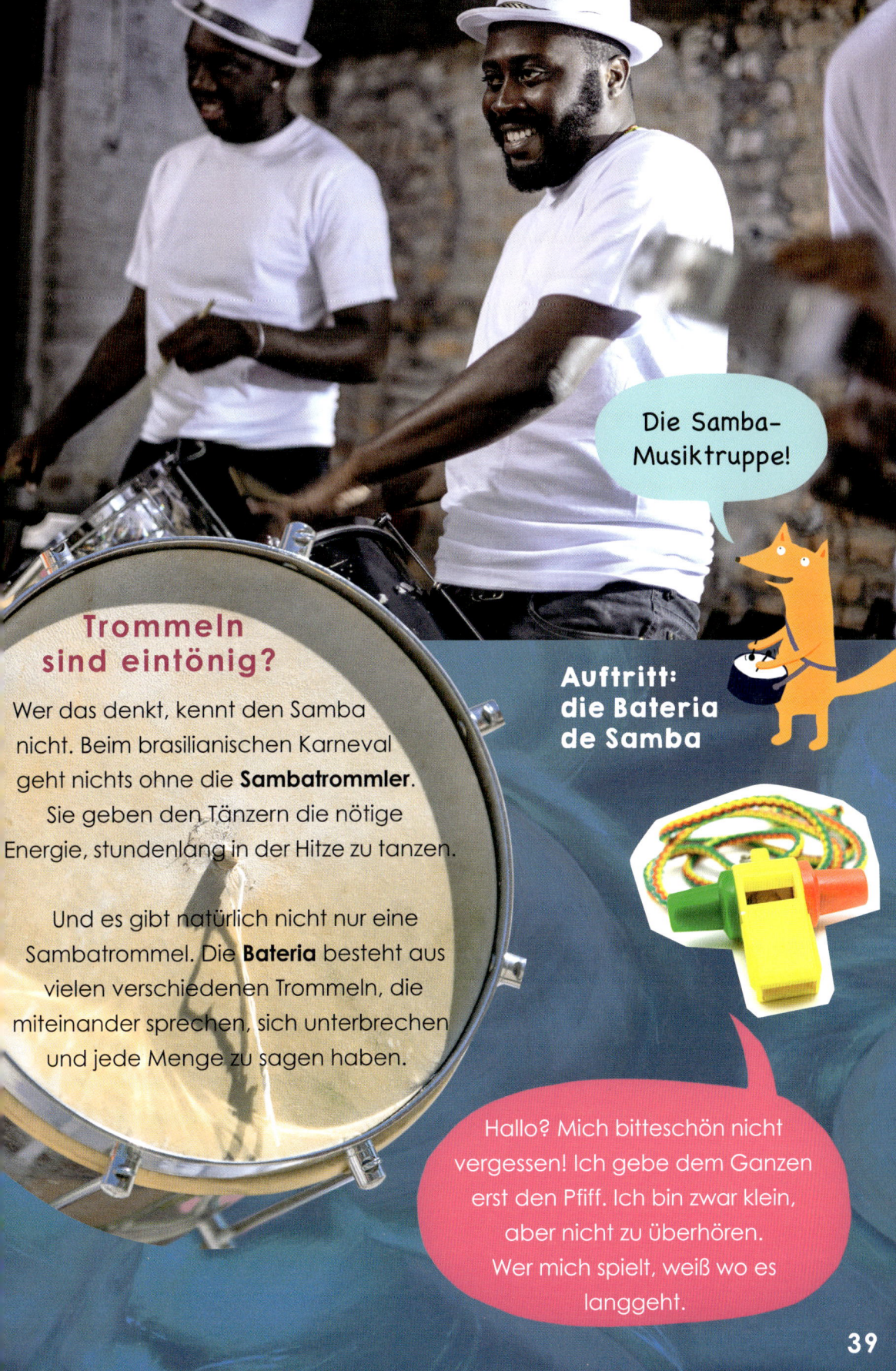

Die Samba-Musiktruppe!

Trommeln sind eintönig?

Wer das denkt, kennt den Samba nicht. Beim brasilianischen Karneval geht nichts ohne die **Sambatrommler**. Sie geben den Tänzern die nötige Energie, stundenlang in der Hitze zu tanzen.

Und es gibt natürlich nicht nur eine Sambatrommel. Die **Bateria** besteht aus vielen verschiedenen Trommeln, die miteinander sprechen, sich unterbrechen und jede Menge zu sagen haben.

Auftritt: die Bateria de Samba

Hallo? Mich bitteschön nicht vergessen! Ich gebe dem Ganzen erst den Pfiff. Ich bin zwar klein, aber nicht zu überhören. Wer mich spielt, weiß wo es langgeht.

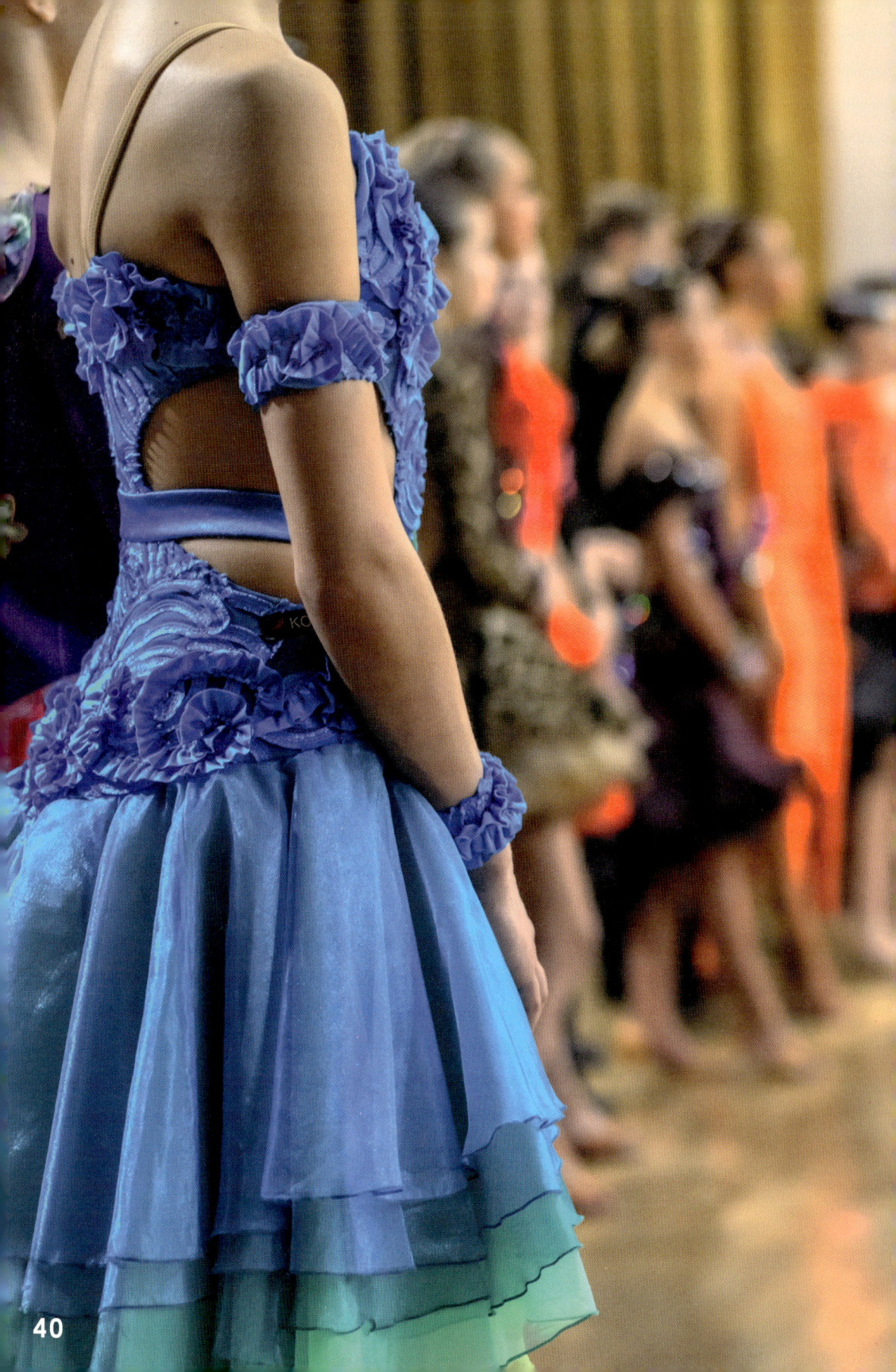

ZEHNKAMPF

Zehn Tänze

Ist Tanzen Sport? Na klar.
Im Turniersport gibt es viele Wettbewerbe.
Und klar festgelegte Regeln.
Getanzt wird in zwei verschiedenen Sektionen:
Standard und Latein. Also zweimal fünf Tänze.

Beim Wettbewerb

Acht oder sogar mehr Tanzpaare erscheinen
gleichzeitig auf der Tanzfläche. Jedes Paar will den
besten Tanz hinlegen und sich im besten Licht zeigen.
Da wird auch schon mal geschubst und versucht,
die anderen wegzudrängen. Jeder der fünf Tänze
einer Sektion dauert ungefähr zwei Minuten. Alle
fünf Tänze werden hintereinanderweg getanzt. Bei
manchen Wettbewerben sogar alle zehn.

DIE ZEHN TURNIERTÄNZE

Der erste Tanz: **Langsamer Walzer.**
Harmonisch und elegant soll er
aussehen. Dafür kommt es auf den
richtigen Schwung an.

Der **internationale Tango!**
Immer im Wechsel: Mal ganz schnelle
Bewegungen, dann wieder langsam
und zärtlich. Und alles Beinarbeit.

Standard

geschlossene Tänze
immer an der Hand

Wiener Walzer: kommt aus Wien.
Ja, klar. Er ist doppelt so schnell wie der
langsame Walzer und hat es ganz schön
in sich. Vorsicht, Drehwurmgefahr!

Slowfox ist englisch und heißt
langsamer Fuchs. Es ist ein ruhiger Tanz.
Mit eleganten Drehungen schweben
die Paare durch den Raum.

Beim **Quickstep** rennen-schweben die
Paare ganz schnell über die Tanzfläche.
Achtung! Nicht ins Publikum reinsausen!

Samba: Hier wird's wild. Auch die Männer müssen tolle Hüftschwünge draufhaben.

Beim **Rumba** zeigt man sich romantisch. Mal nah, mal weit voneinander weg.

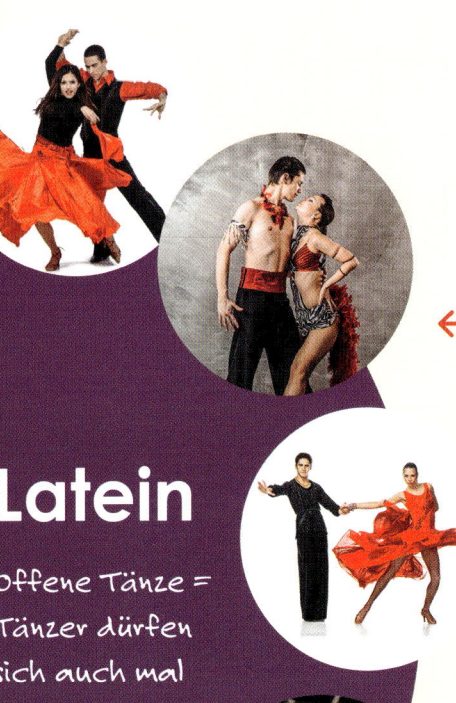

Latein

Offene Tänze =
Tänzer dürfen
sich auch mal
rennen

2-3-spiel-mit-mir. **Cha-Cha-Cha** macht einfach Spaß.
Man überrascht das Publikum mit unerwarteten Bewegungen.

Paso Doble = der mit dem Stier tanzt.
Hier ist der Mann der Torero
und die Dame das rote Tuch. Es wird stürmisch gekämpft. Gekämpft? Getanzt!

Name: **Jive**, sprich mich: Dschaif.
Der letzte der Latein-Tänze. Außerdem der schnellste und der anstrengendste.
Gesprungen, gekickt, gedreht – alles zu Musik, die noch mal extrawach macht.

Internationale Meisterschaften Rollstuhltanz

Sie zähmen den Stier beim Paso Doble aus dem Rollstuhl heraus.
Sie legen einen schwungvollen Jive aufs Parkett
und schwingen die Räder beim romantischen Rumba.

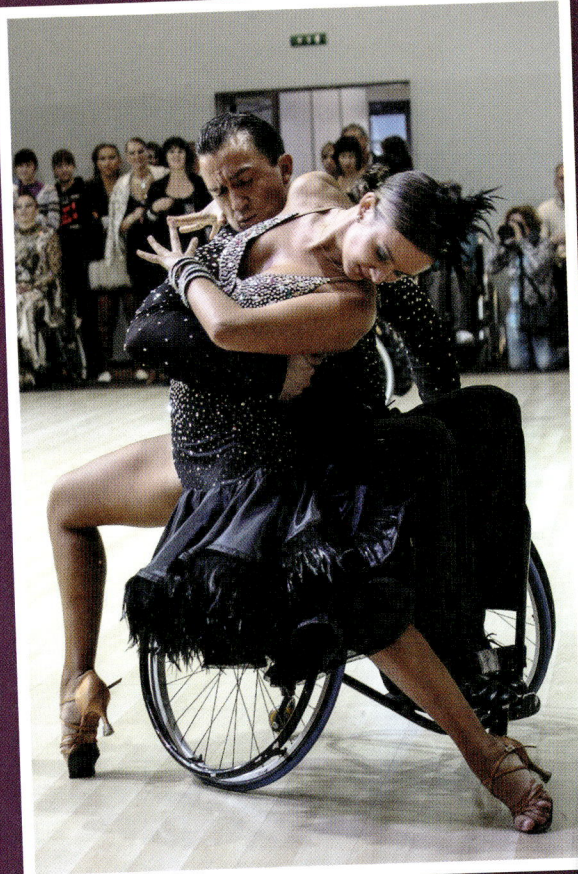

Unglaublich, was man mit einem Rollstuhl alles machen kann! Tanzen, um sich herauszufordern und Spaß zu haben: Rollstuhltanz ist eine atemberaubende Show.

Alle zwei Jahre finden im Wechsel die Europa- und Weltmeisterschaften der Rollstuhl-Tänzer statt. Es gibt die Sektionen Standard, Latein und Freestyle.

Maksim und Svetlana
tanzen Latein

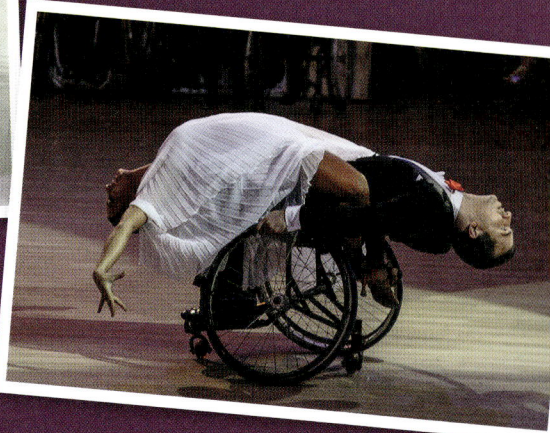

NIEMALS AUFGEBEN

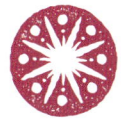

MAKSIM UND SVETLANA:
DIE EUROPAMEISTER IN DER SEKTION FREESTYLE

Schule Nr. 616

Maksim Sedakov ist Sportlehrer.
Er arbeitet an einer Schule für
Kinder mit Behinderungen in
Sankt Petersburg in Russland.
Zusammen mit seiner Partnerin,
Svetlana Kukushkina.

Beim Turnier

Maksim und Svetlana sind
außerdem eines der weltbesten
Paare in den Sektionen Latein
und Freestyle.

Alles geht!

Bei einem Unfall verlor Maksim
ein Bein. Das hielt ihn nicht davon
ab, tanzen zu lernen. Sein Motto:
Niemals aufgeben. Mit dieser
Einstellung schafft er Unmögliches:
Breakdancing inklusive Kopfstand
im Rollstuhl.

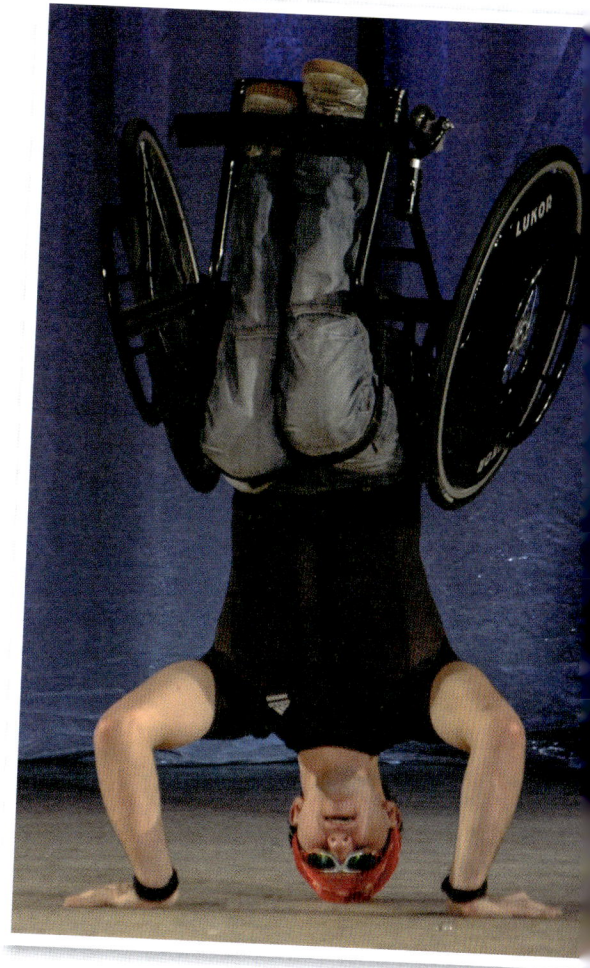

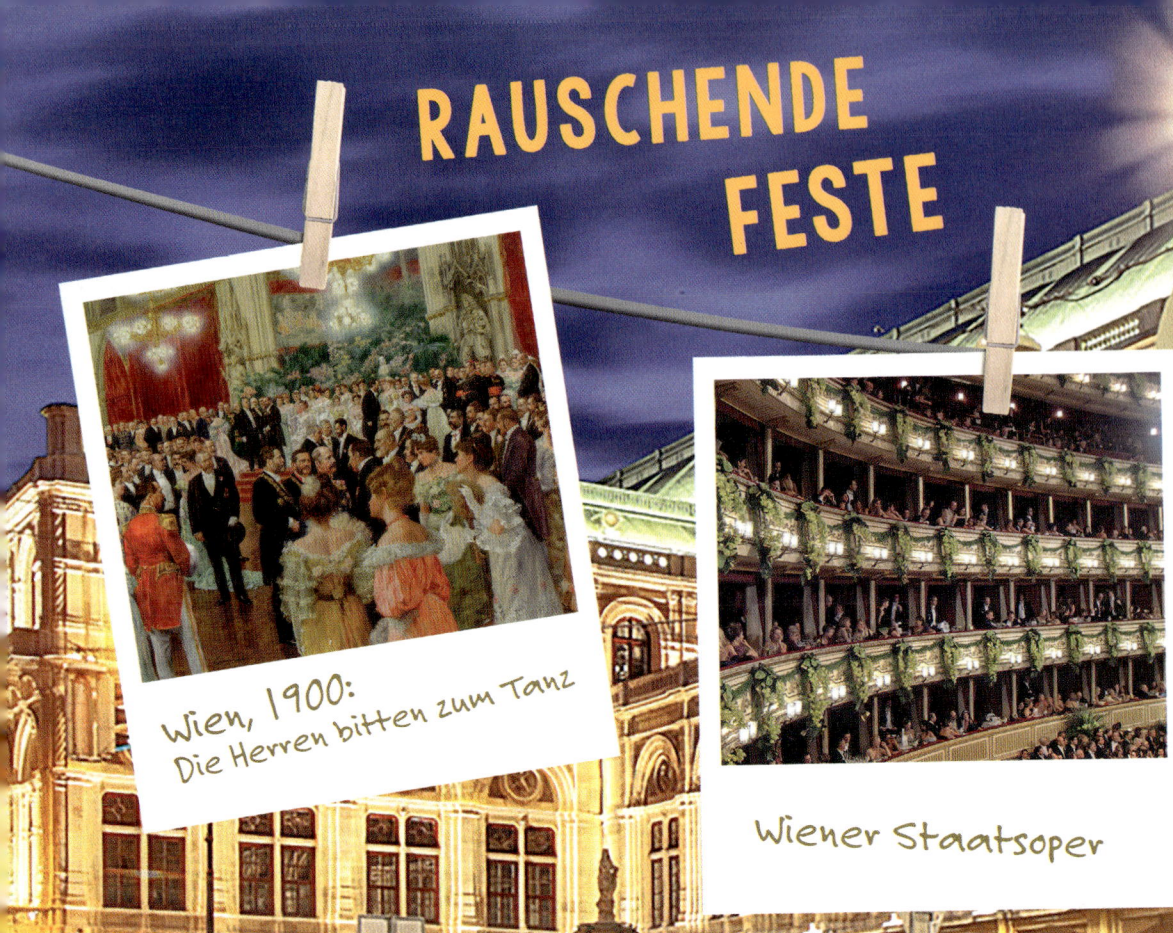

RAUSCHENDE FESTE

Wien, 1900:
Die Herren bitten zum Tanz

Wiener Staatsoper

WIENER OPERNBALL

Eines der berühmtesten Tanzfeste ist der Wiener Opernball. Bereits vor fast 200 Jahren fanden die ersten Bälle in Wien statt. Bis heute ist der Wiener Opernball ein spektakuläres Ereignis. Besucher aus der ganzen Welt kommen im Februar nach Österreich, um beim Opernball dabei zu sein.

Schnelle Verwandlung

Einmal im Jahr wird die Wiener Staatsoper kurzerhand umgebaut und in einen riesigen Ballsaal verwandelt. Allein die Tanzfläche beträgt 850 Quadratmeter. Das ist gut so, denn jedes Jahr werden bis zu 12.000 Besucher erwartet. Zuerst zieht der Bundespräsident in seine Loge. Dann erklingt die Europahymne: **Freude, schöner Götterfunken**.

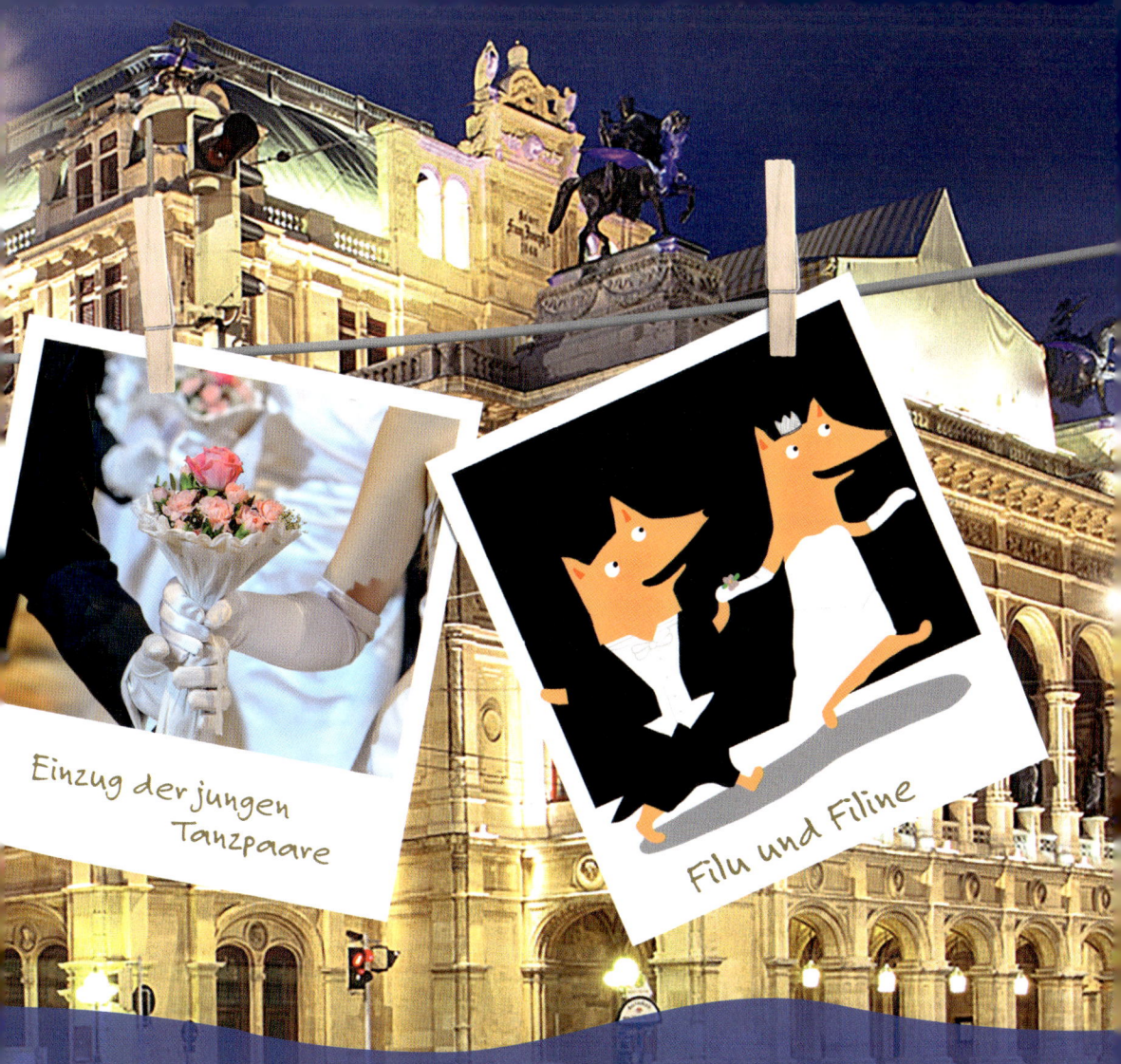

Einzug der jungen Tanzpaare

Filu und Filine

Das Jungdamen- und Jungherrenkomitee

Und dann kommen sie:
Einzug der ungefähr 180 jungen
Tanzpaare, auch das Jungdamen-
und Jungherrenkomitee genannt.
Die Mädchen tragen weiße
Ballkleider, die Jungen schwarze
Fräcke.

Alles Walzer

Die Tänzer und Tänzerinnen sind
alle zwischen 17 und 24 Jahren alt.
Sie müssen den Linkswalzer perfekt
beherrschen und tanzen Monate
vorher vor. Denn jeder darf in
seinem Leben nur ein einziges Mal
den Wiener Opernball eröffnen.
Mit den Worten „Alles Walzer"
laden sie die Gäste auf die
Tanzfläche ein. Und dann wird
gefeiert bis morgens früh um fünf.

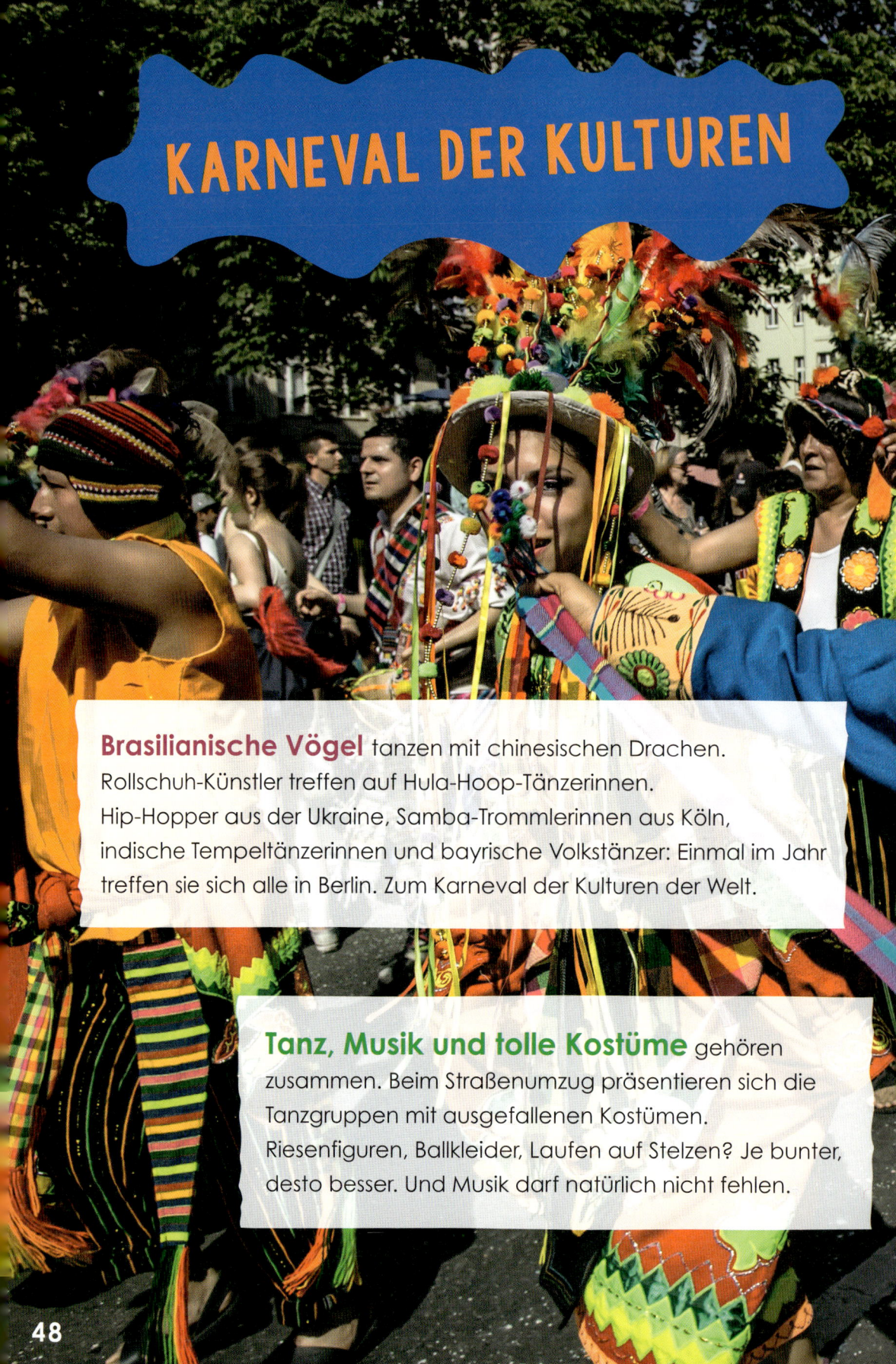

KARNEVAL DER KULTUREN

Brasilianische Vögel tanzen mit chinesischen Drachen. Rollschuh-Künstler treffen auf Hula-Hoop-Tänzerinnen. Hip-Hopper aus der Ukraine, Samba-Trommlerinnen aus Köln, indische Tempeltänzerinnen und bayrische Volkstänzer: Einmal im Jahr treffen sie sich alle in Berlin. Zum Karneval der Kulturen der Welt.

Tanz, Musik und tolle Kostüme gehören zusammen. Beim Straßenumzug präsentieren sich die Tanzgruppen mit ausgefallenen Kostümen. Riesenfiguren, Ballkleider, Laufen auf Stelzen? Je bunter, desto besser. Und Musik darf natürlich nicht fehlen.

48

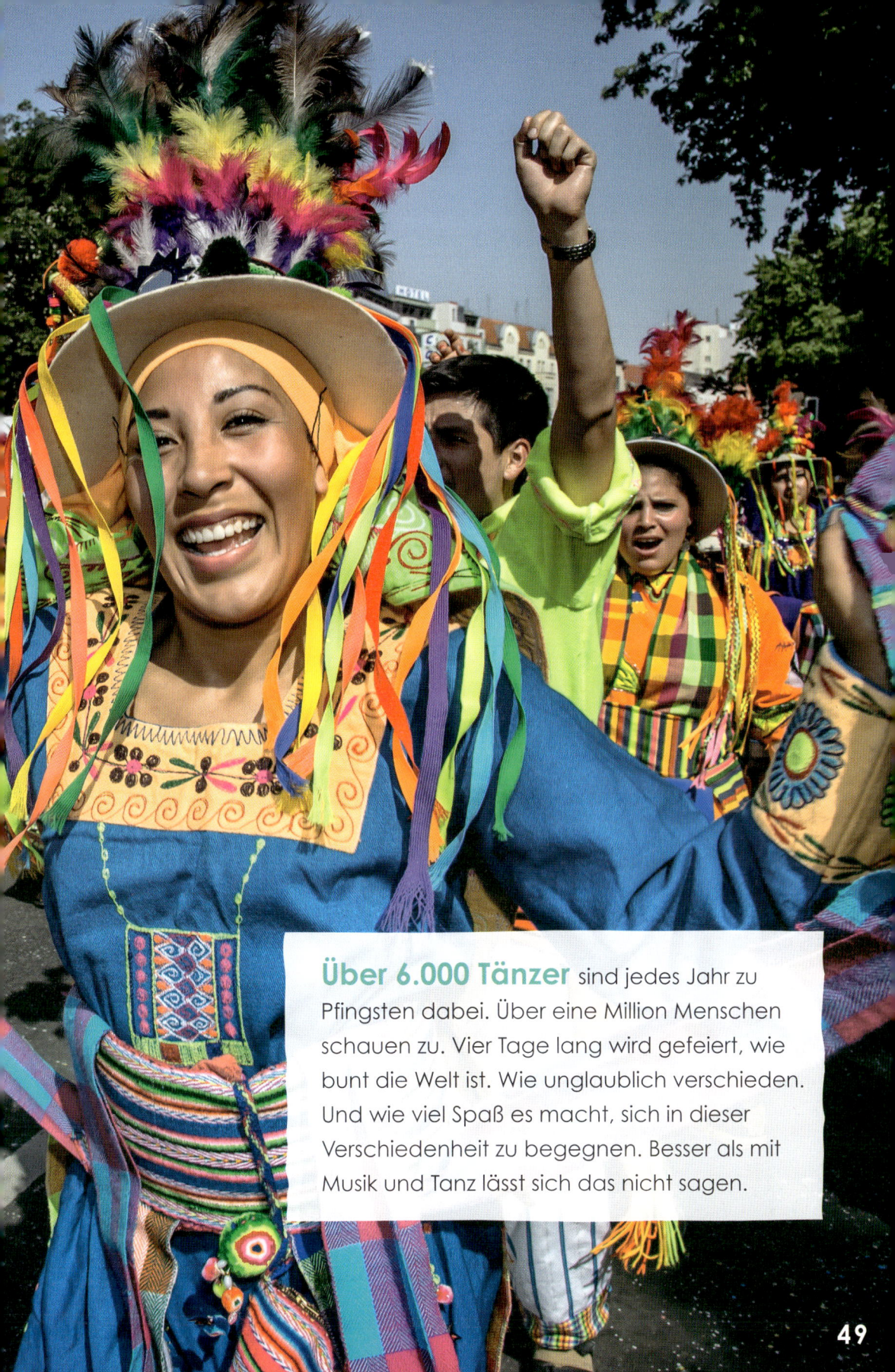

Über 6.000 Tänzer sind jedes Jahr zu Pfingsten dabei. Über eine Million Menschen schauen zu. Vier Tage lang wird gefeiert, wie bunt die Welt ist. Wie unglaublich verschieden. Und wie viel Spaß es macht, sich in dieser Verschiedenheit zu begegnen. Besser als mit Musik und Tanz lässt sich das nicht sagen.

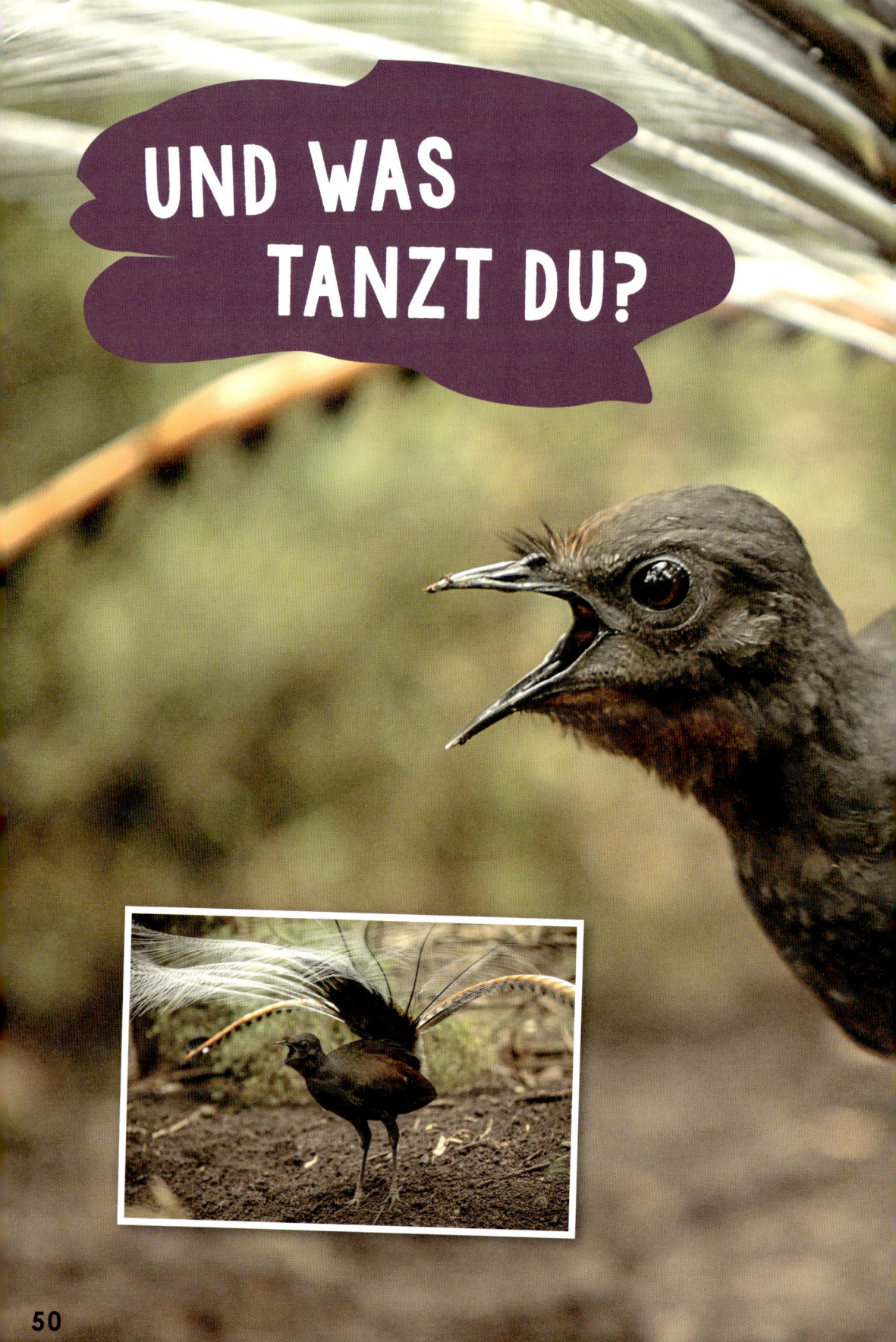

UND WAS TANZT DU?

Interview mit einem Meistertänzer

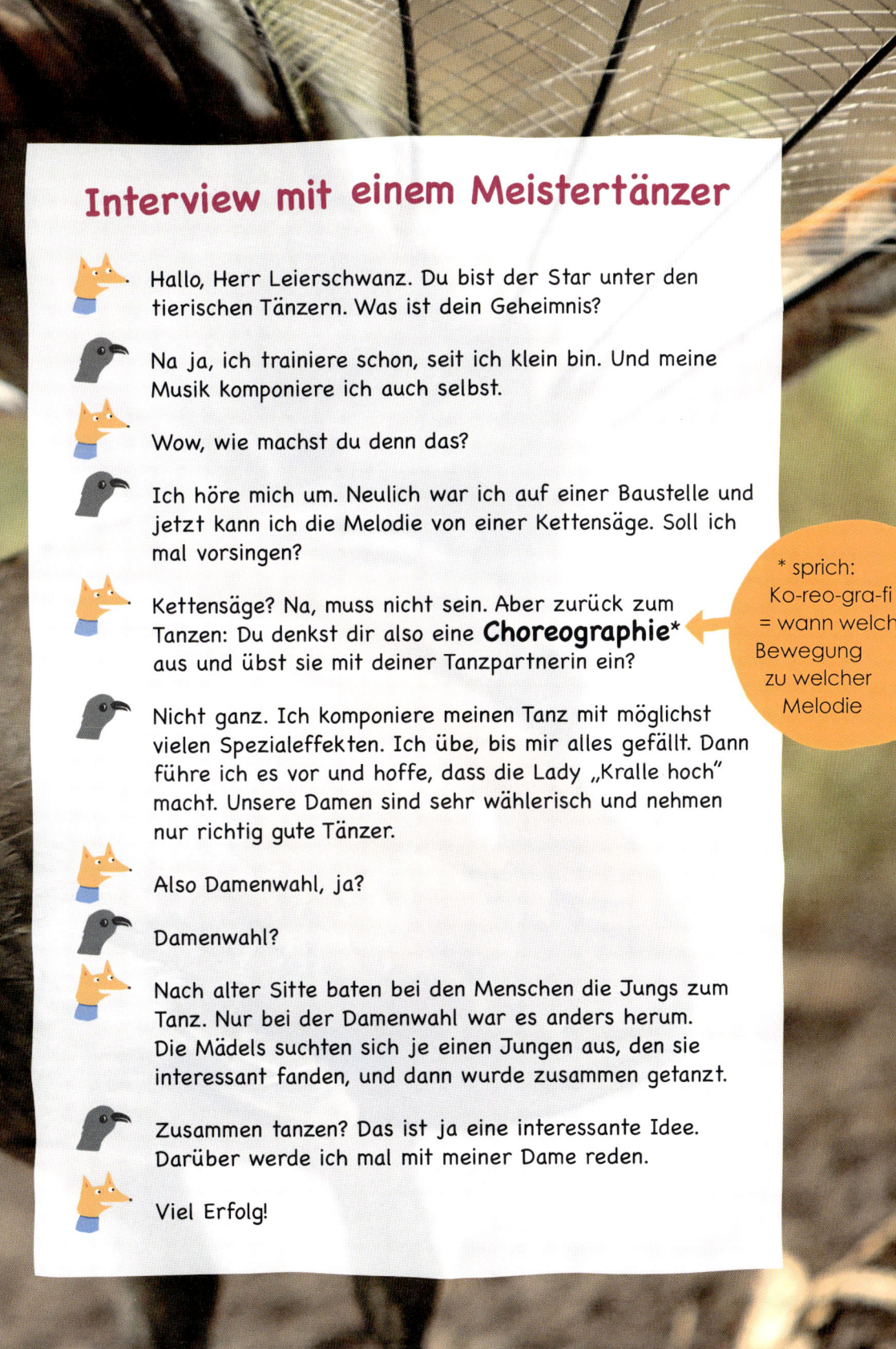

Hallo, Herr Leierschwanz. Du bist der Star unter den tierischen Tänzern. Was ist dein Geheimnis?

Na ja, ich trainiere schon, seit ich klein bin. Und meine Musik komponiere ich auch selbst.

Wow, wie machst du denn das?

Ich höre mich um. Neulich war ich auf einer Baustelle und jetzt kann ich die Melodie von einer Kettensäge. Soll ich mal vorsingen?

Kettensäge? Na, muss nicht sein. Aber zurück zum Tanzen: Du denkst dir also eine **Choreographie*** aus und übst sie mit deiner Tanzpartnerin ein?

* sprich:
Ko-reo-gra-fi
= wann welche
Bewegung
zu welcher
Melodie

Nicht ganz. Ich komponiere meinen Tanz mit möglichst vielen Spezialeffekten. Ich übe, bis mir alles gefällt. Dann führe ich es vor und hoffe, dass die Lady „Kralle hoch" macht. Unsere Damen sind sehr wählerisch und nehmen nur richtig gute Tänzer.

Also Damenwahl, ja?

Damenwahl?

Nach alter Sitte baten bei den Menschen die Jungs zum Tanz. Nur bei der Damenwahl war es anders herum. Die Mädels suchten sich je einen Jungen aus, den sie interessant fanden, und dann wurde zusammen getanzt.

Zusammen tanzen? Das ist ja eine interessante Idee. Darüber werde ich mal mit meiner Dame reden.

Viel Erfolg!

51

Party!

> Tanzen muss nicht immer so eine komplizierte Angelegenheit sein wie bei Herrn Leierschwanz. Es kann auch einfach Spaß machen.

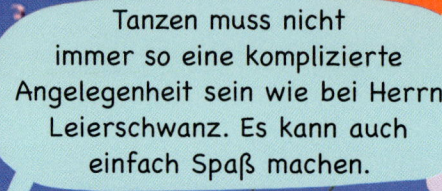

Der Zeitungstanz

Spielbar: Wo immer es Zeitungen gibt.

Teilnehmer: Tänzer mit Kindergeburtstags-erfahrung, 1 DJ

So geht's: Bei 10 Tänzern liegen maximal 8 Zeitungen auf dem Boden. DJ legt los und spielt Musik. Tänzer tanzen.

Höhepunkt: DJ lässt sich nicht anmerken, wann er die Musik anhält. Plötzlich ist sie aus und die Tänzer müssen sich Platz auf einer Zeitung suchen.

2. Akt: Eine Zeitung weniger. Und weiter geht's mit Musik und Tanz. Dann wieder Schluss und Zeitungssuche. Egal ob allein, zu zweit oder dritt: Hauptsache man steht auf der Zeitung. Wer nicht drauf ist, ist raus.

3., 4., 5. Akt: Siehe 2. Akt

Ende: Wenn alle vor Lachen von der Zeitung fallen.

Der Ballontanz

Anlass: Geburtstag, Party, wann immer man Spaß haben will.

Zutaten: Aufgeblasene Luftballons, nicht aufgeblasene Paar-Tänzer, 1 DJ

Ablauf: Hände auf den Rücken!
Ballon zwischen die Tänzer.
Musik ab und tanzen.
Hände bleiben auf dem Rücken!

Aus: Ballon auf dem Boden? Aus für den Ballon.
Aus für das Tanzpaar. – Bis zur nächsten Runde.

Tanz im Reifen

Benötigt werden: Hula-Hoop-Reifen, Tänzer, 1 DJ

Vorbereitung: Je zwei Tänzer in einem Hula-Hoop-Reifen.

Hände können benutzt werden: zum Klatschen,
zum in die Höhe strecken,
zum Umarmen,
NICHT zum am Reifen festhalten!

Los geht's: Und tanzen!
Gemeine DJs stellen auch mal Extra-Aufgaben wie zum Beispiel: Augen zumachen oder mit beiden Händen schnipsen.

Und raus: Fällt der Reifen zu Boden, kann man sich kurz für die nächste Runde erholen.

Anleitung für einen Flashmob*

* Flashmob: Viele Menschen kommen wie aus heiterem Himmel zusammen, machen schnell was zusammen und trennen sich wieder.

Man braucht

- ❤ Lust auf eine spektakuläre Aktion
- ❤ möglichst viele Freunde
- ❤ einen Song, zu dem sich gut tanzen lässt
- ❤ eine Person, die sich um Musik kümmert
- ❤ eine Person, die ein Handy-Video macht

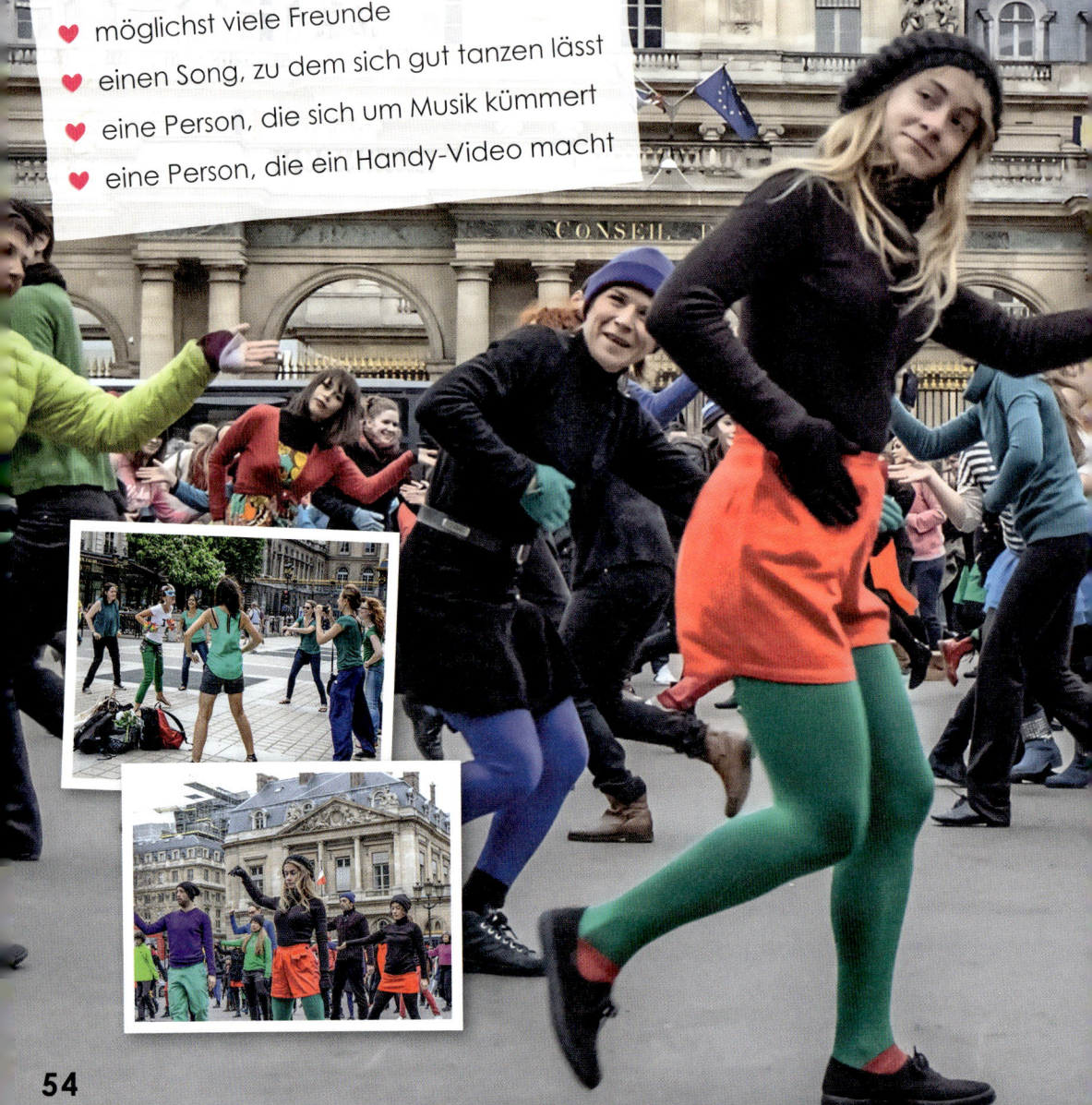

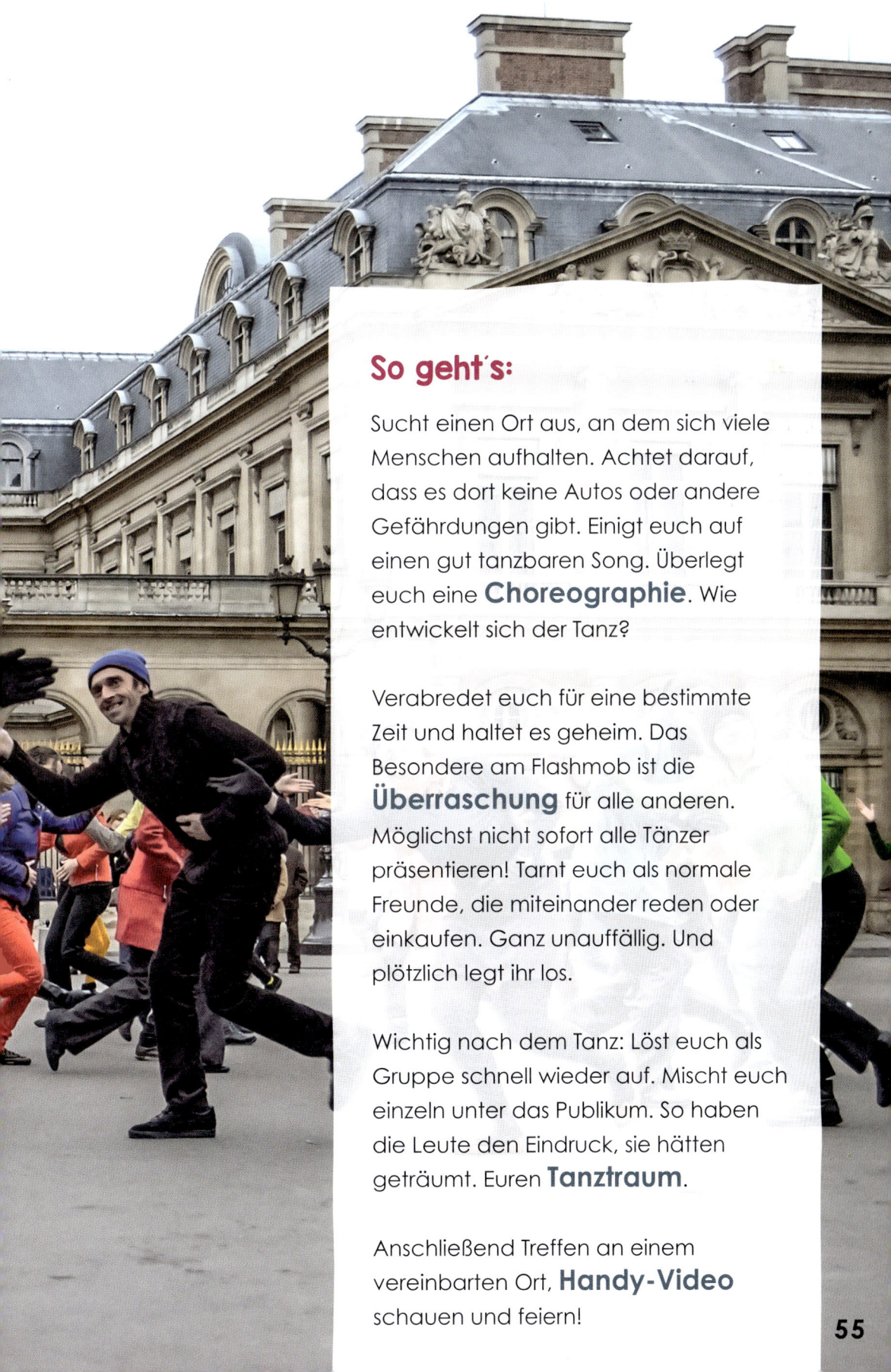

So geht's:

Sucht einen Ort aus, an dem sich viele Menschen aufhalten. Achtet darauf, dass es dort keine Autos oder andere Gefährdungen gibt. Einigt euch auf einen gut tanzbaren Song. Überlegt euch eine **Choreographie**. Wie entwickelt sich der Tanz?

Verabredet euch für eine bestimmte Zeit und haltet es geheim. Das Besondere am Flashmob ist die **Überraschung** für alle anderen. Möglichst nicht sofort alle Tänzer präsentieren! Tarnt euch als normale Freunde, die miteinander reden oder einkaufen. Ganz unauffällig. Und plötzlich legt ihr los.

Wichtig nach dem Tanz: Löst euch als Gruppe schnell wieder auf. Mischt euch einzeln unter das Publikum. So haben die Leute den Eindruck, sie hätten geträumt. Euren **Tanztraum**.

Anschließend Treffen an einem vereinbarten Ort, **Handy-Video** schauen und feiern!

DAS QUIZ

FÜR TOLLE TÄNZER

Macht euch bereit ja

Noch schnell eine Pirouette gedreht. Oder ein Rad geschlagen. Und schon geht's los mit dem großen Tanz-Quiz! Gerne auch mit Rückwärtssaltos in die einzelnen Kapitel.

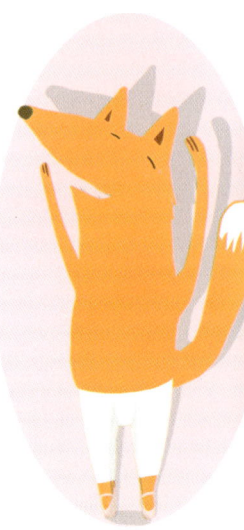

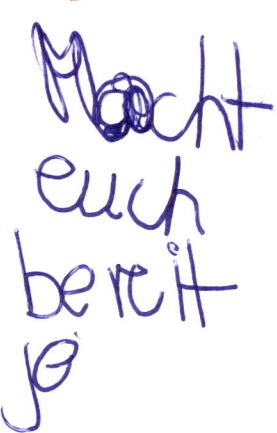

1. Technik, Training und Tutus

Bringe die Sätze mit den passenden Tänzern zusammen.

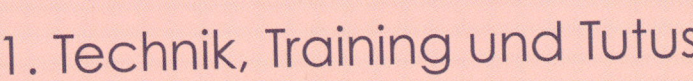

a Primaballerinen tanzen die Solotänze im Ballett.

b Der französische Sonnenkönig gründete die erste Ballettschule. Deswegen haben die meisten Schritte und Positionen französische Namen.

c Bei der Arabesque steht die Tänzerin auf einem Bein. Beziehungsweise auf der Fußspitze. Das andere Bein ist weit nach hinten gestreckt.

2 c

3 b

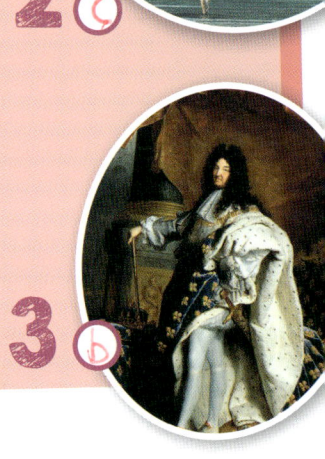

2. Die stolzen Tänze

Was gehört zu welchem stolzen Tanz?

a ein Paar
b Gitarre
c Händeklatschen
d der feste Blick in die Augen

Tango

Flamenco

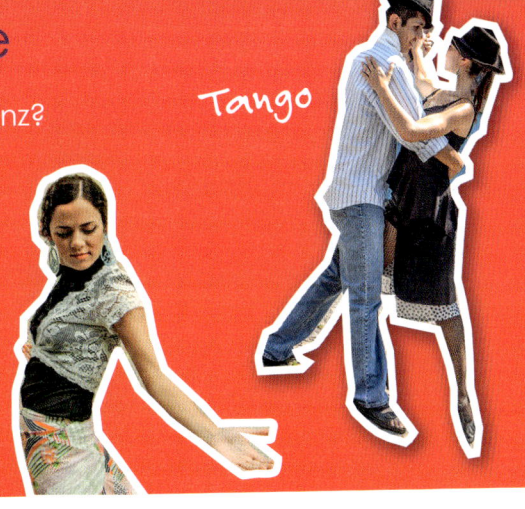

3. Bollywood

Was sind Bollywood-Fakten und was stimmt einfach gar nicht?

		RICHTIG	FALSCH
1	In den Bollywood-Filmen tanzen nur die Frauen.	✓	☐
2	Beim Bollywood-Tanz spielen die Hände immer eine Hauptrolle.	✓	☐
3	Pro Jahr entstehen in Indien rund 900 neue Bollywood-Tänze.	☐	✓
4	In Bollywood-Filmen geht es um Liebe, Gerechtigkeit und den Sieg des Guten über das Böse.	✓	☐

4. Bei Angriff Tanz

1 Wer erfand die Capoeira in Brasilien?
 a die afrikanischen Sklaven
 b die portugiesischen Eroberer

2 Was darf im Capoeira-Orchester nicht fehlen?
 a die Trillerpfeife
 b die Berimbaus

3 Was ist das Wichtigste bei Capoeira?
 a ahnen, was der andere als Nächstes macht
 b wissen, wie man kämpft

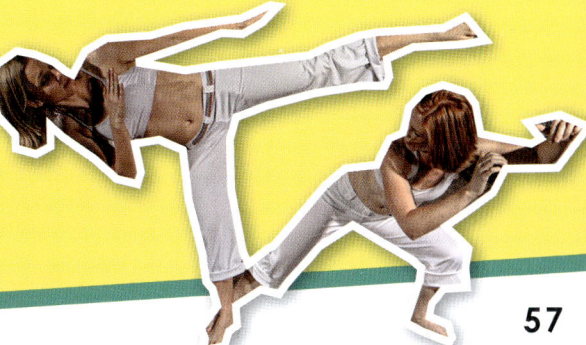

5. Hip-Hop

Bist du ein echter Hip-Hopper? Dann weißt du, was wahr und was falsch ist.

		RICHTIG	FALSCH
1	Hip-Hop entstand zuerst in Brasilien.	☐	☒
2	Breakdancer, Locker und Popper sind alle Hip-Hopper.	☑	☐
3	Bei einem Battle fliegen nur Arme und Beine, keine Fäuste.	☑	☐
4	Rapper mögen keine Reime.	☐	☒

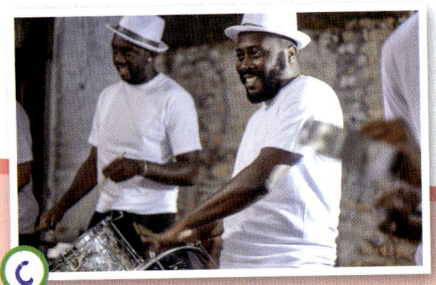

1 c

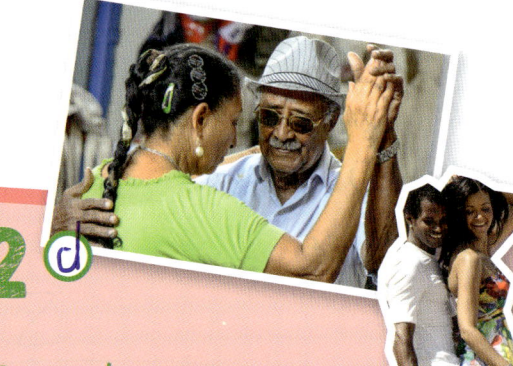

2 d

6. Heute schon Latein getanzt?

Bringe die Sätze mit den passenden Tänzen zusammen.

a In diese Soße sind verschiedene Traditionen eingerührt. Spanische Gitarrenklänge mischen sich mit afrikanischen Trommelrhythmen.

b Der verspielte Paartanz hat seinen Namen vom Wechselschritt. Man zählt die Schritte: Schritt-Schritt-Wechselschritt.

c Bei diesem brasilianischen Tanz geht nichts ohne die Trommler.

d In Lateinamerika tanzen Männer und Frauen in jedem Alter.

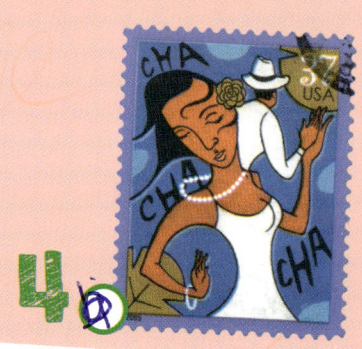

3 a

4 b

7. Zehnkampf

Bei den Turniertänzen sind die Schritte durcheinandergeraten. Finde die fünf Standard- und die fünf Lateintänze.

L	A	F	K	E	R	Z	I	Q	U	A	M	A
U	T	R	Y	P	A	W	E	U	W	E	I	R
J	I	P	C	H	F	S	J	I	V	E	U	B
C	H	A	-	C	H	A	-	C	H	A	B	L
H	U	S	T	O	E	M	W	K	C	H	F	A
U	F	O	C	H	R	B	A	S	H	U	I	R
M	I	*	G	Z	B	A	L	T	O	I	L	U
M	N	D	K	E	S	T	Z	E	V	F	U	M
S	L	O	W	F	O	X	E	P	I	X	L	B
E	U	B	B	I	C	G	R	X	M	A	U	A
L	Z	L	U	T	R	T	A	N	G	O	B	R
W	I	E	N	E	R	*	W	A	L	Z	E	R

8. Rauschende Feste: Berlin

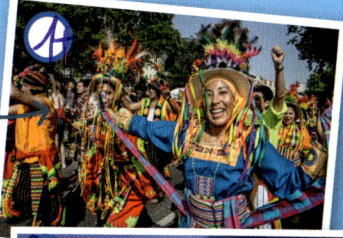

Wien oder Berlin? Ordne die Sätze dem richtigen Fest zu.

1 Über 6.000 Tänzer sind jedes Jahr zu Pfingsten dabei.

2 Die Tänzer sind alle zwischen 17 und 24 Jahren alt.

3 Jedes Jahr werden bis zu 12.000 Besucher erwartet.

4 Brasilianische Vögel tanzen mit chinesischen Drachen.

Wien

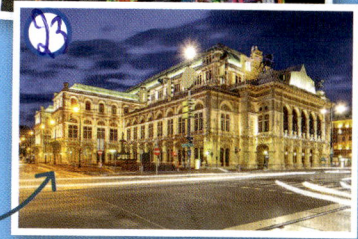

URKUNDE

8 Jahre **für**

tolle Tänzer

1. platz

Naomi Newell
NAME

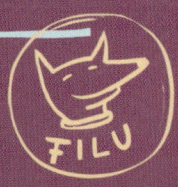

2014 geboren

60

Kennst du
das schon?

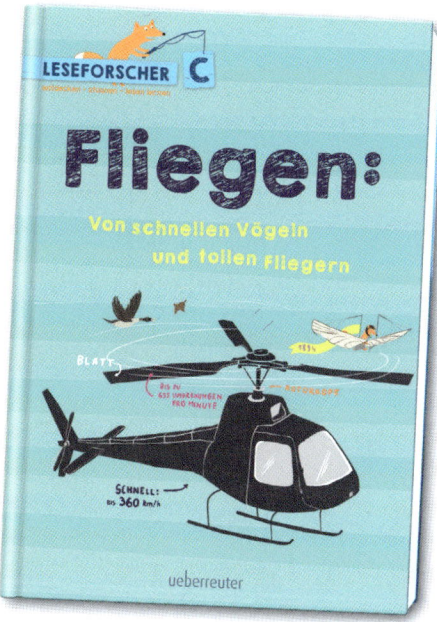

Was ist ein Ramp Agent?

Wieso können Vögel eigentlich fliegen?
Wie klappt beim Flugzeug die perfekte Landung?
Und was ist ein Ramp Agent?
Spannende und unglaubliche Fakten rund um
Flugzeuge, Fallschirmspringer, Raumschiffe und
was sich sonst noch durch die Luft bewegt.

- Für fortgeschrittene Leser
- Verblüffende Details, spannende
  Hintergrundgeschichten
- In cooler Magazinoptik

Kathrin Köller, Julia Dürr
Fliegen:
Von schnellen Vögeln und tollen Fliegern
64 Seiten · Hardcover
ISBN 978-3-7641-5062-4

Herzlichen Glückwunsch!
Du bist ein echter Tanzexperte.
Trage deinen Namen auf der Urkunde ein.

Auf www.ueberreuter.de kannst du
dir die Urkunde auch herunterladen.

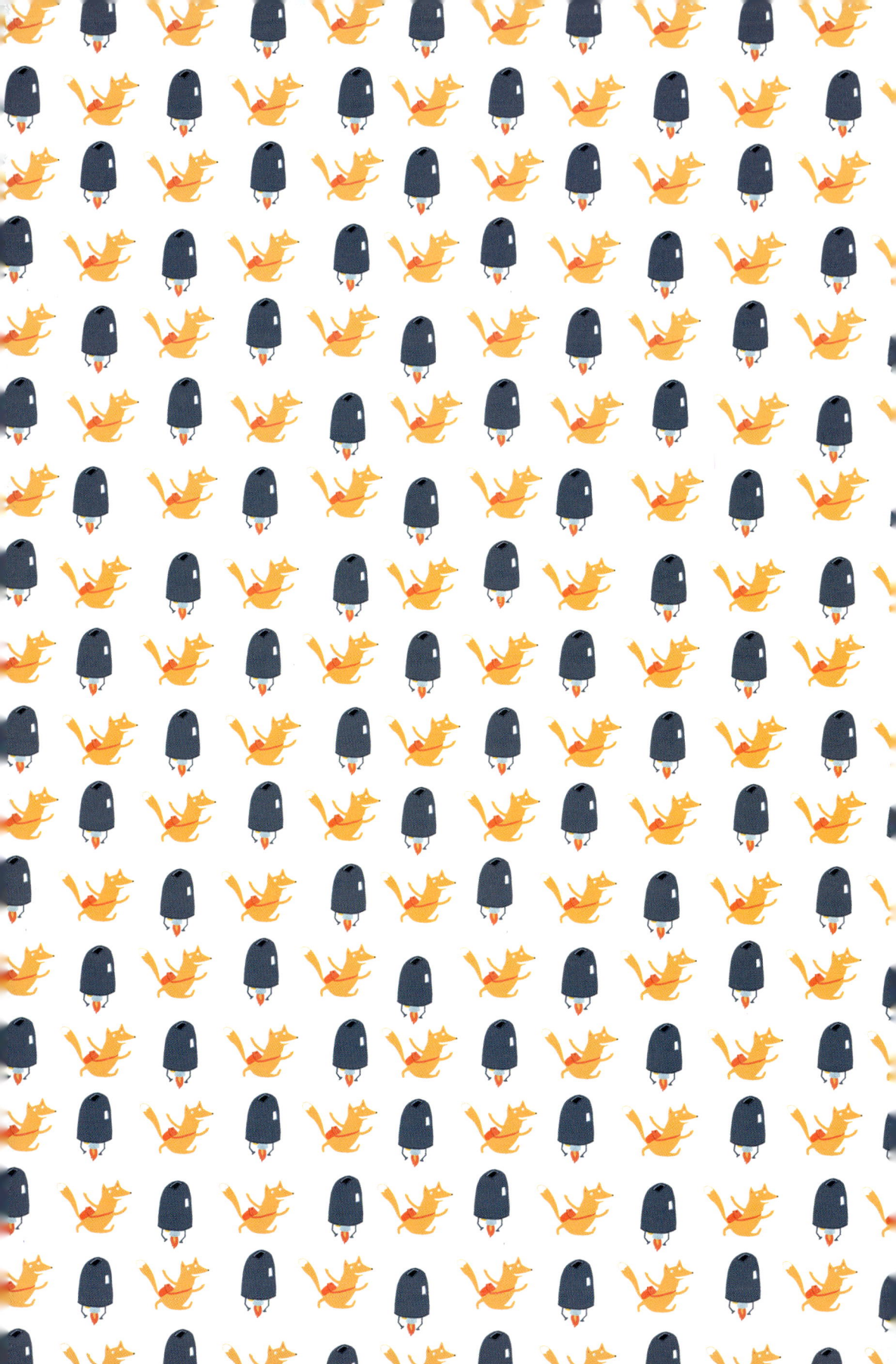